DIETING MAKES YOU FAT

Geoffrey Cannon

2 4 6 8 10 9 7 5 3 1

Virgin Books, an imprint of Ebury Publishing,
20 Vauxhall Bridge Road,
London SW1V 2SA

Virgin Books is part of the Penguin Random House group
of companies whose addresses can be found at
global.penguinrandomhouse.com

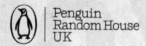

Penguin
Random House
UK

First published in the United Kingdom by Virgin Books in 2008
This edition published in the United Kingdom by Virgin Books in 2018

www.penguin.co.uk

A CIP catalogue record for this book is available
from the British Library

ISBN 9780753553824

Printed and bound in Great Britain by Clays Ltd, Elcograf S.p.A.

Penguin Random House is committed to a sustainable future
for our business, our readers and our planet. This book is
made from Forest Stewardship Council® certified paper.

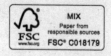

MIX
Paper from
responsible sources
FSC® C018179

Some work in progress towards this book has previously been published in
*Public Health Nutrition, Asia-Pacific Journal of Clinical Nutrition, British
Journal of Nutrition, Scandinavian Journal of Food and Nutrition*, and
other journals. Some information was previously published in the first
version of this book.

DIETING MAKES YOU FAT

Other work by Geoffrey Cannon

Books

The New Nutrition Science (chief editor) (with Claus Leitzmann)
The Fate of Nations. Food and Nutrition Policy in the New World
Superbug. Nature's Revenge: Why Antibiotics Breed Disease
Food and Health: The Experts Agree
The Good Fight. The Life and Work of Caroline Walker
The Politics of Food
Fat to Fit
The Food Scandal (with Caroline Walker)
Dieting Makes You Fat (first version) (with Hetty Einzig)

Reports, projects

'Food, Nutrition, Physical Activity and the Prevention of Cancer:
a Global Perspective' (chief editor)
'*Guia Alimentar para a População Brasileira*' (initial drafts of official
national dietary guidelines, for federal government of Brazil)
'*Alimentos do Brasil*' (Foods of Brazil)
(for government of Brazil)
'Food, Nutrition and the Prevention of Cancer: a Global Perspective'
(project director, chief editor)
STAR°RANK (road and track running standards, records and rankings)
'Getting in Shape' (fitness project for the *Sunday Times*)

Organizations

The New Nutrition Science project (co-convenor)
World Health Policy Forum (co-founder, secretary-general)
Public Health Nutrition (associate editor, columnist)
Brazilian government (member, delegation to World Health
Organization Executive Board meeting)
World Health Organization (representative, Earth Summit on
Sustainable Development)
UK government (member, delegation to International
Conference on Nutrition)
UK government (member, National Nutrition Task Force)
National Food Alliance (now Sustain) (co-founder, previous chair)
Soil Association (previous board member)
Guild of Food Writers (previous secretary)
Caroline Walker Trust (co-founder, previous secretary)
London Road Runners Club (co-founder)
Serpentine Running Club (founder)

For Raquel and Gabriel

O that this too too solid flesh would melt,
Thaw, and resolve itself into a dew!

William Shakespeare

The problem nowadays always turns on how we shall decide to live.

Edward Hoagland

CONTENTS

Part 1
The dieting disaster

*In which I tell some stories of my struggles, confusions and
adventures with food and drink, physical activity, the ups and*

downs of my own weight, and in particular with dieting, from when I was a child and then an adult, until now.

This process gradually started to lead me towards the full meaning of health and wellbeing and the wisely led life. On the way, I began to realize that dieting is not part of the solution, but part of the problem.

2   The fabulous dieting business

Dieting is a booming business. As more and more people become overweight and obese, a correspondingly vast number of dieting regimes have been marketed, often claiming that at last they contain the unique answer.

Like processed foods and drinks, dieting regimes seem wonderfully varied. But however cleverly branded and marketed, they are almost all based on one idea: restrict dietary energy and you will reduce weight. But what then?

3   Why dieting makes you fat

Dieting causes the condition it is meant to cure. The more that we endure cycles of dieting, the more our bodies become trained to seek out food, slow down vital functions, and conserve built-in energy in the form of body fat.

Sedentary people who consume industrialized diets are at high risk of disagreeable, disabling and deadly diseases, whatever their weight – normal, overweight or obese. Continual cycles of dieting increase these dangers.

Part 2
Conscious wellbeing

It is not just dieting that makes you fat, of course. There are four types of reason driving our choices, with roots in human evolution, history and ideology. These basic causes are biological, economic, social, and environmental.

Usually it is not food that makes us fat, but what is done to food, in its production, preservation, processing, and promotion. Obesity makes money. There is no big official, commercial, or medical business interest in wellbeing.

In which I tell some stories of the value of food and drink, as a personal and shared pleasure and a centre of family and social life, as well as protection of our health and enhancement of our wellbeing. We can act on this knowledge now.

In this 21st century it is time to revive the value of food as a precious resource, thinking and acting as customers, consumers and citizens, and as members of one species with special responsibilities within the whole living and physical world.

Here is how: the system for you to enhance your positive good health and also to reduce excess body weight and fat. These seven golden rules incorporate the most reliable knowledge and wisdom on the best quality food and drink.

Good health is not just physical; it is an aspect of the good life, which includes the enjoyment of food and drink. Here is the way to protect your wellbeing and that of your family and children, of future generations, and of the planet.

*The science of food and nutrition is now being born again, in
a form fit for the 21st century. This new nutrition is designed
to develop and maintain positive health and wellbeing, and to
protect the human, living, and physical world.*

*Here are detailed notes meant to illuminate and develop the
themes of the main chapters. These include references to some
of the books and papers used, and also a guide to more
sources of information and inspiration.*

INTRODUCTION
HOW TO USE THIS BOOK

What 'dieting makes you fat' means. What you will find here. What you will not find. This is not a dieting book. It includes the seven golden rules for lifelong wellbeing, which also work if you want to reduce body fat.

This book addresses you as a citizen as well as a consumer. Eating and living consciously protects you against disease. It also creates positive health and wellbeing in the living and physical world of which we all are a part.

Enjoyment of food and drink is part of the joy of living. It is hard to have a good relationship with food or with life if it seems that what you are eating and drinking is making you more and more overweight. All the more so, if all your efforts to reduce weight lead to hunger and craving and to an increase in weight back to or beyond where you were before, and a sense that even when you eat and drink less you still become heavier or flabbier.

Extra body fat often leads to obesity, which may be debilitating, and is associated with increased risk of various serious and even deadly diseases. But what's just as bad is the sense that your body is out of your control, even alien, the sense of failure that this creates, and the fear – often justified – that at least some people in your life see you as somebody who is feeble, lazy or greedy, who can't or won't get a grip. Being and staying the weight and shape you want to be isn't just about protecting yourself against disease, it's about your whole health and wellbeing.

These days, bookshops are stuffed with dieting books. Half or more of the advice on 'health and wellbeing' on websites now is about how to be and stay slim. Business in slimming drugs is booming. At the same time, rates of overweight and obesity among children and young people as well as adults are rapidly increasing, all over the world. We live at a time when food and drink is cheapened and fatness is feared. What's happening? One reason is that advice on what to eat and drink for good health is mostly incomplete, misleading, or wrong, as is advice on what to eat and drink in order to get rid of body fat. A purpose of this book is to show you the right way, starting with why dieting is the wrong way.

DIET AND DIETING

The term 'diet' is ambiguous. Now it usually means all of what we eat and drink, although this is not what 'going on a diet' means. 'Diet' once was a great concept. Dietetics was originally the philosophy of the wisely conducted life in all its aspects – physical and also mental, emotional and spiritual – within which the appreciation and celebration of food and drink, including everyday meals, and the feasting and fasting meant to mark special occasions, is one part. Diet in this broad sense is part of Chinese, Indian, Egyptian, Greek, Roman, Mayan and Arabic teaching, and of worldwide oral tradition, as it was in Europe and the Americas until the rise of science in its modern sense. (For more on 'diet' and 'dieting' see the notes to this introduction, at the back of the book.)

Here is what I mean by 'dieting makes you fat'. The terms 'dieting', as in 'dieting books', and 'diet', as in 'going on a diet', are used in what is now the usual sense. This does not mean occasional prudence or restraint in what you eat or drink, or avoiding specific foods and drinks you think are bad for you. It also does not mean the one time in your life when you transform the quality of what you eat and drink, become more physically active, reduce body fat, get in shape, and maintain this change always – which is what I recommend in Chapter 6. It means the occasional or regular temporary following of regimes that restrict energy intake from food and drink, with the intention of reducing a substantial amount of body weight, after which you resume your 'normal' pattern of eating and drinking.

These qualifications, which are important, exclude only a small proportion of people who go on diets. Some dieting regimes claim not to involve restriction of energy – measured as calories or kilojoules – but as you will see, practically all of them actually do, whether they say so or not.

Now for 'makes you fat'. Of course it is not only dieting that makes you fat. Typically, people 'go on a diet' for the first time because they want to get rid of unwanted body fat and weight that has accumulated for some other reason. But the first part of this book shows that the process of dieting itself increases body fat and body weight – and why. The more severe the regime, and the more often dieting is repeated, the greater is this unintended and unwanted effect.

People who follow the advice given in dieting regimes do not become heavier and fatter at the moment the regimes are completed. Of course not! If dieters really do consume less energy than is used by their bodies, then they will for sure reduce their weight and also their body fat – although less, and often a lot less, than most champions of popular dieting regimes claim or assume. Measured at that point, dieting works. What I mean is the whole effect of dieting, including what happens immediately after the regime is completed, and then a couple of weeks later, then in the next year or two, and long-term.

Not everybody who goes on a diet becomes fatter afterwards. There are people who do keep off all or some of the weight they have shed. But this is most unusual. Generally such people are one of four types. Some use drugs or undergo surgery to maintain their new weight. Others stay on the regime – or a variation – for ever. Some become a lot more physically active.

And yes, some people do confront the cravings dieters suffer after the regimes end, and prevent some, or even all, of their weight rebounding by what is usually called willpower. Most of them become much more careful about what they consume, are sensitized to the addictive qualities of some foods and drinks, and are unusually active. Their examples have informed the seven golden rules in chapter 6.

Nevertheless, dieting makes you fat. A display of dieting 'success stories' is much the same as a display of lottery winners – some people occasionally do beat a system that is stacked against them. Another analogy is with feats of endurance: there are some remarkable people who can swim long distances in icy waters because of their exceptional temperament, or biochemistry and physiology, and after intense training. But for almost all sedentary people, usually the only way to keep off the body weight and fat shed by dieting is by going on another and then another dieting regime. These will progressively strip away lean tissue and make the dieter increasingly flabby. The process is like that experienced by increasingly addicted gamblers who seek yet another system that really will beat the odds this time, although experience tells them that it will only increase their misery, dependence and despair. I know. I have been there.

WHAT IS HERE?

This book shows that dieting is an important cause of fatness. It explains how to stop overweight and obesity before it starts. It outlines ways to get in good shape, enjoy life more, regain wellbeing, and to feel better in your body and in the world. It has two parts within which there are six chapters. The chapters begin with quotations indicating their scope and flavour.

The first part, *The dieting disaster*, shows you what not to do. It has three chapters. In chapter 1, *Confessions of a retired dieter*, I recount some of my own experiences and reflect on what these may mean. Chapter 2, *The fabulous dieting business*, is a tour of the main types of dieting regime: magic ingredient, manipulated macronutrient, and 'be sensible and go easy', and the new wave of 'don't diet' dieting books. Chapter 3, *Why dieting makes you fat*, may be the chapter you turn to first – but you need the context of the whole book. It explains how and why dieting is self-defeating, and how and why continual dieting is itself damaging and dangerous.

The second part of the book, *Conscious wellbeing*, shows you what to do. It begins with chapter 4, *Everything else that makes you fat*. This summarizes the forces in the world now that make us fat. The good news begins in chapter 5, *The place of food in our world*. This includes stories that put food and drink and meals back into the centre of our lives, respecting the living and physical world of which we are a part.

Chapter 6, *Your seven golden rules*, is a system for you and for every able-bodied person, including those who want to reduce their body fat. It distils what I have learned about the value of food and nutrition over the last quarter of a century. When you follow the rules, you are most likely to improve and maintain your health and overall wellbeing and, as you involve them, that of your family, friends, and community. This final chapter is also for you as a citizen concerned for the new generation of children, and the future of our planet.

After the main text there are two extra sections. Annex 1, *The new nutrition*, outlines the revolution that is now making sense of nutrition as a science in this 21st century.

Annex 2, *More insights*, includes detailed notes referring back to the main text chapter by chapter, starting with this introduction. These take the book's thesis further and are designed as a resource whenever you want to know more. Thus the notes to this introduction include more information on the ancient and traditional concept of 'diet', define 'overweight' and 'obesity', explain body mass index (BMI), and explain (kilo)calories, kilojoules, and other weights and measures. The notes also include references to relevant and useful books, reports, articles and papers.

Who knows best?

In this book I have summarized evidence trawled from specialist journals and from experts in energy metabolism, obesity, and associated disciplines. The book also includes observations and reflections of thinkers and teachers from times gone by, and from outside current conventional science.

For much of my professional life I have worked with scientists with the purpose of making sense of their work and making it more meaningful. This involves identifying the most relevant and useful evidence and explaining what it means in the world outside research centres. I have due respect for orthodox scientific research, and am also aware of its limitations. Just as war and peace are too important to be left to soldiers and politicians, disorders and health are too important to be abandoned to physicians and scientists.

Also, I have come to realize that observant and conscientious people who have thought long and hard about the human condition may be better guides than research teams whose findings often give exact answers to unhelpful questions. Faced with the mass of information on any topic now available on the internet, it's worth remembering that knowledge may drive out wisdom.

WHAT IS NOT HERE?

You should also know what is not here. Again, this is not a dieting book. It contains no proposals for quick fixes. The closest I get to 'a new you in seven days' is chapter 6, my system for six or seven months and then for always, designed to enhance and maintain your wellbeing. Yes, if you want to reduce your body fat, you can use the seventh rule for this purpose.

You will not find 'success stories' here featuring the author's clients or friends who, thanks to following the recommended regime, together lost the weight of a tipper truck, have become irresistibly attractive, and now all play hockey at international level, direct *Fortune* Top 500 companies, and eat six pastries a day, while remaining slim, rejuvenated and energetic.

You will also find little here about resistant starch, fatty acid fractions, phytochemicals, neuropeptide Y gene expression, leptin and ghrelin, or the Ad-37 adenovirus. These keep the wheels of academic research, as well as of the dieting business, turning. But you don't need to know much about such stuff. Not much has practical relevance.

There are no recipes here. Highly geared entrepreneurial dieting book authors often hire recipe writers to rustle up a hundred or so dishes and meals that follow their formulas. I do not agree with dieting recipes. The only dishes and meals you will fully enjoy are those made to share with your partner, family, friends and colleagues. If you like to cook and prepare food, use the recipe books derived and adapted from traditional cuisines from those parts of the world where overweight and obesity are – or have been – uncommon. A word of warning, though: most cookbook recipes are for show or feast food. Seek out recipes for simple everyday meals.

WHAT CAN AND CAN'T BE DONE?

What if you are very overweight? It is one thing to prevent weight increase, overweight and obesity. Controlling and reducing excess weight is another matter. There are also likely to be big differences between people who are overweight, those who are obese but otherwise able-bodied and evidently healthy, and those who are disabled or severely obese.

If you are obese, especially if you have been sedentary for many years and want to shed a great mass of excess body fat, there is no easy way, especially if you are not able-bodied. You know this already. Severe obesity is practically intractable. Drastic treatments using drugs or surgery have their own dangers. Dieting is characteristically just as self-defeating for obese and very obese people as it is for overweight people. This said, the seven golden rules in chapter 6 will benefit everybody.

The way to whole health

Dieting has a context. Anybody who expects to reduce weight and then simply and only for this reason gain health is bound to fail. Health in its full sense means not just absence of disease, but positive physical, mental, emotional and spiritual wellbeing, and involves us with our families and communities, within the living and physical world. Excess body fat is a condition that involves our whole beings, not just our physical dimension.

This implies a deep approach, including investigation of the evolutionary, historical, economic, social and environmental causes of malaise and wellbeing. Dieting is a sign of the times. These include misunderstanding of the sources of human happiness and fulfilment, and of our place in the world.

This book is for all the hundreds of millions of people who are fatter than they want to be, who have tried dieting, and who have found that dieting does not work, and especially for those who want to know why. It is also for everybody who wants to know why obesity has rather suddenly become a global public health emergency. Further, it is meant to bring obesity and dieting out of the closet and into the light, as warning signs that we humans are moving in the wrong direction. There are no immediate answers to what is now the global epidemic of obesity. However, I believe that if all the lessons of this book were followed everywhere, obesity with all the problems it brings would eventually again become uncommon.

Achievement of whole wellbeing involves an earned sense of self-responsibility, self-mastery and self-fulfilment, all part of our purpose here on the planet. Once we are on the way to realizing our own personal potential, we are better able to support others.

The first people to think about are children and young people, and those not yet born: they need not repeat our mistakes. We all now have a responsibility to ensure our children can rejoice in their physical being, enjoy delicious food and drink, and become in harmony with the whole world.

A PERSONAL NOTE

Chapter 1 is about my times on and off and on and off dieting regimes, and other chapters include stories of my own experience of the quality of food and drink and their effect on health and wellbeing. This book might have been written impersonally, or relied only on research and interviews with others. However, my personal experiences and my professional work tell me that any thesis, no matter how well backed with evidence, is a point of view. Also we can all learn and support others as a result of becoming more conscious of, and reflecting on, our own lives. You may find that what's most helpful is to bring to mind what you know already.

Having lived in Britain since I was a child, I decided in 1999 to begin the new century by living and working elsewhere. I no longer felt able to understand any international public health issue as long as my knowledge of the world elsewhere was limited to trips. Rudyard Kipling's line 'What do they know of England, who only England know?' applies to all countries. I felt I might better understand the issues of Europe and Northern America and other materially rich societies from a different perspective. In 2000 I chose Brazil.

Until the 1980s and 1990s obesity was not a big issue in middle-income countries like Brazil and South Africa, or low-income countries like India and China, and dieting was not big business outside high-income countries. Now both are worldwide blockbusters, as are the even bigger issues of population increase, depletion of resources, and climate change; and all of these are related. It helps to know what goes on elsewhere, to take a long view, and to see the big picture.

Body fatness and dieting are also about the place of food and drink in our lives. You may want to know how to reduce excess body fat permanently, either personally, or on behalf of people in your life, or as a public health issue. This is best done by acting in the light of awareness of the value of food and drink and physical activity to you, and also to everybody you know, to humanity, and to the whole world. Such connections are much more obvious these days.

What's here is what I believe, based on what I have learned. I hope it is helpful. For you, best is what you explore, discover, record, enact, and thus wholly experience, on your way to fulfil your potential.

Juiz de Fora and Cabo Frio, Brazil,
London, UK, and Washington, USA

NOTE
WHAT'S NEW

This is a completely new book, written for this 21st century. If you have already heard that dieting makes you fat, the reason is that the first version of this book, written in the 1980s, was a bestseller in the UK and in many other countries.

The first version of *Dieting Makes You Fat*, which I co-authored with Hetty Einzig, was a number one bestseller in the UK, and was published in many languages and editions throughout the world. What it said and showed inspired countless people, and shook the dieting industry, which afterwards focused rather less on 'calorie cutting' and rather more on the quality of food and the value of physical activity.

Key points in the first version have shaped the new generation of 'don't diet' dieting books, some of which are rather good. Some rightly point out that on dieting regimes, weight reduction is at first mostly of water, and then of muscle and other lean tissue as well as of body fat, and that after such regimes end, the body of a sedentary person characteristically becomes flabby, relatively fatter and usually also absolutely fatter. Some rightly say that dieting switches on the body's built-in biological processes designed to endure and survive famine conditions. One or two dip a toe in the deep water and say something like 'so sometimes some diets can even have the effect of making you fat'. But such caution is mistaken. As a rule, dieting makes you fat, period.

What's different?

The basic thesis of this book remains the same as the first version. That said, this is a completely new book. As one example, the first version was all about personal health and wellbeing. As you can see from the contents list, this version also discerns the big picture, of dieting and body fatness in wider – including economic, social and environmental – dimensions. Reducing body weight and fat, gaining good health, and contributing to a better world, are all part of a greater whole, and each supports the others.

Once you gain and maintain positive health and whole wellbeing, and help to encourage the people in your life to do the same, you will become a drag on the trade of many businesses and institutions, as well as being an unsuitable case for treatment.

The bigger picture

The first version was a book of its times – the 1980s. It was centred on the self of the person who just wants to know about dieting and fatness. Then it seemed appropriate to write only for individuals who wanted to know how to shed body fat and how to become energetic, fit and healthy.

The world as we now experience it in the early 21st century is transformed from that of the late 20th century. Now individuals – including you, and me too! – are best placed in the context of our families, friends, colleagues and communities, and of our human species as part of the whole living and physical world. We all are not alone.

PART 1
THE DIETING DISASTER

Candy says, I've come to hate my body, and all that it requires, in this world.

Lou Reed

The aspects of things that are most important for us are hidden because of their simplicity and familiarity. (One is unable to notice something – because it is always before one's eyes) . . . We fail to be struck by what, once seen, is most striking and most powerful.

Ludwig Wittgenstein

PART II
THE DIETING DISASTER

1. CONFESSIONS OF A RETIRED DIETER

We hold that folk on no account should vary
Their daily diet until necessary;
For as Hippocrates doth truly show,
Diseases sad from all such changes flow.

School of Salerno

We have been taught to neglect, despise, and violate our bodies, and to
put all our faith in our brains. As a consequence, we are at war with
ourselves – the brain desiring things which the body does not want, and
the body desiring things which the brain does not allow; the brain giving
decisions which the body will not follow, and the body giving impulses
that the brain cannot understand.

Alan Watts

In which I tell some stories of my struggles, confusions and adventures with food and drink, physical activity, the ups and downs of my own weight, and in particular with dieting, from when I was a child and then an adult, until now.

This process gradually started to lead me towards the full meaning of health and wellbeing and the wisely led life. On the way, I began to realize that dieting is not part of the solution, but part of the problem.

Now that overweight and obesity have become global epidemics, and so many children and young people are fat, we need to know that dieting is a disaster, and why, and what to do. This is vital information for parents, consumers, citizens, health professionals, and policy-makers. It is essential guidance for everybody who has ever 'gone on a diet', then increased in weight and body fat, and who feels that they have failed. The fact is that dieting is a cause of the condition it is supposed to cure.

You may be one of those people who eat and drink whatever they like and whose body fat never increases. Perhaps you are one of those unusual people who have found their own ways to be rid of and keep off excess body fat permanently. You may carry a lot of body fat and rejoice in your size. Or – and I guess this is more likely – you are worried about your own body fatness, or that of members of your family, or of friends or colleagues.

These days overweight and obesity affect us all, one way or another. The second part of this book puts obesity and dieting – two sides of the same coin – into the broad context of how we all live now. Modern life has gone wrong in some ways that we personally can help to put right, starting in our own lives. This world in which so many people are now obese is also the world in which farmers and growers in Africa are exploited, the earth's living treasures are being plundered, the soil is becoming degraded, sources of water and energy are running out, the polar icecaps are melting, and the climate is changing. One theme of this book is that these personal, social and environmental issues are all related to one another. Chapter 6 shows how you can gain and maintain good health and wellbeing, and – if you want – also reduce body fat; not as an isolated individual, but as somebody who is increasingly conscious of the place of humans in this world, now and in future. But that's for later.

You may well already be aware that as a rule dieting, meaning restriction of energy from food and drink, does not work. In this first part of this book I look at dieting from three points of view. The next chapter anatomizes the dieting business, now a colossal global industry. The third chapter spells out the science showing that dieting makes you fat, and that dieting may itself be dangerous. In this first chapter I tell my own story which, if you have 'been on diets', may have some resonance with your story.

DIETERS AS FAILURES

The covers of some dieting books feature pictures of authors with sparkling teeth and smiles and burnished complexions. Do what I say and you can look like me – or attract somebody like me – is the message. Such books are usually written by men, some of whom have patented their own brands of supplements and potions. Other dieting books feature an older man with a serious expression dressed in a white coat. This lets you know that the author has a medical degree. The message is one of authority: trust me, I'm a doctor. Another approach is to use shots not of the author but of a model, a slim, pretty, winsome and unthreatening young woman, maybe eating and smiling at the same time. These books are usually written by women. This could be – will be – the new you, is this message.

Well, I am not a physician, nor a girl next door, nor am I sun-lamp toasted easy side over, and for most of my life I have not embodied the message of this book. The first time I was fat was when I was a child, and ever since I have tended to be overweight. Like Christian in *Pilgrim's Progress*, I have been beguiled by Vanity Fair and stuck in the Slough of Despond.

While every human story is different, mine may have points in common with yours. Further, since publication of the first version of *Dieting Makes You Fat*, I now have plenty more experience and learning, including of more mistakes, and here is the result: stages of my pilgrimage.

Many of the decisions I have made and have not made in my life have been affected by my weight, which has influenced my opinion of myself. Failing to keep off weight shed on dieting regimes has made me lose self-confidence – if I can't do that, can I be sure that I can do anything? It's even more demoralizing when dieting regimes are advertised as easy, or else just a matter of willpower.

After the first few days I have generally found that dieting is easy. Dieters do shed weight on any serious regime. It's what happens afterwards that causes misery. Failure as a dieter feels like failure as a person. What's wrong with me? What's worse is when you don't know what is happening.

All people who are fat or liable to be fat have their own story of when, how and why they got fat in the first place. Getting fat and dieting and getting fat, and then dieting and getting fat, has been a feature of my life. Sometimes I forgot about it or blanked it, sometimes I decided to get a grip and shed weight. Some of the stories here may be peculiar to me. I guess that some will resonate for you, especially if you have already been on a number of dieting regimes.

Did it ever occur to you that dieting was the worst thing you could have done? Like somebody who agreed to a surgical operation that went wrong, I live with that thought, for similar reasons. At the time the decision seemed right and inevitable, and there seemed to be no choice. There was – oh, there was – but the damage is done. Like people who persist in keeping their savings in dud shares, veteran dieters have a big investment in continuing to believe that dieting is safe and healthy and that it works – or should work.

Voluptuous women and massive men were models of beauty and authority in times gone by, and in some cultures people who are big as well as tall are still considered the most attractive. Some people enjoy being overweight, and some obese people are happy about their size. This was never my case. Carrying excess body fat has always made me feel bad. As an adult I knew the time when as a child I first became fat, but it took me a long time to understand some of the reasons why. It was when I was between eight and eleven years old; I know because of pictures here at home now, some of which I found in my parents' records of me after they died.

Here I am aged eight sitting on a wall outside Coventry Cross, the flats in Bromley-by-Bow in London's East End where my father's parents lived. Here I am in the same year in a block of head-and-shoulder Polyfotos taken at the long-gone Gamages department store in Holborn, as organized by my mother. Slim, if that's the right word for a boy. And then, here I am aged eleven in a formal framed portrait taken in my new secondary school uniform, pudgy, a right little porker, maybe 15 pounds or 7 kilograms overweight. It's evident that my personality had changed. In the earlier pictures I am open, looking outwards; in the later picture I am guarded, looking inwards. Why? What happened?

Recently I realized why, after an exchange of opinions with a colleague who is a big-shot US National Cancer Institute executive. He was saying that fast food is not fattening just because of being prepared and eaten quickly, and that a calorie is a calorie. In reply I disagreed, and said that the term 'fast food' needs definition – as it does – but that the convenience and circumstances of fast food, as well as what it's made from and its typically high energy density, do make it fattening.

YOUNG SUPER-SIZER

Fast food . . . and then it all came back to me. I'm inside me aged eight to eleven, in the ABC fish and chip shop on the Seven Sisters Road in Finsbury Park, north London. The sight, smell and sound of the chips (French fries) sizzling gets my juices flowing. This is my regular take-away trip on cold evenings. Waiting in the queue between men and women in long overcoats and scarves, I feel important. In those days of pounds, shillings and pence, my order is two big 1s 3d portions of cod and 4d packets of chips irrigated with Sarson's malt vinegar, plus a drift of salt from the grenade-size aluminium shaker, plus the treat, three 2d wallys (pickled cucumber) forked up from a great jar on the counter above my head.

The fish and the chips are fried to order. Through the glass front of the counter I watch the cook take up the fish fillets tail end first and slap, slap them on the egged flour, and then shovel the chipped potatoes, sling them in their wire cages, and plunge them into the boiling oil, which hisses and fizzes. The third wally is my secret. This I ask to be wrapped separately so I can wolf it as I walk back. And now I sense me savouring its taste and the aroma of hot oily batter soaking through yesterday's newspapers and onto my hands, as I hurry back along the Seven Sisters Road and round the corner to the apartment in Wilberforce Road where I live with my mother.

My mother didn't eat food for comfort; indeed, I don't remember her finishing her meals. I devoured my man-size portion, crispy bits and all. She ate most of her fish but not much else. When I was much younger and she fed me, she used to say, 'Just the stuff to give the troops!' to tempt me to eat another spoonful, meaning that meals should be finished. Now it was a few years later, with my father living else-where, and after finishing my meal I dug into her leftover batter and chips. (There are more details on the caloric wallop delivered by processed potatoes in the notes to this chapter.)

Tizer ('the appetizer') was a favourite soft drink for London street kids in those days: an early rocket fuel, bottled, sugared, flavoured red fizz. Plus I had started to wear glasses, and knew it would be smart to get top scholarship marks in the primary school examinations that kids then took at age eleven. So I ran around and roller-skated a lot less, and sat and studied a lot more. When I arrived at my secondary school I was conspicuous, as the one boy in my house and year who was fat.

So, why did I get fat? We all know the physiological reason: too much energy in, not enough energy out. 'Fortunately, all that a patient needs to know, and indeed must know, is that obesity arises only as consequence of taking in more energy in their food than is expended in the activities of their daily life,' says a standard textbook. In the misleading jargon, I was in 'positive energy balance'.

Suppose aged eight to eleven, in contrast to when I was younger, I was averaging 200 calories (840 kilojoules) a day more from food, and 150 calories (625 kilojoules) a day less from exercise. Assuming I was previously in energy balance for a growing child, a 'positive' balance of 350 calories a day is 3,500 calories every ten days. Given that there are 3,500 calories in a pound of fat, and given these mathematics, I would have put on an extra 36½ pounds a year or 109 pounds (50 kilograms) in three years. Obviously such theoretical calculations are wrong, for I had not become a Michelin boy. But I was fat.

Any physiological account does not answer the real question 'why?' The obvious biological reason was because I was often eating for two, and many of my meals had become replaced by energy bombs and rocket fuel – energy-dense fast food takeaways and sugared water. But this was not just a matter of biology. It was also because my mother was not able to be both father and mother to me, and I fended for myself in the one way I could, by getting top marks, the route to security. My parents' divorce, and with it the loss of family meals, also affected me. If my parents had been happily married my story would have been different in a number of ways.

This story of long ago seems to me to resonate with how children very often live now, including those with both parents at home. The common factor is the replacement of family meals by pre-prepared packaged foods and drinks, which people in the family often eat alone, and the replacement of regular physical activity by sedentary ways of life, and these days in particular television viewing and other hours a day spent using computers. Overweight and obesity have emotional, economic, social and other dimensions.

THE NIBBLE DIET

What I did then, in my second term at my boarding school, was go on a diet of my own invention. It was time to stop being fat and feeling miserable, isolated, and powerless. So I stopped eating meals.

In the vast dining hall in which almost a thousand boys and masters were sat, the boys around me scoffed lots and lots of stodge. There were mounds of bread with margarine and jam, sweetened tea served in big bowls, sausages, breaded herring, meat pies served in vast tin containers, another main dish known as 'anti-tank rubber' sliced into servings, 'frogs' eyes' (sago puddings), and more bread, margarine, jam, and tea. Plus in morning breaks a third of a pint of milk and 'squashed fly' biscuits with embedded dried fruit. Plus 'tuck' – confectionery and biscuits and individual fruit pies and jams and fizz bought at the school shop or sent in big tins by parents.

But I was on the Nibble Diet. Finally I was in control. The writer of the standard textbook would have been pleased with me. He goes on to state: 'If the diet is restricted so as to supply less energy than is being used, then the body has to draw upon the stores in adipose tissue and weight is lost. Eating and physical exercise are behavioural activities and so controllable by willpower, and hence obesity is a behavioural disorder.'

Pull your socks up, get a grip! I have proof of the results. My school, Christ's Hospital, played a part in early 20th-century nutrition policy. Observations and experiments carried out by G E Friend, the school doctor from 1913 to 1946, communicated by him to government, led to the national fortification of margarine with vitamins A and D. Dr Friend's successor, the school doctor in my time, continued the practice of weighing and measuring all the inmates at the beginning and end of terms, to prove that the school food was raising big, strong, tall boys.

In the twelve weeks of my second term I dropped a stone (14 pounds, 6½ kilograms). The doctor was disbelieving at first, and then interrogated me. My line on his chart was the only one going down, in the wrong direction for him. I had messed up his epidemiology! Perhaps he rubbed out my record. But it was 14 pounds, I remember. That was my goal and I achieved it, and was pleased with myself. Any other excess fat was used up as I grew, and in PT (physical training) and rugby football, and running, and I was never fat again at school. I wasn't much good at sports but I had a good time and kept fit.

At the end of my first year at Oxford University, a bunch of us drove to Venice and then caught the boat to Cavtat on the Dalmatian coast just south of Dubrovnik, swam, sunbathed, flirted, lived mostly off tomatoes, melon, yoghurt, and slivovitz (plum brandy), and hitchhiked back to Paris on a diet of baguettes, butter, cheese, paté and wine. I arrived back bronzed and in great shape. Maybe that was the one time in my life that I was lean.

THE MIND-BODY PROBLEM

But then at university my weight increased, as I settled into some new ways of living, including buttered salted cucumber sandwiches, the white bread diagonally quartered, in the afternoons. This was on top of regular meals, including mounds of white toast and margarine plus bacon, fried eggs and sausages at breakfast in my college hall, and lager and curries in the Dildunia, Walton Street, served with chips (French fries) and processed peas.

Already positioning myself as an intellectual, I had the idea that athletes were thickos, and that a way to prove intellectual status was to be indolent. Exercise was confined to the occasional punt up the Cherwell River on sunny days with companions and a hamper full of breads, butter, meats, pies, cheeses, fruits, salads, wines, and other goodies from the Oxford covered market.

One of my subjects was philosophy, and I wrote essays on what was then – and maybe still is – known as 'the mind-body problem'. This started with René Descartes, the 17th-century French philosopher who worried about how to prove that he existed, as introverts may, and decided that the answer was *'cogito, ergo sum'* ('I think, therefore I am'). Having identified himself with the intellectual faculty of his brain, he decided that the physical being is complex clockwork. In which case, how does the human mind relate to the human body? This is 'the mind-body problem' that was still foxing Oxford philosophers when I was a student.

The obvious answer is to toss Descartes in the trash. But Cartesian thinking became the basis of Newtonian physics, which in turn generated increasingly effective machines used in war and peace to create the supremacy of the European powers, the age of 'the Enlightenment', the rise of the British Empire, modern science as we still know it, and the world in which we live now. Descartes was a 'given'. Everybody 'knew' that the mind is separate from the body, despite all the difficulties of maintaining this position (hence the 'problem'). In case you feel I am drifting from the point, the notion that our bodies are machines that will always do what in our minds we want them to do is one reason for the disaster of dieting.

As a student I identified me with my mind and pretended my body was invisible and irrelevant. My body was the container for me. The formal photograph of me as I was getting married in my last year at Oxford shows me plump, features blurred. Getting married when you don't like the look of yourself is a bad move. It means that you don't believe anybody who says nice things about you, unless they are admiring your style or your mind.

THE JAFFA DIET

In 1967 my family included three children and, as when I was aged eight to eleven, what worked for me was work, all day and much of the night. True, I needed to work overtime to earn enough money, but was driven to work into the night anyway by obsessions with mass media, in particular magazines, graphic design, and rock'n'roll. There was no way to succeed in these worlds while looking blowsy. So for me mid-1967 was the summer not of love but of dieting.

From my time on the Dalmatian coast, I had an idea what to do. I ate tomatoes again and also Jaffas – the big oranges whose peel comes off in one piece if you plunge in your thumb and then are careful – and not much else. This diet regime would have supplied around 500 calories (2,100 kilojoules) a day, and so would be categorised by experts as a VLCD (very low calorie diet), but I wasn't counting. Plus water of course. Dunkin' Donuts – which had just opened maybe its first London branch near the junction with Fleet Street – I now saw as the devil's den for journalists craving the connection with their sugar dealer.

After three days or so I was not hungry, and felt wonderful. Light-headed, sure, but this was professionally helpful – although it was wise to check the traffic a few times before crossing a road, and to hold the rail when descending stairs. Mind over matter again! I was dreaming dreams and seeing visions without any external chemical aids. After a while, ten oranges or so a day gave me sore lips.

In those days I knew nothing about nutrition. But I seemed to be an example of the guidance written in that standard textbook. 'The majority of patients . . . have a tendency to relapse that can be overcome only by strong motivation and willpower,' it stated, and: 'If the patient is well motivated and is persistent in following medical advice, she should be able to lose up to about 15kg (33lb) in two or three months without undue difficulty . . . the prognosis for a person only moderately obese and well motivated is therefore good, provided she follows advice.'

Without seeing myself as a patient and without benefit of a physician, in three months I dropped 41 pounds (18½ kilograms), from 13 stone 3 (185 pounds or 84 kilograms) to 10 stone 4 (144 pounds or 65½ kilograms). My reward was a cream suit and a cream silk tie, which I bought in a boutique on the super-trendy King's Road in Chelsea. After changing in the shop, I got on a double-decker bus, flaunted myself on its open platform, and was admired by a stranger. 'You *are* slim,' she said, or was it he, and I bounded off the bus in bliss. Maybe that was the one time in my life when I was thin.

After two days off the diet I could not zip up the suit trousers, and they hung in my wardrobe unworn for 15 years, a souvenir of the two days in my life when I was super-slim.

LITTLE HELPERS

At the end of 1968 I moved out of my marriage and in 1969 became a BBC executive, replete with a hospitality cabinet, an expense account, and a company car which I morphed into a personal taxi account. Now I really was super-busy I was locked into twelve-hour days with long lunches where the deals were struck; after-hours office lubrication of staff, visitors and self; and a felt need to be driven to and from all the street doors I entered and exited.

In 1970 I was worrying about my weight again. In my wardrobe there were four suits, bought one after the other: the memorial cream suit, the realistic slim suit, the plump suit, and the fat suit, the one I could wear, which was becoming snug. Horror! After directing the Palermo Pop Festival for RAI, the national Italian state television network, I had lunch in Rome with the fabled music director Tony Palmer, who recently had dropped a vast amount of weight. 'How come?' I asked. He ordered a huge ice cream. 'Watch,' he said, reached into a pocket, produced and opened a phial, knocked a pill onto his palm, and dropped it on the cream on top of the ice cream. 'Here is how,' he said. 'Ponderax. If you want, see Tibor Csato.' He gave me a telephone number.

Tibor had consulting rooms in Great Cumberland Place, close by Marble Arch. Hungarian, or maybe Romanian, licensed to practise medicine in Britain, he spent time only with patients who interested him. Medicine was incidental to conversation and ping pong, at the end of which he prescribed what he thought might be useful, or what you wanted. He was not a Dr Feelgood, he simply believed in 'do what you will'. This encouraged his patients to take responsibility for their own choices. I exchanged my scrip for the appetite suppressant and metabolism stimulant Ponderax (fenfluramine) half-heartedly, because I have always been suspicious of drugs, and did not repeat my request.

ME AND THE DIETING DOCTORS

When you are fat you avoid being photographed. A picture taken of me at the second Isle of Wight pop festival in 1970 showed what I had been in denial about: a football-up-the-jumper belly. Around that time I was confronted by Huw Wheldon, the charismatic managing director of BBC television, a man who came to the point. 'You have become fat,' he declared. 'Being fat does not suit you.' So I went on my own version of the high-protein, very low-starch and very low-sugar regimes of John Yudkin and Irwin Stillman.

Knowing nothing about nutrition or energy metabolism, I was interested only in being and staying slim. My instructions to myself on what to eat and drink every day, no more, no less, I listed on a folded note kept in my wallet as if a talisman. These were:

2 eggs boiled or poached, 4 ounces of lean meat or boiled fish; 1 slice bread, 2 water biscuits; ½ ounce butter (level dessertspoon); ½ ounce sugar (level dessertspoon); 1 ounce milk (enough for two coffees); 2 ounces hard cheese. In any amount: water (3 pints at least); tea, coffee; pickles, dry spices; peppers (only 'fruit' allowed); lemon; chemical sweeteners. All else is forbidden, including butter (+½ ounce), sugar (+½ ounce); alcoholic drinks; and fruit or fruit juice.

My target was 10 stone 10, because this is 150 pounds. In the first days I recorded a spectacular initial weight loss with ignorant pride, and after twelve weeks my weight reduced from 13 stone 8 (190 pounds or 86½ kilograms) to 10 stone 9 (149 pounds or 67½ kilograms): an average of 3½ pounds or over 1½ kilograms a week. I was impressed. Dieting obviously worked. I dived into my wardrobe, but the zip of the cream trousers jammed.

Checking out that regime now, I reckon it adds up to something like 500 calories (2,100 kilojoules) a day. Even if I had wolfed pickles I can't see it adding up to much more than 600 calories a day. Assuming that I was in energy 'deficit' by maybe just under 2,000 calories (8,400 kilojoules) a day, and bearing in mind that, as we all know now, initial fast weight loss is mostly water, the restriction of energy intake pretty much explains my results.

In 1972 Tibor handed me a *Unit Eating Guide*. This was a handy little fold-out 'diet sheet' distributed to physicians by Servier Laboratories, manufacturers of Ponderax. Apparently over 250,000 copies were produced. It listed foods in three groups. One list was 'eat as much as you like' foods, described as 'quite ordinary'. These included butter, cabbage, cockles, cod, cooking oil, courgettes (zucchini), cream, duck, flathead, ginger, leatherjacket, liver paste, margarine, okra, olives, oysters, pumpkin, processed cheese, salad oil, snails, suet, and tripe. Another list was printed on red paper. 'Danger! Avoid if possible' was blazoned across the top, rather like the road signs that warn of falling rocks. This list of 'foods that are rich in carbohydrate, and don't contain much in the way of nutrients' included ale, bread (brown), bread (white), cereals, bun, chocolate, flour, fructose, gin, grapes, honey, ice cream, macaroni, oatmeal, plum pudding, potato, sago, sugar, taro, yam, yoghurt (flavoured), and Yorkshire pudding. There was a time when I knew these lists almost off by heart. Their alphabetization appealed to me. Meals of garfish, mayonnaise, pepper, sea slugs, shrimps and skate were In, whereas meals of port, teff, toffees, tonic water, treacle and vermicelli were Out. This was the stuff of limericks.

However, between 1971 and 1974 I put on over 30 pounds (14 kilograms), despite a few quick intermediate purges in which I went down and up around 10-12 pounds. In 1974 I went on the high-protein diet again. This time I decided to obey doctors' orders, so I more or less banned processed sugar and starch and butter, but added fruit, vegetables, tuna with oil drained, diet soda (tonic water), and mustard. One sin was allowed: a glass of red wine a day. Without butter and sugar and with vegetables and fruits, this added up to something like 650-700 calories a day.

From 13 stone (182 pounds or 82¾ kilograms) my weight dropped by 10 pounds in 2 weeks, 20 pounds in 4 weeks, 25 pounds in 6 weeks. Then after 9 weeks, once again I broke the 150-pound barrier, and held steady at 146 pounds (10 stone 6, or 66½ kilograms) between weeks 12 and 16. The cream trousers were still too tight. They had been tight even in those two days seven years before. Besides, I had a feeling that the broken zip was trying to tell me something. This was the end of my time as a success story on this type of dieting regime. On the last day of 1975 my weight was back up to 180 pounds (82 kilograms) again.

OH! MISERY!

My New Year's resolution for 1976 was to go for a water-only fast. My one sin was coffee with milk. After 10 days I dropped 15 pounds (7 kilograms). In the next 3 months I put on 16 pounds (7½ kilograms).

Between 1967 and 1975, including other half-hearted efforts that I gave up after a short while, I shed at least 200 pounds (over 90 kilograms). If all my diets had worked, on New Year's Day 1976 I would have weighed about minus 20 pounds.

The dieting regimes mentioned so far were pretty radical. These were the ones I recorded. At other times I just ate less or a lot less of what I normally ate and drank. These regimes were ineffective, but the after-effect was the same: as soon as I started to consume more of what I usually ate and drank, I immediately developed a raging appetite, and the weight all went back on again. But what could I do? Craving food, I ate and grew fat. The records I kept as attempts at self-encouragement were full of notes like 'halfway there!' and then 'failed', and 'failed again'. Most of my life now was spent backsliding from dieting. Why could I not 'get a grip'? Why was I always 'letting go' of myself?

Food, hunger, appetite, desire, craving, my body: these were all my enemies. Increasing weight and getting fat was an inward weakness, an intractable problem, and a sign of a general failure that I could not keep secret. Anybody could see that I was out of shape and so didn't shape up. Also I was scared that if I did not go on (and on and on) dieting regimes I really would look like the Michelin man. My father became fat when he was a young man, and that scared me too. The genes, the genes! When I dared to weigh myself and found that yet again I was above 13 stone (182 pounds or 83 kilograms) a combination of self-hatred and self-respect took charge, and I went on yet another dieting regime.

It was obvious to me that failure to keep shed weight off was *my* failure. This is what 1,001 dieters, mostly women, said when interviewed in the late 1970s for the UK consumer magazine *Which?* They confessed to 'lack of willpower and determination'. One said how I felt: 'I know how to lose weight. I know I can lose weight. I lack the willpower to keep at it for what amounts to a lifetime, because whenever I give up on the programme, I put it on again.' A report on obesity published around that time in the UK said: 'The problem is one of motivation, which is a very personal matter.' Gee, thanks! When asked why people become fat by a 2006 national Pew poll conducted in the USA, 59 per cent of respondents said the reason was lack of willpower.

Now trained as an expert dieter, I was good at inter-office 'lose-weight' competitions. Some time in the mid-1970s the challenge was between me and my colleague Russell Twisk, for three weeks. The bet was £1 a pound. After two weeks Russell was 2 pounds ahead, and feeling confident. Heh heh. In the third week I did six days on a water-only fast, on the last day drank not a drop of water, and spent all the last night in the Jermyn Street Turkish Baths, now closed, in those days used by boxers and jockeys just before a fight or race. At the final weigh-in the scales first showed I was the winner by 2 pounds. Then I took the 7 pounds of butcher's weights I had purchased for the occasion out of my pockets: I was the winner by 9 pounds and £9. Russell, a racing man, pointed out that horses run with weights, and I accepted £2. Reminiscing with Russell recently, he reminded me that at the celebration blow-out at Le Lavandou in Marylebone High Street immediately after the weigh-in, I was helped to my seat by the head waiter, who thought I was wasting away.

GETTING IN SHAPE

In 1977 a long-term relationship broke up, and I joined one of London's first health clubs: Debenham's Gym'n'Tonic, now long gone, then in Welbeck Street. There was also a professional motive. Tony Morgan, the Olympic yachting silver medallist, had been appointed the BBC's youngest governor; he wanted to get the lowdown on the machinations of the corporation's executives from an insider, and he was a member of Gym'n'Tonic. So I turned fink: we met in the early mornings in the sauna and plotted.

After six months on the Nautilus machines, I could do 200 sit-ups (and on one occasion with an audience, 300). I asked Mike Welton, the trainer in charge, to give me a reason why I was doing this. 'To keep fit, sir,' he replied respectfully. 'That's not a reason,' I said. He leaned forward confidentially. 'When you are fit,' he said, 'you can eat all day, drink all evening, and make love all night.' (Except he didn't say 'make love'.) 'Thank you, Mike,' I said, 'that's a reason.'

In 1978 I went to Hyde Park, watched the first *Sunday Times* National Fun Run, and realized that I had become a spectator of my own life, not a participant. So I started to jog. By the summer of 1979 I was running the 4½ miles (7.2 kilometres) round Hyde Park and Kensington Gardens, slowly, but without stopping.

That summer I also took a holiday in the Cyclades, ate lots of fish, salad including feta cheese and olives, and rough bread, all washed down with the local retsina, walked a lot and swam a bit, came back from holiday 8 pounds (3½ kilograms) lighter, and decided that my dieting days were ended.

Russell and I challenged one another to run the New York marathon, which we did in 1980. We remember one training run. The night before there had been a big snow dump, and I cycled in the dark to his house in Ealing. He opened the door in his pyjamas and dressing gown and asked me if I was mad. 'Russell,' I said, 'this is one to tell to our grand-children.' So we ran through Gunnersbury Park to Kew Bridge, along the Thames towpath, and round Richmond Park, making new tracks all the way. On the way back as we approached the huddled commuters by the Kew High Street bus shelter, I stripped off my singlet, waved it round my head, and accelerated. That morning I was at my desk at the *Sunday Times* before my colleagues arrived. Ah, mastery. This was better than dieting.

But I was puzzled. In those days exercise was discounted as a way to lose weight. John Yudkin said: 'To dispose of a good business lunch, you would have to play squash for eight hours.' Irwin Stillman said: 'No amount of exercising will reduce you if you overeat.' Herman Tarnower, whose Scarsdale Diet was first published in 1979, said: 'It is extremely difficult to lose significant weight by exercise.' In 1982 the British Code of Advertising Practice said: 'A diet is the only practicable self-treatment for achieving a reduction in excess fat . . . claims, whether direct or indirect, that weight loss can be achieved by any other means, are not acceptable.'

Just like when I was a boy, I tended to become fat for what seemed obvious reasons: being sedentary and eating and drinking a lot, often in restaurants. Thinking about this now, what kept my shed weight off, at school and later in the 1970s, was physical activity, more or less to the level of an average person in the days before machines took over the physical work that humans are designed to do.

What I did not pay attention to then though, was that when I became physically fit my weight did not decrease a lot: instead I shed body fat and gained lean tissue. As a result, at a fit 165 pounds (75 kilograms) my waist measurement was 5 inches (12½ centimetres) less than it was at a fat 176 pounds (80 kilograms). That's a big difference.

THE STANFORD REVELATION

It began to dawn on me that the dieting books were wrong, and I started to take a professional interest in dieting. I began to see the light as a result of observing the effects of my own physical activity, as I wrote about the joys of jogging in *Running* magazine, which I did in my 'Fun Runner' column for a decade, as a result getting interested in exercise physiology and a literature unknown to the dieting doctors.

Thus, when Derek Miller, Professor Yudkin's colleague at what is now King's College London, said that to work off the energy contained in a hearty meal you would have to walk up and down Ben Nevis, Britain's highest mountain, he was referring to studies done of people walking on treadmills whose energy expenditure was measured while they were exercising. But everybody who is physically active knows that after exercise, the body is warmer for some time, which means that energy is also being used after the activity has finished. Further, what about the cumulative effect of getting in shape, as a result of which relatively inactive body fat is essentially replaced by lean tissue – muscle – that when used is more metabolically active all the time?

The dieting doctors, who seemed to be a desk-bound bunch, knew nothing about this. Indeed, it was only when the jogging boom started, in the USA in the 1970s and in the UK in the 1980s, that exercise physiologists had an abundant resource of initially sedentary people who had decided to start running, and whose responses to moving from being fat to being fit – including changes in energy requirements and turnover – could be measured. In the summer of 1981 I decided to check all this out, and visited Stanford University in Menlo Park, just south of San Francisco. The people I went to see were Jack Farquhar, William Haskell and Peter Wood, of the Stanford heart disease prevention programme; this included aerobic physical activity, running in particular.

Yes, they confirmed that physical activity increases the amount of energy the body uses after the activity is completed. Yes, physical training, as a result of which body composition changes to less fat and more muscle, results in the body needing more energy all the time. This is very important, I said. They agreed.

Then I realized that the dieting books were wrong in another way. 'What about dieting?' I asked. They explained that energy restriction causes a lowering of metabolic rate, sometimes dramatic, usually in proportion to the severity and length of restriction. The effects of exercise on energy turnover are underestimated, and those of energy restriction are overestimated. There is a whole literature on this, they said. When sedentary people go on diets they lose muscle and other lean tissue, some of which is not replaced after the dieting ends. The weight increase is mostly fat. So in that case, I said, jumping a couple of steps ahead of the logic, dieting makes you fat.

Yes, was the answer. Then there was a pause. One of them said something like 'Gee. That's a bestseller!' I was elated. So that was why my dieting regimes had never worked! The Stanford team generously copied for me a case-load of salient academic papers, I flew back to London, and wrote a feature for the *Sunday Times* with the title 'Dieting makes you fat', published in the post-Christmas issue. Gail Rebuck, who with Anthony and Rosie Cheetham had just launched the Century publishing house, bought my book proposal, telling me that it would be the first number one bestseller in the first Century list in the summer of 1983, which it was.

HARD TIMES

For me personally that first version of *Dieting Makes You Fat* was meant as a requiem for my dieting days. Physical activity, that's where it was at, plus the sparkling new nutritional orthodoxy of diets high in fibre, and low in fat, saturated fats, sugars, salt and alcohol.

Dieting Makes You Fat made a lot of positive waves. Afterwards, most dieting regimes acknowledged exercise, and many got the point that with food and drink it is quality rather than quantity that counts. A new wave of books merged diets that they said would cause reduction in weight with those that would also reduce the risk of heart disease, cancer, and other chronic diseases. The dieting wars of the 1990s and 2000s have been, and still are, between champions of high protein, high fat and low starch and sugar, for quick weight reduction, and champions of regimes high in wholegrains, vegetables and fruits, and low in fat and sugar, for general good health as well as, they say, to shed weight. All the same, though, every year calorie counting and energy restriction becomes bigger and bigger business.

And me? As long as I kept on running, I stayed more or less the same weight and shape. Encouraging myself by encouraging others, in 1981 I had formed London 1982/50, a group of 50 citizens who had decided to train to complete the marathon distance in 1982, which they did. This in turn led to the creation of the Serpentine Running Club and sister clubs in north and south London.

Something I learned from those days is that in a sedentary society, amount of weight is equated with amount of fat. It is assumed that the more you weigh, the fatter you are. But weight and fat are not the same. For example John Walker, a 1982/50 and Serpies stalwart, who is about the same height as me, weighed 83 kilograms before his marathon training and 84 kilograms after the race. These are weights at which I have been conspicuously fat. But John, an infantryman who served in the Falklands, was what we called a 'brick shithouse' type: solid muscle which, with its much higher water content, is heavier and more compact than fat, as well as being in the right places. The most important measure to make when you increase your physical activity is not of your weight but your waist. More on this in chapter 3.

My ninth and last marathon, in New York in 1984, I ran – and jogged and walked – over an hour slower than my best time. After that, running round parks lost its glamour. In the later 1980s I became full-time engaged in food and nutrition policy, stopped being particularly physically active, and my weight and waist increased again; but not so fast as in the days when I dieted. I retained some fitness by regular runs round Hyde Park and Kensington Gardens.

Then I made a mistake. Caroline Walker, then my partner, later my second wife, was diagnosed with cancer in early 1985 and died in late 1988. In such circumstances the healthy person has a responsibility to stay in shape. But in a process of perverse sympathy I neglected myself, and entered the 1990s a lot less fit, and more fat, than had been my plan and vision a decade earlier.

PLAN JAMS

My records of the early 1990s are jammed with plans. I joined health clubs, bought and sometimes rode a 15-speed racing bicycle, ran sporadically, sometimes gave up alcoholic drinks, tea and coffee, ate lots of vegetables, and usually bobbled around between 172, 161 and 172 pounds (78, 73 and 78 kilograms). Then I made another vow, that my weight should always be under 11 stone 11 pounds (165 pounds, 75 kilograms). For two months I went wholefood vegan, for the craic. This regime ended when, after running along the towpath of the Grand Union Canal in west London carrying a chapter of a new book, I fainted in the foyer of my then publisher, fell against the edge of a metal table, and cracked a couple of ribs. This was predictable; my blood pressure tends to be low, and drops rapidly when I restrict what I eat and drink. Afterwards my weight steadily increased.

At the end of 1996 I was up to 13 stone 3 (185 pounds or 84 kilograms), and a candid friend commented on my paunch. Ouch. So on New Year's Day 1997 I joined the Porchester Baths health club at the bottom of Queensway in west London, near where I lived, and signed up with Paola, one of the personal trainers. Noticing that some of the advice given to members was adapted from *Dieting Makes You Fat*, I stayed incognito. My plan was to eat just over 2 pounds (a kilogram) of vegetables and fruits every day and once again to ban alcoholic drinks. After 14 weeks of aerobic training on stairs and cycles, plus anaerobic training on the resistance machines, together with my diet plan, I had dropped 25 pounds and reached my target weight of 11 stone 6 (160 pounds or 73 kilograms). This checks out as a body mass index (BMI) of 22 which, according to the World Cancer Research Fund report I was then directing and editing, was exactly where as a population member I should be.

This figured: my aim was to use around 1,000 calories a day more than I was consuming, which allowing for a lighter body needing less energy from food to stay in balance, predicted a drop averaging around 6 pounds or close to 3 kilograms a month.

Before and after moving to Brazil in 2000, my weight drifted upwards again. Between April and June 1999 I was bingeing for the one time in my life. I had a reason for self-destruction, and this horrible time coincided with business trips and hospitality in Italy where I was necking a lot of pasta, fruit tarts, and red wine, more even than my chunky Italian colleagues.

In those three months my weight shot up; I must have put on more or less a stone (14 pounds, or 6½ kilograms). This taught me a lesson for life. Sometimes when you undereat or overeat, your body protects you, and the decreased or increased weight is not what the usual calculations of energetics predict. This time something I was consuming had an unexpectedly dramatic effect, and I had become fat again.

THE WOUNDED HEALER

Since 2003 I have been writing 'Out of the Box', a column in the journal *Public Health Nutrition*. In 2004 I decided to explore fasting. My motive was not to shed body fat, but to find out and record what prolonged fasting felt like. I thought then – and now – that warnings against radical fasting forget that humans are evolved to adapt to food insecurity and famine, and that fasting is a feature of seriously observed philosophies and religions, a way to remember the hard times. I blanked on the fact that radical fasts have the same effect as dieting.

So I fasted three times for periods of seven to ten days: one fast of fruit only, one of grapes only, one of water only. Just like the books say, your body quickly gets the message that there is no food available, your brain as well as the rest of your body feeds off your built-in energy stores, and you become enlightened.

Now I make my confession within this confession. In 2004 I came out of dieting retirement. In 2004 I prepared to get married, and for me this time was not going to be a fat wedding. My first wedding had been a register office job. This third wedding was billed as a Brazilian extended family *festa*, every adult guest with a digital camera. No hiding place.

Impressed by the effect of fasting, I wanted a quick result, so I went on a two-week water-only fast, twice, this time in order to reduce weight. A few days before the big day I was exactly where I wanted to be. Yes, yet another target achieved, this time 11 stone (154 pounds, or 70 kilograms) making a body mass index of 21.5; and I celebrated in town by buying my wedding gear: a cream suit and a white Panama hat.

Six months later I had put back all the weight I had shed, and more. Once again I organized my trousers into the cream, slim, get real, and fat pairs. I could still get into the Panama hat. All this connected me with me as a younger man. Over the next three years I realized it was time to write *Dieting Makes You Fat* all over again.

Personally I now realize that I will always tend to be fat. Perhaps this tendency 'runs in the family' on my father's side. But if instead of growing up in Britain I was a rural worker in India – or indeed a manual labourer anywhere – it's practically certain that I would have stayed lean, at least as long as I remained active. More to the point though – because I am not an Indian peasant or a manual worker, and probably nor are you – I made two mistakes when I was a child. One was to stop running around as kids are designed to do, and instead to stay indoors and behave like a little office worker, sitting down almost all my waking time, and also consuming a lot of fat and sugar. Two, the big mistake, was to semi-starve myself, and in this way to train my body to retain and to increase its store of fat as soon as I had stopped my self-invented nibble regime. If I had not done this and instead had played games and joined in sport at school and regained a zest for natural active life, I would have been less likely to have developed the appetites that made me fat as a young man.

This lesson from long ago is not just personal. When I was a boy few children were fat. Now childhood obesity is common, and not only in materially rich countries. One reason is that these days, children as well as adults have become sedentary, and also consume a lot of fat and sugar, now mostly as contained in energy-dense highly processed foods and drinks. Another reason is because now even young children are being put on energy-restrictive dieting regimes in the belief, urged on parents by health professionals, that dieting will help children not just to reduce weight and body fat, but also to stay slim. It will not. Dieting makes children fat too.

Professionally I have for many years been in a privileged position to think these issues through. As well as the early knowledge I gained in writing the first version of this book, since the mid-1980s my main work has been interrogation and interpretation of the findings of biological science. Since the early 1990s I have worked with some of the world's leading nutrition scientists, many of whom have given me information and shared opinions that support the thesis of this book. During this time I have also gained increasing respect for broader fields of study, and for the testimony of experienced and thoughtful observers. Since around the year 2000, I have paid special attention to the evolutionary, historical, economic, social, environmental as well as biological determinants of disease and health – and of overweight and obesity.

At the same time, at first as a journalist and then as an author, executive, campaigner, and occasional delegate at United Nations assemblies, I have come to understand at international as well as national level, the title of one of my books, the politics of food. As they say, I have been inside the belly of the beast. Industrial food systems are not designed to improve your health, but to make money, and the most profitable products are usually bad for your health. No UN agency, national government, or established expert organization is ever likely to admit this.

In this book my main task has been to explain why dieting makes you fat, to outline what else makes you fat, and to show how we can gain good health and wellbeing, which includes escaping out of the dieting trap.

It seems to me now that quite a lot of what is written here is plain common sense, once you know how to set aside what now amounts to a colossal food, drink, dieting, and medical industry whose products are generally unhealthy and whose messages are mostly wrong. You also may find that some of what is here is surprising. For example, as told in chapter 3, something you won't find in any book on nutrition or dieting is that for 2,500 years pig breeders have known that the most effective way of fattening their animals is first to starve them. But I am jumping ahead – the next chapter is all about the fabulous dieting industry.

WHY WE EAT

These confessions and reflections – apart from this last passage – were drafted at our holiday home in Cabo Frio, two hours north of the city of Rio de Janeiro. Leaving, we drove out and south in the dark, and then west on the spectacular highway through the Atlantic forest up and over the mountains of Petropólis, towards the state of Minas Gerais and the city of Juiz de Fora where we live most of the time. I insisted on stopping at Barrakin, which serves great snack meals.

The *mandioca frita* (cassava chips/French fries) at Barrakin are bliss. For native Brazilians the *mandioca* root is central to their religion as their source of life, as is maize (corn) for the Mayan people. Scores of families live on cleared land out of sight of the highway, and sell their *mandioca* and bananas by the roadside, and to the Barrakin cook, fresh out of the ground.

But why did I need to stop? Was it the girls? Three young women, maybe sisters, bring the drinks and serve spit-grilled meat, sausage and chicken to truckers on the road driving into the interior of this vast land, sitting in the open thatched eating area. They all have style, and one is like a thin, fey, wild, shy young Julia Roberts. No, that wasn't the reason. I ordered *mandioca frita* and ordered a beer. Also a *vinaigrete*, which in Brazil is marinaded chopped onions, peppers and tomatoes, and we took the food back to the car in tinfoil containers. I was not driving.

Aromas wafted in the space inside the car as we drove towards Minas. After a while the fat chips were all eaten, and I scooped up the last crispy bits and crunched them and sucked the grease and vinegar off my fingers. Then I realized what it was that I had needed, and still need now: I was, as I am now as I write, me as a child, walking alone along the Seven Sisters Road in the dark, wanting what my mother wanted also, a home.

Hunger and appetite, and the reasons why we do what we do, are deeper and more complex and compelling than we may suppose.

2. THE FABULOUS DIETING BUSINESS

The Holy Grail of Western medicine is a safe and comfortable way to lose excessive body fat. This fruitless search has been the basis of an almost endless array of 'reducing diets' that have tantalized the fat folks and enriched the publishers and the medical businessmen. The reducing diets have been disappointing – some would say, a medical disaster.

George Mann

Around the world, obesity is concurrent with the increased incidence of these things: TV, mobile phones, cars, multi-storey buildings, computers, pornography, credit-card use, cocaine use, binge drinking, celebrity gossip, images of extremely slender female models, images of male models with six-pack stomachs, media driven by advertising, depression . . . and supermarkets with upwards of 20,000 products under the same roof.

William Leith

Dieting is a booming business. As more and more people become overweight and obese, a correspondingly vast number of dieting regimes have been marketed, often claiming that at last they contain the unique answer.

Like processed foods and drinks, dieting regimes seem wonderfully varied. But however cleverly branded and marketed, they are almost all based on one idea: restrict dietary energy and you will reduce weight. But what then?

Methods of shedding weight, such as purging, vomiting, exercise, sweating, bleeding, fasting, the taking of medicinal waters, the use of stimulants, anorectics, emetics, diuretics, and yes, reducing diets, are as old as urban society. Baths built around mineral water springs were centrepieces of ancient Greek and Roman cities.

After Europe became industrialized, spas became used less for general healing and rejuvenation, more for weight reduction. In the early 20th century Baden-Baden and Wiesbaden both offered the 'grape cure' – nothing but grapes for two weeks, starting with 2–3 pounds (up to a kilogram and more) a day, working up to a daily heroic 8–12 pounds (3½–5 kilograms). Marienbad was maybe the first fat farm, patronized by Edward VII and his entourage. When leaving Marienbad the King-Emperor always issued instructions that his waistcoats be taken in; but his valet always refused, knowing that the imperial paunch would soon swell again.

THE OBESITY BOOM

Until the mid-20th century obesity was uncommon, except among materially rich people who enjoyed their food and drink and who did not engage in physical work. But now almost all people in high-income countries lead largely sedentary lives and have plenty to eat and drink, and the world is getting stuffed.

Since the 1980s, rates of obesity have rocketed. This was foreseen in the preface to a compendium of academic papers published in 1978, which stated: 'The study of obesity is alive and thriving. The chapters in this volume attest to this fact and promise a bright and rewarding future in this area.' Half or more of all adults in most European countries including western Russia, and in North America, are now said to be overweight, of which roughly one-third are said to be obese. In 2005, the US Federal Aviation Authority increased the weight of its Standard Passenger (used to calculate the centre of gravity of airliners, speed needed for takeoff, and fuel requirements) by 8 per cent for males and 18 per cent for females. In-flight magazines and telephones are being removed to save weight and to accommodate bellies and, according to a report in the *Guardian,* so are life-vests. Wags have suggested that check-in areas should include people-measurers with the warning: 'if you cannot fit in here we will put you in the hold'.

Sweeping statements are made on the impact of overweight and obesity on health. 'More than one million deaths . . . annually are due to diseases related to excess body weight,' claimed a European Charter issued from a ministerial conference in collaboration with the World Health Organization, held in Istanbul in late 2006.

In Britain, super-size school uniforms are now being produced, including shirts with 17½-inch (44.5cm) necks and trousers with 42-inch (107cm) waists. Young obese girls may become sexually mature at the age of ten, which predicts a surge of pre-teen pregnancies. Three-year-olds are now being treated for obesity. In late 2007, a Foresight report produced for the UK government included a bold projection of current trends, suggesting that by 2050 most British adults will be obese. The number of severely obese adults in the USA is reckoned to have quadrupled between 1986 and 2000, from 1 in 200 to 1 in 50.

Overweight and obesity is not a phenomenon just of materially rich countries. In Brazil between 1975 and 2000, the percentage of underweight people decreased from 25 to 4, while overweight people increased from 16 to 40.5 per cent, and obese people increased from 4.7 to 11 per cent. That is to say, about half the Brazilian adult population is now overweight, of which roughly a quarter are obese, women more than men.

This very rapid shift from underweight to overweight has occurred in most middle-income countries and also in the cities of low-income countries. Between 1975 and 2005, rates of obesity in urban India increased fivefold. Around the year 2000 among the middle class in New Delhi, one-third of men and half of women were obese by the standards used in India, as were one in seven slum-dwellers in northern India. The only countries where on average people are reducing body fat are those beset by famine, war or blockade.

In the USA the Institute of Medicine, whose task is to advise and guide the federal government, concluded in 2007 that 'childhood obesity is a nationwide health crisis'. Rates of overweight and obesity in children and young people in many materially rich countries have increased three- or fourfold since the 1980s. In the USA, the average weight of girls aged between 12 and 17 increased between 1966 and 2002 from 54.5 to 59 kilograms (118 to 130 pounds); of boys in the same age range, from 57 to 64 kilograms (125 to 141 pounds). In the UK, the average weight of 12-year-old girls increased from 41.5 kilograms (91½ pounds) in 1977 to 49 kilograms (108 pounds) in 2007, and their average waist measurements increased by nearly 9½ centimetres (over 3½ inches). For 12-year-old boys the figures were 40.4 kilograms (89 pounds) in 1977 and 47 kilograms (103½ pounds) in 2007, with waists increasing by an average of nearly 8 centimetres (over 3 inches).

Bariatrics, the branch of medicine concerned with obesity, was invented in the mid-1960s. Obesity can be treated by surgery that restricts the capacity of the stomach or bypasses some of the gut. This is a major procedure; it uncommonly results in death, but post-operative 'complications' are very common, and the chance of failure is quite high. In the USA in 2003 over 100,000 people underwent such bariatric surgery; in 2007 around 180,000. Brazilians also favour surgery; in 2006 around 25,000 operations were carried out. In other countries such procedures are less common. A bariatric surgeon has suggested to the House of Commons Health Committee that around 1 million people in the UK are suitable cases for surgical treatment.

THE DIETING INDUSTRY BOOM, BOOM

The world is also getting stuffed by the dieting industry, which is now a colossal business. In Europe and the USA, two leading marketing firms give evidently valuable advice to the industry: their annual reports cost around €3,000 and $US5,000, respectively. Datamonitor, one of these firms, sees 'phenomenal growth in the market for weight loss products'. In the early and middle years of the 2000s the reports estimated the total value of the USA dieting industry – meaning food, drink, and supplements – at $US46 billion (yes, thousand million) a year. The estimate for Europe was €93 billion. It is safe to say that the figures for 2010 will respectively be well over $US50 billion and €100 billion.

The annual sales of the dieting industry altogether are a lot more than those of Nestlé, the world's biggest food and drink manufacturer. A media release issued by one of the marketing firms was headlined: 'Keeping dieters dieting the key to market growth'.

It is said that in any one year, around two-thirds of women and one-half of men in North America and in the materially richer European countries try to reduce their weight. Few keep shed weight off. A representative of the European marketing organization expressed concern: 'Overall, only approximately 1 per cent of dieters achieve permanent weight loss.' But this is no cause for commercial concern. Indeed, what could be better than an industry whose products do not work, or work only as long as you use them, for as long as you live, but whose customers believe that they have no other choice? If you get worried about the stability of banks you can put your savings into property or under your mattress. People who try but fail to reduce weight on a dieting regime typically see no alternative but to try a new regime.

The dieting book bonanza

When I first planned this book, I did not intend to anatomize the global dieting industry, but thought to include a chapter summarizing dieting regimes available to anybody with access to the internet. Ha! Impossible! A check on Amazon.com using the key words 'weight loss' generated 43,833 entries, of which the first 200 – and for all I know the first 1,000 – are almost all different books.

Just half an hour digging beneath the US version of my email home page gives me the Atkins Diet, the Better Sex Diet, the Blood Type Diet, Bob Greene's Best Life Diet, the Cabbage Soup Diet, the Chewing Gum Diet, Crazy diets (lots of these), Diet Busters (foods and drinks to avoid when on a diet), diets of the stars (many of these), the Doctors' Crash Diets (several of these), the Dr Phil Diet, the Fat Flush Diet, the Fat Smash Diet, the 5 Factor Diet, the Grapefruit Diet, the Great Abs Diet, the Green Tea Diet (big with Oprah Winfrey), the Juice Fast Diet, the LA Weight Loss Diet, the Martha's Vineyard Diet, Nutri-System, the SlimFast plan, religious diets (including the Hallelujah Diet, the Maker's Diet, the What Would Jesus Eat Diet), the Sonoma Diet, the 3 Hour Diet, the 3 Hour Diet for Teens, the Ultimate New York Diet, the Ultra Metabolism Diet, the Weight Watchers Diet, and the Zone Diet.

Later I found the Philosopher's Diet, the Brain Food Diet, the

Shangri-La Diet, and many, many more. In late 2007 I browsed the Barnes and Noble store in Georgetown: the 'Health', 'Trends in Health', 'Medical Reference', 'Choose Your Diet', and 'Diet' sections, altogether filling an entire aisle, were mostly dieting books.

Ah well, you might think, that's just the USA. Not so. The numbers of dieting regimes have rocketed all over the world, in parallel with the soaring rates of overweight and obesity. For example, business is booming in Brazil, as I noted when looking round the bookshop at Belém airport in the summer of 2007 at the end of a tour in Amazonia. There was a whole section devoted to dieting books. Here are their titles in Portuguese – some are mentioned above. Two were named after places (*Dieta de Sonoma*, *A Dieta de South Beach*); one was time-based (*A Dieta Das 3 Horas*); there was a one-food dieting book (*A Dieta do Mel* – honey); an eponymous dieting book (*A Dieta Perricone*); two based on the notion that French women don't get fat (*As Mulheres Francesas Não Engordam*, *A Não Dieta Dos Francescas*); two based on biochemical theses, one orthodox (*A Dieta Do Indice Glicêmico*), one unorthodox (*A Dieta do Typo Sanguineo*); and one whose title in English is *Ten Habits That Mess Up a Woman's Diet*. There were more, but my flight was called.

Jeez! It's unlikely that Kennedy, Heathrow or Schiphol bookshops stocked as much choice 25 years ago. There are few obese people in the streets and markets in Belém, and I saw none in the countryside, except one broken-down truck driver. However, it was a different story in the Belém Hilton hotel restaurant, where breasts billowed, bellies bounced, and backsides biffed my breakfast off my table; and here, I suppose, were the airport shop customers.

To comment even briefly on just the leading current dieting regimes would take a whole book – and there are such compilations, designed along the lines of A–Zs of movies, music or museums. You can surf for dieting regimes. Maybe you do.

It's all about branding

Then I saw the light. Dieting regimes – the successful ones – are branded products, just like mass-marketed snack foods. The British writer William Leith describes himself browsing a 'library' of savoury snacks in a New York supermarket. 'I could have full-fat snacks or low-fat snacks or no-fat snacks. I could have Wheat Thins or Crisps or Bits or Ritz or Hits or

Twigs or Snaps or Pops or Chips or Dips or Chewys or Crunchys or Munchies or Lunchies. I could have Frites or Ruffles or Pringles or Singles or Doubles or Mingles; I could have Chunkys or Funkys or Baldies or Garibaldis or Grahams or Lays or Frito-Lays or Newtons, or Cheddars or Cheese-urns, Fritos, Doritos, Cheet-ohs, Tostitos.' Maybe he invented some of these brand names, but even so, on, and on, and on. Trade magazines state that in the USA over 15,000 new food and drink products are introduced every year, of which several thousand are new packaged snacks.

Here is the connection. If you have some knowledge of food chemistry and technology, when you look at the labels of snack products you will see that most of them are variations of just a few homogenized master ingredients: 'refined' starches and sugars, hydrogenated fats, hydrolysed protein, and sodium compounds, mixed up and made savoury, crunchy, munchy, tasty, tempting and moreish, sometimes with sprinklings of 'natural' ingredients like powdered milk, egg or cheese, and practically always with sophisticated combinations of cosmetic and other additives. The same applies to packaged baked goods like biscuits and cakes, and to ice cream and confectionery. They taste different, but the master ingredients are again much the same, except there are more sugars, processed from cane, beet, or corn. The variety is in the packaging and presentation. The products are mostly made up from the cheapest – often subsidized – ingredients on the market. The magic and the profit are in the branding.

Throughout history around 7,000 plant species are known to have been used for food by human societies, says the socio-biologist Edward O Wilson. Now, nine-tenths of the world's food comes from 20 species. Four-fifths of the world's population relies on a few varieties of four staple crops – wheat, rice, corn, potatoes. Similarly, within what seems to be a vast array of dieting regimes, there are three basic different types. Almost all either rely on magic ingredients (items claimed to have special slimming qualities), or else manipulate the proportions of 'macronutrients' (protein, fat, carbohydrate and alcohol), or else are 'sensible' – these advocate 'enjoy a balanced varied diet but watch your weight'. Plus there are now the 'don't diet' dieting regimes, some evidently influenced by the first version of this book and the evidence that continues consistently to support its thesis.

Almost all have one feature in common. Just as the main secret of branded snacks is processed starches, sugars and fats, plus chemical additives, the main secret of branded dieting regimes of all types, whether they admit to this or not, is restriction of energy from food and drink. This is basically how they all work – as long as you are on them. Here I touch on just a few, including some I have tried myself.

First though, here is a general remark. There is a lot of sanctimonious hostility to dieting regimes. Influential health professionals and their representative organizations can be quick to condemn claims made – for instance for the special properties of some fruits, or animal foods high in protein, or dietary fibre, or certain herbs, or for fasting – saying that these are nonsense or even fraudulent. Physicians, nutritionists and dietitians often warn that dieting deprives the body of energy – of course it does! – and that most dieting regimes are nutritionally unbalanced – of course they are!

No doubt people have died as a direct result of dieting, but the numbers will be a tiny fraction of those killed directly or indirectly by prescription drugs or by hospital infections. Zeal against dieting regimes would be better directed towards scrutinizing claims made for prescription and other legal drugs and, when appropriate, denunciation of their ill-effects.

Further, sometimes claims made for dieting regimes, including some that have from time to time been denounced by medical or nutritional establishments, have turned out on investigation to have some sound foundation. Many if not most dieting regimes do contain good bits, the equivalent of the cheese or eggs, nuts or seeds in snack foods. Indeed, some snacks are nourishing as well as delicious, especially when prepared and served fresh; and likewise some dieting regimes are healthy in themselves. Their eventual effect on the weight and the body fat of the people who follow them is another matter, as you will see in the next chapter.

MAGIC INGREDIENT DIETING REGIMES

Magic ingredient dieting regimes, like those featuring green tea, chewing gum, or cabbage soup, are appealing for the same reason as antibiotic drugs: they are a 'magic bullet' approach to weight reduction. Furthermore, when the claimed active ingredient can be synthesized, it is also often marketed in the form of pills, powders or potions.

The papaya and potato diets

A classic magic ingredient dieting regime is the Beverly Hills Diet. In its first stages this restricts dieters to papaya, which 'softens body fat', pineapple, which 'burns it off', and watermelon, which 'flushes it out of the body'. Mango is also recommended. This works as long as you stay with it, because an average-sized woman would have to eat something like 5 kilograms (11 pounds) of any of these fruits a day to achieve energy balance.

The principle is identical with that of the venerable grape cure. Any single-food regime will almost certainly work while you are on it. Denis Burkitt, the Irish surgeon who became the great evangelist for dietary fibre, once organized 23 young men from Galway to eat ten large potatoes baked in their skins every day for three months. Every day, but only after they had eaten all ten potatoes, they were free to eat and drink anything else they liked. Most shed weight.

Why? A large potato weighs around 200 grams or close to half a pound, so ten might altogether weigh 2 kilograms or around 4½ pounds. Potatoes are mostly water and therefore bulky; ten leave room for little if any other food. The energy in 2 kilograms of boiled or baked potatoes is something like 1,500 calories (6,300 kilojoules) a day: a lot less than relatively active young men need to stay in energy balance. If the experiment had allowed them to add fat or oil to the potatoes, and so perhaps double or treble their energy density, the result would have been different and the Galway volunteers would have increased in weight.

Dieting regimes based on one or a few foods rely on you becoming full up or fed up or even nauseated before it or they have supplied enough energy to keep your body in energy balance. The more bulky such foods are, the less of them you will be able to eat before feeling sated.

Mrs Eyton's green bananas

Being grossly overweight already (in the nine pieces of luggage sense, nothing personal), I didn't buy any dieting books in Belém, but I had done so at Sydney airport a few weeks previously. One of them was Audrey Eyton's new F-book.

Mrs Eyton's *The F-Plan Diet*, best known in the UK, was first published in the early 1980s and sold millions globally. With her the magic ingredient is not papaya or mango, but dietary fibre. In 2006 she followed up with *The F2 Diet*.

F2 is a snappy book: 100 pages of text and 100 pages of lists and recipes. 'Unbeatable for fast weight loss' are its introductory words. As a former popular journalist and founding editor of *Slimming* magazine, she does not resist a gimmick. 'Eat at least one medium-size green banana each day,' she says. 'Buy the greenest bananas you can find, just a few at a time.'

'Get slim fast and feel fantastic in *days*!' say the cover selling lines. '*New* super-slimming tactics.' The cover picture is of a pretty girl-next-door type with a winsome smile, wearing a loose white halter-neck, and unbelted blue jeans that look as if they are about to fall off – as presumably have her excess pounds, thanks to *F2*.

Nutritionists who care about transit times, poo consistency, and gut health, will look kindly on any bestseller that boosts consumption of foods containing a lot of dietary fibre. Mrs Eyton now tells the glycaemic index and resistant starch stories, which when demystified amount to recommending minimally processed plant foods that the body digests at a natural speed. She also points out that fibre is munchies for friendly flora, the gut bacteria that protect our health. Plus she recommends reduction of dietary fat and alcoholic drinks.

However, on examination the F-books are really standard energy-restricting regular-weighing dieting regimes. Thus in *F1* she says: 'Allow yourself 1,500 calories daily if you are male, of at least medium height, and more than 7 pounds overweight ... allow yourself 1,000 calories daily if you are female and less than 14 pounds overweight.' Having said (mistakenly) that one pound of body fat equals 3,500 calories, she goes on to say mistakenly that 'with a daily deficit of 1,000 calories you could expect to reduce around two pounds a week'.

She is against physical activity. In *F2* she says, 'It is exceedingly difficult to shed any significant amount of surplus weight by exercise alone ... this would require a very great deal of time, effort, persistence and patience'. As in *F1*, calorie cutting is the way, and 'on a high-fibre diet you will shed fat faster than any other diet of the same number of calories. This is well-proven scientific fact.' This time, though, she evidently reckons that if you consume more fibre and less fat, the calories will look after themselves. What about sustainability? 'That phrase "this is a diet you can follow for the rest of your life" somehow fills me full of profound depression.' She braces readers to expect to increase their weight after completing her regime.

Mrs Eyton's general approach is more or less in line with current conventional consensus dietary guidelines, especially for gut health, but she does not understand physical activity. The claims made in *F2* range from reasonable to incredible. The chances of *F2* followers keeping shed body fat off long-term after the regime has ended, is, as with all energy-restricted diet regimes – and especially those that neglect physical activity – practically nil.

MACRONUTRIENT MANIPULATION DIETING REGIMES

Chemically, foods and drinks are made up from macronutrients, supplying energy, and micronutrients – also essential for health and life – which do not supply energy. Proteins, fats and carbohydrates are macronutrients, as is alcohol (ethanol); vitamins and minerals are micronutrients. The chemical approach to food, nutrition and health, which displaces foods and drinks in favour of their chemical constituents, has generally proved to be a disaster – more on this in chapter 4. One result has been scores, maybe hundreds, of macronutrient manipulation dieting regimes.

Dr Atkins's prime ribs

In the first half of the 2000s, the best-known dieting programme in the USA and worldwide has been that of the highest-profile 'dieting doctor' Robert Atkins, whose *Diet Revolution* was first published in 1972. His *New Diet Revolution*, a chunky paperback of 445 pages, published in 1992 and updated in 1999, has broken all records. Global Atkins book sales are estimated at up to 20 million, and it's said that just before he died in 2003 around one in ten adults in the USA and UK were 'doing Atkins'.

Just in case you don't know, Dr Atkins's diet regime is comparatively very high and absolutely high in animal protein and animal fat, very low in carbohydrates (foods containing substantial amounts of sugars or starches) and – although he liked to portray himself as a gourmet and played this down – low in alcoholic drinks. His main claim is that carbohydrates make you fat. In his first phase all carbohydrates were Out:

'Super Don'ts. Put these out of your life and your recipes. Bread, cereal, corn, ice cream, ketchup, macaroni, milk, potatoes, pulse vegetables, rice, spaghetti, sugar, sweets/chewing gum, water biscuits. Note: one piece of chewing gum can spoil the whole metabolic balance.' In his second phase he narrows his attack: 'When I speak of carbohydrates, I'm referring to the unhealthy ones – sugar and white flour, milk and white rice, processed and refined foods of all kinds, junk food and the like.'

He enjoyed provoking the nutritional and medical establishment, which since the 1970s in the USA and the 1980s worldwide has generally agreed that healthy diets are comparatively low in fat, saturated fat, protein, and red meat. Thus he says: 'Juicy broiled New York sirloin steak? English cut roast prime rib of beef? Poached salmon with *béarnaise* sauce? Crispy duck in a Chinese restaurant? Pan-fried chicken? Dig in.'

Do carbohydrates make you fat?

The rationale of Robert Atkins's method, not clearly explained in successive editions of his book, is that the virtual elimination of all types of carbohydrate from food and drink forces the body to exhaust its own store of immediately available energy from carbohydrate, which is stored in the muscles in the form of glycogen bound up with water. This done, the body liberates energy from its stores of fat. Plenty of protein from food is then reckoned to reduce (or 'spare') loss of protein from the body's lean tissue.

He also claims that 'his' regime works almost irrespective of the amount of energy consumed from the recommended foods: 'Many of you will be able to lose weight eating a *higher* number of calories than you have been eating on diets top-heavy in carbohydrates.' He says that carbohydrates (or 'refined' carbohydrates, or foods made with sugar and white flour – again, he is unclear) raise levels of serum insulin, whose purpose is to store dietary energy preferentially as body fat, whereas fat and protein do not have this effect. So, he says, carbohydrates, not higher-energy fats, make you fat.

The phenomenal success of the Atkins Diet has caused a cascade of high-protein, low-carbohydrate books. Among these I admire the key words in the title of *The New High Protein Healthy Fast Food Diet*; and *The Delicious, Doctor-Designed Foolproof Plan for Fast and Healthy Weight Loss*, the subtitle of *The South Beach Diet*.

Brillat-Savarin's summer seltzer

Robert Atkins did not invent the basic idea of 'his' dieting regime. Nor did the other US 'diet doctors' Herman Tarnower and Herman Taller, who preceded him, and nor did the British psychiatrist Richard Mackarness, or nutritionist John Yudkin who preceded them.

Dieting regimes that allow many fresh animal foods, some dairy foods, and non-starchy and salad vegetables, and restrict or prohibit foods containing starch or sugar, were advocated by Jean Anthelme Brillat-Savarin in the early 19th century in France, before the chemical approach to food was invented. He begins in a tone of thunder and lightning, familiar to anybody who has looked through the more magisterial modern dieting regime books. 'Very well then; eat! Get fat! Become ugly, and thick, and asthmatic, and finally die in your own melted grease: I shall be there to watch it.' And then this philosopher and gastronome continues: 'But what do I see? A single phrase has convinced you. It has terrified you, and you beseech me to hold back my lightning. Be assured; I shall map out a diet for you, and prove to you that there are still a few pleasures left for you here on this earth.'

He states that carnivorous animals never become fat: 'Think of the wolves, jackals, birds of prey, crows, etc.' He further states that free-ranging herbivorous animals rarely get fat except sometimes in old age, but when intensively reared 'they gain weight quickly . . . when they are forced to eat potatoes, grains, and any kind of flour'. And thus, 'all animals that live on farinaceous foods grow fat whether they will or no; man follows the common rule'. He also observes: 'Obesity is never found either among savages or in those classes of society which must work in order to eat, or which do not eat except to exist.' By 'work' he means manual labour.

Bingo! 'A more or less rigid abstinence from everything that is starchy or floury will lead to the lessening of weight.' His advice to a 'charming fat lady' includes: 'You love soup, so have it made *à la julienne*, with green vegetables, cabbages, and root vegetables. I must forbid you to drink it made with bread, starchy pastes, and flour.' Veal and poultry should be preferred. 'Shun everything made with flour, no matter in what form it hides; do you not still have the roast, the salad, the leafy vegetables?'

Writing at a time when consumption of sugar, even among wealthy people, was very much lower than it generally is now, of obesity he says: 'Starch produces this effect more quickly and surely when it is mixed with sugar.' And he notes the effect on appetite: 'The mixture of sugar with flour is all the more active since it intensifies the flavour,' and: 'We seldom eat sweetened dishes before our natural hunger has been satisfied.'

If you must eat bread choose that made from rye, because – he says – this is the least pleasant bread. He also favours some special foods and drinks: he commands 30 bottles of Seltzer water during the summer, with white wine from Anjou, and says: 'Shun beer as if it were the plague, and eat often of radishes, fresh artichokes with a simple dressing, asparagus, celery, and cardoons.' He apparently saw no need to follow his own advice and died a few months after he published his book, so he did not get rich. (If you want to know about cardoons, see the notes to this chapter.)

The first drinking man's diet

Any diet low in carbohydrates, meaning starchy and sugary foods, has to be high in protein, fat or alcohol. In the early 1860s William Banting, a prosperous undertaker who constructed the Duke of Wellington's coffin, took the advice of his physician William Harvey. In his mid-60s he dropped 48 pounds (22 kilograms) of excess weight, was delighted, and in 1862 published an account of his regime that became a mid-Victorian smash hit. He has passed into history – *The Oxford English Dictionary* still includes 'banting' (not altogether accurately) as 'the treatment of obesity by abstinence from sugar, starch, and fat', and 'banting' is still the general word for dieting in Sweden. He recorded what he consumed every day:

> *Breakfast*. 4–5oz of beef, mutton, kidneys, broiled fish, bacon, or any cold meat except pork; a large cup of plain tea; and a little biscuit or 1oz of toast.
>
> *Lunch*. 5–6oz of any lean meat or fish, any vegetable except potatoes, 1oz of dry toast, some cooked fruit, any kind of poultry or game, and 2–3 glasses of good claret, sherry, or madeira.
>
> *Tea*. 2–3oz of fruit, a rusk or two, and a cup of plain tea.
>
> *Supper*. 3–4oz of meat or fish as at dinner, and a glass or two of claret.

Night-cap. A tumbler of grog (spirits/liquor), or a glass or two of claret or sherry.

His self-prescription banned milk, butter, beer and sugar, and he severely restricted consumption of all sugary and starchy foods. Of these 'insidious enemies' he reckoned sugar was worst, and observed that just 5 ounces (140 grams) increased his weight by a pound (just under half a kilogram).

Overall the Banting diet is similar to the Brillat-Savarin commandments, and includes over a pound or 450 grams of meat and other flesh food a day. It also includes around the equivalent in alcohol of a bottle of wine, depending on the size of the glasses. This 'drinking man's diet' is relatively very high in protein and high in alcohol. 'A glass or two' is vague, but a guesstimate of the whole diet is around 2,000 calories (8,400 kilojoules) a day, of which around 500 calories (2,100 kilojoules) is from alcoholic drinks.

DIET, DIETING, AND HEALTH

Until the beginning of the 1970s, the medical profession generally did not take overweight and obesity seriously. By the second half of the 20th century obesity had become fairly common, especially in middle-aged people living in materially rich countries. It was not seen as a disease, but the consequence of ways of life and personal habits that are not the business of physicians. The medical establishment tended to dismiss dieting as quackery, or else as ancillary treatment to be carried out by dietitians as instructed by physicians.

This all changed when obesity was agreed to increase the risk of heart attacks, identified as the biggest single cause of death in those countries where rates of obesity were highest. In the 1970s and 1980s, governments of many countries came to a general agreement – after being pressed by physicians who had the ear of politicians – on what nutrients and foods cause heart disease. Those targeted were total fats, saturated fats, dietary cholesterol, and fatty foods. It also seemed sensible to act on the assumption that restriction of such nutrients and foods would prevent heart disease. The foods targeted were usually relatively fresh. For example, a 1982 World Health Organization report on *Prevention of Coronary Heart Disease* recommended to 'de-emphasize' high-fat meats from domestic breeds, high-fat dairy products such as 'whole milk, cream, cheeses', 'whole eggs' and 'commercially baked products'.

Fatty highly processed foods were never much mentioned in such reports, perhaps because it was felt that it would be too complicated to list them, perhaps because the physicians and other experts who were responsible for the recommendations felt that this was a job for dietitians, or perhaps because being distinguished and busy men, they did not often visit supermarkets.

This general agreement then developed to include prevention of diabetes (type 2), high blood pressure and stroke, gut and bone disorders and diseases, dental caries, and some cancers. The idea is that all these chronic diseases – individually, and some grouped as 'syndrome X' or 'the metabolic syndrome' – are caused in large part by diets high in total fat and saturated fat, and also added sugars and salt, and low in dietary fibre, or else by aspects of such diets.

Further, the idea is that all these diseases can be prevented and controlled by 'healthy' diets, defined as being low in total fat and saturated fat, high in relatively unprocessed cereals (grains) and vegetables, fruits, pulses (legumes) and dietary fibre, and relatively low in added sugars and salt. Physical inactivity is also seen as a cause of most of these diseases, and regular physical activity as a way to prevent them.

This ambitious, even audacious, general theory also includes prevention, control and treatment of increase in weight and overweight, and of obesity, which itself became classified as a disease. This is when obese people became identified as suitable cases for treatment.

Does fat make you fat?

So as a main cause of weight increase, overweight and obesity, carbohydrates were out, and dietary fat was in. Orthodox medical and health professionals generally agreed that fat makes you fat. This position was not, and is not, based on what scientists call 'hard evidence' accumulated from the results of relevant types of research studies. It has been more a matter of deduction and what seems common sense.

The reasoning goes like this. First, given that diets high in fats and saturated fats are a cause of heart disease, and given also that obesity is itself a cause of heart disease, it remains generally agreed, if only for the sake of consistent public health messages, that the same dietary recommendations should apply to both prevention and treatment of obesity, and to prevention of heart disease.

Second, in itself dietary fat is the most energy-dense macronutrient, supplying roughly nine units of energy for any given weight, compared with roughly seven for alcohol and four for protein and carbohydrate. Although we consume foods and drinks, not isolated macronutrients, it seems common sense to indict fatty foods as the most important dietary causes of weight gain, overweight and obesity. And third, well – fat is fat. Probably the most compelling argument against fat is the simplest. Here is fat in food. Here is fat in the body. One makes the other. That's the idea.

Official and other authoritative guidelines generally agree that fat makes you fat. They also agree that the best way to reduce body fat is to consume diets that are now recognised to be protective against chronic diseases, but less of them – a return to 'count the calories'. This 'be sensible but go easy' approach is now generally accepted and promoted by orthodox physicians and nutritionists, other health professionals, their representative organizations, and the mainstream media.

The dieting wars

Since the 1970s, the medical and nutritional establishment has condemned dieting doctors who continue to preach low-carbohydrate, high-fat regimes. In 1973, the year after Robert Atkins launched his regime, it and he were denounced by the American Medical Association. A report issued by the Royal College of Physicians of London in 1983 stated magisterially of dieting: 'The old concept of reducing only carbohydrates is nutritionally and medically inappropriate.'

It was in this context that Nathan Pritikin developed his general theory, a radical version of what is now the conventional wisdom. He stated that everybody in materially rich countries is at risk of chronic diseases. Therefore, he said, disease can be prevented and symptoms of disease treated with diets very high in cereals (grains), vegetables and fruits, and thus in dietary fibre, and very low in meat, fats, sugars and salt. He also advocated wholefoods. His programme was given a boost by the support of the dietary fibre evangelists Denis Burkitt and Hugh Trowell.

Nathan Pritikin's ideas have been independently developed in the USA by the cardiologist Dean Ornish, whose dieting book *Eat More,*

Weigh Less also states that symptoms of chronic disease often fade on diets radically low in meat and fat and high in starchy foods.

So, as from the 1980s, macronutrient manipulation dieting regimes have been mostly of three types, all opposed to one another: the Atkins type, the 'sensible' type, and the Ornish type. Like snack foods, these all have variations.

Studies made of all types of dieting regime – whether or not they specify 'cutting calories' – evidently show that they supply less energy than the body needs to stay in balance, so on any regime the weight of dieters drops, if only for this reason. Claims that 'you can eat as much as you like' are, it seems, misleading, simply because it is hard to achieve energy balance on any regime that radically cuts down entire types of macronutrient. Again, what happens after any regime has ended is another matter.

My opinion is that recommendations for good health, for protection against disease – or for reduction of weight and body fat – that focus on the chemical composition of foods and drinks are all wrong. Macronutrient manipulation does not work. The right approach, certainly for positive health and wellbeing, is to pay attention to the foods and drinks we consume, not to their chemical constituents. Again, see the next chapter on this point.

'DON'T DIET' DIETING REGIMES

What I also found in Belém airport was an example of the 'don't diet' dieting book (*A Dieta Sem Dieta*). At Sydney airport I had already purchased two more books that sounded like 'don't diet' dieting regimes: *Never Say Diet Again*, and *The Don't Go Hungry Diet*.

There are two types of 'don't diet' dieting books. One claims that certain foods or nutrients are so satisfying that when you eat lots of them you will stop increasing and start decreasing weight and body fat. Thus you will reduce your energy from food without 'counting calories' or any conscious sense of restriction. Some other dieting regimes say this too, without being branded as 'don't diet'. The other type states that the main issue is not too much food and drink but not enough exercise, and that it's best to become a lot more physically active, and thus use more energy and become in higher energy balance. As you will see in the following chapters, I agree.

Naturally I was curious to see if 'don't diet' dieting books repeat points made in *Dieting Makes You Fat* or intermediate sources. Indeed they do. 'Dieting can cause the body's metabolism to slow down . . . This mechanism protected our ancestors from famine . . . but is not so useful to us now,' says *Never Say Diet Again*, and: 'Dieting can actually make you fat, as a sluggish metabolism can trigger the yo-yo syndrome. When you lose weight you lose it as fat and muscle but, when you regain it, it only comes back on as fat.' 'After six years of dieting, I'd gained 40 kilos! I had dieted myself fat,' says *The Don't Go Hungry Diet*. And after some brainy stuff about hypothalamic levels of neuropeptide Y, 'we had discovered some of the ways in which dieting can make you fat'.

The word 'can' here has two functions. One is to avoid categorical statements and so stay in your comfort zone. To be somewhat cynical, the other is the Low Tar ploy: other grotty old dieting regimes (can) make you fat, but this sparkling new dieting regime will make you 'reduce weight and keep it off forever', as most dieting books claim. And indeed, it is possible to do this, but not if you rely on dietary energy restriction – see chapter 6.

Never Say Diet Again is compiled by a team of dietitians at the Sydney Royal Prince Alfred (RPA) Hospital Weight Management Program. It suggests that when you feel hungry, instead play with your pet, paint your toenails, mow the lawn, or begin a craft activity. It accepts *The Australian Guide to Healthy Eating*, whose recommendations include a range of 90–300 grams of protein a day, which at the upper end implies that roughly half of all energy can come from protein. It cites five food groups: carbohydrates, protein, vegetables and pulses (legumes), fruits, dairy. It recommends strengthening calf muscles: 'Lift up and down on your toes. Balance yourself by holding on to a wall or a piece of furniture.'

Despite its title, this isn't a 'don't diet' but a 'sensible' dieting book. There are masses of these now, published in the USA, the UK and continental Europe, often issued by professional associations or with their stamp of approval. My guess is that the RPA Hospital Weight Management Program dietitians work mostly with middle-class, middle-aged, very fat ladies, with a policy of 'be careful with fat, sugar and alcohol, try to be active, and every little bit helps'. This might prevent further increase of weight and fat, but is most unlikely to lead to significant or permanent shedding of body fat.

Dr Amanda's 12,000 steps

The author of *The Don't Go Hungry Diet*, Amanda Sainsbury-Salis, also from Sydney, once weighed 93 kilograms/205 pounds, which at 1.60 metres (5 foot 3 inches) height, made her BMI around 36 – approaching gross obesity. She says that her own regime, including 'wood-fired pizza *Napolitana* with chilli olive oil drizzled generously on top', doner kebab, and halva, has enabled her to keep off a drop of weight of 28 kilos (62 pounds) for a decade. Blurbed as 'Dr Amanda', she is positioned as 'an internationally renowned molecular scientist', and she does indeed have a substantial list of co-authored papers registered on PubMed – mostly experiments on mice, rats and squirrels.

Like you and me, Dr Amanda is not a squirrel. Her book presents what she has found out for herself and on behalf of clients, apparently mostly obese and grossly obese women who have attended her Sydney clinic. She says 'the only way to lose weight is to eat less than your body needs'. Her three nutritional guidelines are: 'Eat a wide variety of foods ... Eat wholefoods ... Eat mainly vegetables and fruit'. She says: 'It's almost impossible to lose weight *and keep it off* without physical activity,' and prescribes 8,000–12,000 steps at brisk walking pace every day – which as I know from my own daily jogging and walking, will take at least an hour to an hour and a half.

Diets mainly made up of vegetables and fruits, plus more than an hour of moderate physical activity every day, will put most people into 'negative' energy balance – as the phrase is – even if these include some fatty or sugary calorie bombs. The most interesting bit of *The Don't Go Hungry Diet* is what Dr Amanda characterizes as the Famine Reaction and the Fat Brake. She identifies various mechanisms that during and after energy-restrictive dieting 'alter the body's metabolism, enabling it to conserve and lay down fat', because humans are evolved to survive periods of food insecurity and famine by using the body as a larder. That's the famine reaction.

The fat brake is the mechanism designed to stop incessant weight gain which, she says, we wreck by yo-yo dieting, also known as weight cycling. She says we can thwart the famine reaction simply by eating, and by training ourselves to tell when we really are hungry, and that with some servicing and re-lining, the fat brake will burn off extra energy consumed. And she claims that we can re-set our set points to the weight we want to be.

The Don't Go Hungry Diet really is a 'don't diet' dieting book. Dr Amanda recognizes (while understating) the importance of physical activity, but her rigorous regime is realistic, and its intriguing strategy for fooling the 'famine reaction' may well be correct – as you will see in the next chapter.

THE DR GEOFFREY AMAZON DIET

Now you know how to write a dieting book, and if you do you may become rich and famous. Positioning and branding, that's the secret, as with any product.

First, have an idea – any idea – that can be positioned in a title that grabs the attention. You could go for a niche market with *The Whisky Drinker's Diet*, or *The Executive Diet*, or *The Eating For One Diet*. You could go for bigger sales with intriguing titles such as *The Sugar Lover's Diet*, or *Eat Fat and Get Slim*, or *Gorge and be Gorgeous*, or *The Aphrodisiac Diet*. You could look for a food that has not been claimed as the magic ingredient for dieters: maybe *The Ice Cream Diet*, or *The Apple Pie Diet*, or *The Burger and Shake Diet*, or *The Balsamic Vinegar Diet* – but I see from my internet travels that some of these titles have been taken. Another approach is a title that sounds brainy, like *The Homoeostasis Diet*, or glamorous, like *Diets of the Supermodels Revealed*, or cosmic, like *The Fibonacci Diet*, or philosophical, like *The Pythagorean Diet*, or opportunistic, like *The Da Vinci Diet*, or cryptic, like *AAA Diet* (*Action Against Avoirdupois*, which also has the advantage of putting you first in any alphabetical list), or mystical, like *The Essene Diet*. Any or all of these would have an extra line in big type saying that what the book says is Scientifically Proved, or else Reveals Secret Wisdom.

Since I live in Brazil, I would position my dieting book, designed as a shop window for my personal 'get very rich' dieting regime, as *The Dr Geoffrey Amazon Rainforest Diet* (no connection with any existing dieting books or regimes with the word 'Amazon' or 'rainforest' as part of their names). I would have it all ways with the button-pressing subtitle *The Secret Wisdom of the Rainforest now Scientifically Proved that Makes You Slim Forever*. Intriguing, eh? If you saw a bookstore window piled high with a book so positioned, would you go inside and pick up a copy? Sure you would.

DIETING AS A SIGN OF THE TIMES

Walk down any high street or around any shopping centre in most cities and notice the number of outlets for fast foods and for pharmaceuticals. In the USA, pharmacies or 'drug stores' stock dietary supplements, metabolism boosters, fast and junk foods and drinks, and pharmaceuticals, in adjacent aisles. Specialist fast-food and drug chains are separately owned – so far – but their outlets are often next door to one another. Switch on the television and notice the number of shows, whether fiction or 'reality', which are distractions from reality. Uncontrolled weight increase, overweight and obesity, and the fantasies of dieting, are not just a matter of personal and public health. These are symptoms of a deeper malaise.

The immediate dangers of dieting are minimal, unless you are constantly on and off dieting regimes. That's not the issue. The first big question to ask about dieting is: does it work? Read on and you will see what you may well already know from experience: as a rule, the answer is no. Claims made by the dieting industry appeal to our base desires, like the email spam messages that say you have won $US10 million, or can enjoy multiple orgasms forever. The dieting business is fabulous. It sells dreams, and dreams rarely come true.

3. WHY DIETING MAKES
YOU FAT

Venice and Ravenna 1819. Moore found Byron greatly changed, much fatter in figure and puffier in face . . . Byron took his late breakfast standing: one or two raw eggs, a cup of tea with no milk or sugar, a dry biscuit – he was still following his abstemious diet . . . Pisa 1821–2. Not the least of the surprises for Hunt was that Byron had become almost unrecognisably plump.

Fiona MacCarthy

Nothing in biology makes sense except in the light of evolution . . . Seen in the light of evolution, biology is, perhaps, intellectually the most satisfying and inspiring science. Without that light it becomes a pile of sundry facts some of them interesting or curious but making no meaningful picture as a whole.

Theodosius Dobzhansky

Dieting causes the condition it is meant to cure. The more that we endure cycles of dieting, the more our bodies become trained to seek out food, slow down vital functions, and conserve built-in energy in the form of body fat.

Sedentary people who consume industrialized diets are at high risk of disagreeable, disabling and deadly diseases, whatever their weight — normal, overweight or obese. Continual cycles of dieting increase these dangers.

Dieters, nutritionists and physicians – and indeed most of us – usually assume that people become increasingly fat because they have inherited a tendency to 'put on weight', or because they are eating and drinking too much, or because they are physically inactive. These are indeed some of the immediate reasons why people become fat; but they are not the only reasons. Another reason is dieting. If you are sedentary and overweight, and want to get rid of body fat permanently, about the worst thing you can do is to keep on dieting.

People who habitually 'go on a diet' fail again and again, and become frustrated and demoralized. They think dieting works, or should work, and therefore that the failure is their fault. This may be your own bitter experience. But body weight rebound and increased body fat are practically inevitable consequences of the process of dieting itself. How counterproductive and even damaging is dieting? This depends largely on your general state of health and fitness, range of body weight and fat, and your gender and age; and also on the nature and quality of your normal diet and of the dieting regime itself. As a general rule the more restrictive the regimes, and the more often they are repeated, the fatter – note, though, not necessarily heavier – you will become.

FREQUENTLY ASKED QUESTIONS ANSWERED

The idea that dieting makes you fat has been in circulation since the first version of this book was published in many countries in the 1980s. It is now occasionally mentioned in 'don't diet' dieting books and articles, usually qualified in some way like 'so some diets could even have the effect of making you fatter', usually without much explanation. It is a hot topic. Acquaintances who learn that I am the co-author of the first version of this book often tell me that its thesis corresponds to their own experience as dieters. People who resist the idea, despite the evidence – often including their personal experience – do so for any combination of five reasons.

What does 'dieting makes you fat' mean?

The first line of resistance often takes the form of saying: 'But everybody knows that when you go on a diet you reduce weight.' True, you do, if you follow the specifications of practically any dieting regime. But that's not what is meant by 'dieting makes you fat', as already stated in the introduction to this book.

Again, here is what is meant by 'dieting'. Some of my friends and colleagues occasionally notice they have put on some weight, perhaps after Christmas or before going on holiday, and want to drop say 2 or 3 kilograms (4½–7 pounds, roughly). They do so by eating and drinking prudently for a while – maybe by saying no to desserts or cutting down on alcoholic drinks – or maybe by becoming more physically active and using their health club subscription, or by running or swimming. Occasional restrained eating and drinking is not what is meant here by 'dieting'.

The terms 'dieting' as in 'dieting books' and 'diet' as in 'going on a diet' are used here in the usual sense. Dieting here means the occasional or continual following of regimes that restrict energy intake from food and drink, with the intention of reducing a substantial amount of body weight, after which you resume your 'normal' diet and way of life. Whether or not they 'count calories', regimes often are devised to restrict dietary energy to around 1,500 calories (around 6,250 kilojoules) a day; some are more restrictive. Regimes that restrict energy to below around 1,000 calories (4,200 kilojoules) a day are known as VLCDs (very low calorie diets) or 'crash' diets.

Next here is what is meant by 'makes you fat'. Dieting of course is not the only reason why people become fat! As shown in the next chapter, there are many causes of weight increase, overweight and obesity. People 'go on a diet' for the first time because they have decided that they want to 'lose' some body fat and weight they have 'gained' for some other reason.

When dieters really do restrict dietary energy, as specified in dieting regimes, of course their body weight and also their body fat reduces. The big mistake here is to judge the regime at the point at which it is stopped. This is like judging the state of your finances by paying attention to the one time when your bank balance is in the black, and on this basis deciding that you can go on the razzle. The process of dieting includes the day, weeks, months and yes, years after the regime is ended. Reliable judgement of the effects of dieting is based on long-term observation.

Can you beat the system?

The next objection to the idea that dieting makes you fat is that we all know that some people who follow dieting regimes succeed in reducing their weight, and stay that way. Indeed so, but almost always there is more to their success than meets the eye.

Some well-known people are evident success stories. In the USA Mike Huckabee, a Republican presidential candidate in 2008, starting in 2003 reduced from 280 to 175 pounds (129 to 79 kilograms). In the UK Nigel Lawson, former chancellor of the exchequer, in the mid-1990s dropped from 109 to 79 kilograms (240 to 170 pounds). Both wrote books about their success. More generally, in the USA the National Weight Control Registry (NWCR), run by James Hill of the University of Colorado in Denver and Rena Wing of Brown Medical School in Providence, Rhode Island, have records of around 6,000 people who have reduced weight by at least 30 pounds (around 13 kilograms) and have not put this weight back on again.

These stories contain at least two lessons. For a start, they are most unusual. In the USA on the day you read this, tens of millions of people are dieting. The most methodical review of the epidemiological literature, undertaken at the University of California, Los Angeles, and published in 2007 (more on this below) concludes: 'It appears that dieters who manage to sustain a weight loss are the rare exception.' Jules Hirsch of Rockefeller University, New York, a specialist in obesity since the 1950s, has asked the US National Institutes of Health and also US politicians 'to be straight with the American people and tell them that for all practical purposes obesity treatment doesn't work.' With reference to cancer that has spread to other organs or throughout the body, he says: 'The five-year success rates I've seen are of the order of about 5 per cent, which is a rate similar to that for the successful treatment of metastatic malignancy.'

The second lesson from these stories is that after the dieting regimes recorded by the NWCR ended, the people – and also Governor Huckabee and Lord Lawson – did not revert to their 'normal' diet. They changed their eating and drinking habits. They also changed other aspects of their ways of life. A common factor in almost all the NWCR cases is a big increase in moderate and vigorous physical activity, to levels of an hour and more a day. That's different. That's not what's meant here by 'dieting'. Indeed, this approach as part of the way to maintain and improve health, wellbeing and also gradually to reduce body fat is what I recommend in chapter 6. What I do not recommend is dietary energy restriction.

Are there people of iron will who reduce body fat solely by dieting and who stay more or less at the same reduced weight after resuming a 'normal' diet and 'lifestyle'? No doubt there are. They are like successful gamblers. If your aunt went to Las Vegas and won a million dollars on the slot machines, would you believe that anybody who plays the slots can beat the system? No, you would not.

Who gains by telling you?

At this point my quizzical acquaintances may be a bit impressed. The next common question is: 'If this is true, why haven't I heard it before?' (for some people have not). The answer is: 'In whose interest is it to tell you?'

Remember, there is a vast industry out there, dedicated to the proposition that dieting makes you slim. The big money is in dieting. It is a terrific repeat business. Are any of the people in the business, whether commercial or professional, likely to agree or even allow the possibility that dieting makes you fat? That would be like expecting a soft-drink manufacturer to accept that sugared cola and other soft drinks make you fat (which they do). People committed to dieting are not about to tell you that dieting is a disaster.

Who can you believe?

Occasionally I am asked why I should be believed. Well, the thesis of this book is based on a vast amount of work done by others, and is the best fit with the facts. Also, in order to understand the whole field you need to read and think and reason about a whole lot of inter-related topics. Making sense of science is my line of work – it's what I have been doing since the early 1980s. Specialists know a lot more about their own areas than I ever will. But they are no more able to see a big picture than anybody else of comparable general ability and training, unless they are prepared to devote a lot of unpaid time to studying topics otherwise unknown to them.

Does this spell doom?

People who want to reduce their own body fat may well not want to believe that dieting makes you fat because they think that, if true, it means they have been wasting their time and also now are doomed. So the fifth question is: 'So are you saying there is nothing I can do to reduce my body fat?'

My response is that sure, all able-bodied people can reduce their body fat and indeed their body weight if that's really what they want to do, but restriction of dietary energy is not the way. There is now no need to elaborate on the right way, because I can invite them – as I do you – to follow the golden rules contained in chapter 6.

OUR BODIES ARE MORE THAN MACHINES

Much current conventional scientific literature, and therefore much derivative popular writing, is mistaken or confused in its assumptions and assertions about human biology in at least five relevant respects. These errors go a long way towards explaining why most health professionals at all levels, together with the dieting industry, still persist in recommending dietary energy restriction as the most effective method to reduce body fat, despite the mismatch between what they claim or accept and what actually happens.

Here comes the first mistake. All of us who have been educated in the modern 'Western' convention have been induced to think of the human body as a machine – a marvellous and wonderful thing, but a machine nonetheless. Biochemistry, physiology, and conventional medicine, are based on this assumption. It is wrong. Machines are neither alive nor dead. We are alive. When we are alive, waking and sleeping, we are learning, adapting, and changing, consciously and unconsciously, all the time.

Complex machines, like personal computers and the programs they contain, include mechanisms that respond to situations foreseen by their makers, and as extensions of ourselves they enhance our abilities. But computers do not change their nature – their shape or size, or their functions – because of how we treat them. We do. If we overload a computer it may crash, but it does not become physically heavier. We do. If we treat a computer with special respect it does not itself generate new programs that enhance its functions. We do. We are not machines. Among all mammals, *Homo sapiens* is the most adaptable, a reason why the human species has become dominant.

All types of training are processes of adaptation. These may be conscious and deliberate, or they may be unintended or unconscious. Training can have good or bad effects. For example, children who are rewarded with sweets are being trained to associate sticky sugary foods with achievement, and to get into habits that are good only for the bottom lines of the confectionery trade and the bank balances of dentists.

As another example, at rest the bodies of young sedentary people and young physically active people of the same weight may look fairly similar. But inside, their bodies have been altered – trained to function differently in many vital ways. Anybody who is physically fit can probably run for 20 minutes and more without stopping; anybody who is unfit may not be able to manage more than a few minutes. This is not a matter of willpower. For an unfit person, sustained vigorous activity is physically impossible, just as you maybe can sit down at a piano and play Bach or boogie-woogie, but I cannot.

The bodies of people who regularly restrict energy on dieting regimes become physically trained in other ways and respond differently in their responses to food and drink. Jules Hirsch compares the body of an obese person who habitually goes on dieting regimes to the body of a slim person who is starving.

The bottom line here, if you want to get and stay in good shape, is that you need to train and thus adapt yourself appropriately. When you prepare yourself for any substantial task you will be most likely to succeed.

BODY FAT IS DIFFERENT FROM BODY WEIGHT

Practically all you hear or read about body composition, energy balance, health and disease, and dieting, is in terms of body weight. Dieting regimes focus on weight reduction. This is the second mistake. What people who are bigger than they want to be really want to reduce is their body fat. This is different.

It's easy to explain the attention to body weight. It is a simple measure. Scales make it easy for health professionals to weigh people, from birth onwards. Many people have scales in their bathroom and weigh themselves from time to time – I do, and they are a useful check, as long as you realize that level of body weight and degree of body fatness are not the same thing.

It is true that in any population or group of people whose degree of physical activity is much the same, body weight is a reasonably good indicator of body fat. If a group of sedentary people are weighed, and then their body fat is estimated – by taking skin-fold measurements or by more exact and complicated methods – there will be a pretty good correlation *within* the group between body weight and body fat. The same will be true within any other homogenous groups. These might be a bunch of citizens who all run or take other types of regular aerobic exercise; or another group who all train with weights or who do a lot of manual work; or by contrast perhaps a group of sedentary older people who have lost a lot of lean tissue.

But the body compositions *between* these groups will differ. Physically active groups will have more lean tissue and less body fat compared with any sedentary group. An active and lean group of people may have an average weight much the same as or even more than a sedentary flabby group, one reason being that lean tissue is 20 per cent heavier than body fat. An inactive older group, even if their weight is relatively light, are likely to have much higher proportions of body fat relative to their weight compared with any group who are fit and physically active.

Indeed people with a sedentary way of life whose lean tissue diminishes and whose body fat increases, but whose weight stays much the same, will be seriously misled if they rely on weight as a measure of fatness. They will have become fatter. The same applies in reverse. People who become and stay more physically active may weigh much the same or possibly even more when they are fit, but they will be leaner than they were.

Bear in mind that by definition, lean people are physically fit and active, and if they are muscular will be relatively heavy. Light people will be lean only if they are fit; a light sedentary person is likely to be flabby, and may even be fat. The term 'overweight' is misleading: it usually really means 'fat, but not obese', but this applies more to sedentary than to physically active people. The bottom line here, if you want to get into shape, is to pay less attention to reducing body weight and most attention to increasing lean tissue and reducing body fat, by being physically active.

CALORIES ARE FUZZY COUNTERS

Here comes the third mistake. It's about dietary energy – call this 'calories'. One of the most intense debates concerning energy balance, obesity, and weight reduction and increase, concerns how the human body metabolizes foods and drinks. The muddle is caused by confusing calories as disembodied units of energy subject to the laws of thermodynamics, with what happens inside our bodies when we consume them.

Calories (and kilojoules) are units of energy. A calorie – actually a kilocalorie – is the amount of heat needed to raise the temperature of a litre of water by 10°C. A calorie is equivalent to 4.18 kilojoules. The energy value of macronutrients is ascertained by analysing the chemical composition of foods and burning the foods in a crucible, placed within a machine called a bomb calorimeter, surrounded by water. Conventional nutrition scientists, and the dieting regimes that follow their lead, then assume that our bodies work like bomb calorimeters, or steam engines, as they metabolize the energy from food.

This is what is meant by 'a calorie is a calorie'. Thus Marion Nestle of New York University says: 'When it comes to weight loss, it's the calories that count.' Others say that once inside the body a calorie is actually not just a calorie. By this they mean that the body uses the energy contained in different foods and drinks in different ways, depending on the nature of the foods and drinks, and also depending on the conditioning of the body. Thus in discussing foods and drinks absorbed relatively slowly, compared with those absorbed quickly, David Ludwig of the Children's Hospital, Boston, says: 'The concept that "a calorie is a calorie" underlies most conventional weight loss strategies . . . however . . . all calories are not alike.'

David Ludwig is correct. Our bodies are indeed not bomb calorimeters or steam engines. In general, the crucial difference between different types of food and drink is how processed they are: not just their energy content, but the speed of their metabolism, and the extent to which they are satisfying. Highly processed foods are usually energy dense, need little chewing, and are liable to be over eaten. People whose 'normal' diets are mainly made up from processed foods and drinks are more likely to become fat, less likely to reduce weight on dieting regimes (especially if these rely on snacks), and more likely to put back all the weight – and often more – after the regime is ended. David Ludwig and other researchers also find that some types of processed foods and drinks are preferentially converted to body fat. This area remains controversial, partly because manufacturers whose products may well be especially liable to make you fat spend a lot of money commissioning research that seems to show otherwise.

The bottom line here is: forget about counting calories, and prefer fresh and lightly processed foods and drinks. Foods like these that are absorbed relatively slowly are most satisfying, most healthy, and least likely to make you fat.

HUNGER IS NOT JUST FOR ENERGY

Most teaching and writing on food and nutrition assumes that hunger is only for energy from food. The reason for this fourth mistake is that historically food and nutrition policy has focused on impoverished populations, at first within industrialized countries and now mainly in middle- and low-income countries. The Food and Agriculture Organization of the United Nations gauges the state of the world's food and nutrition by estimating the calories from food and drink per head available for consumption in all countries.

But hunger and associated drives like desire and appetite are not just for energy from food. This is another reason why 'counting the calories' is an unhelpful approach to weight control. If you desire sweets or biscuits or cola drinks, your appetite is not for their energy but for their taste and for the rush – their impact on your mood once you have consumed them. In the next chapter I point out that humans have a built-in hunger for sweetness and succulence and therefore for sugary and fatty foods and drinks, independent of hunger for dietary energy or for food in general.

Our sense of hunger and satiety is also affected by the physical bulk of food. Fresh and benignly processed foods, such as vegetables, fruits, pulses (legumes) and wholegrains, contain a lot of dietary fibre and water. They are bulky and make us feel full. Processed foods concentrated in sugar or fat are compact – physically small. They deliver a lot of dietary energy but leave us relatively empty, and are not satisfying.

Hunger is also for nourishment. Farmers who raise free-range livestock in natural conditions know that their animals may seek out corners of fields containing plants that are concentrated sources of specific bioactive compounds. This sense is evidently muted in humans. However, pregnant women often discover strong desires for unusual foods or substances not normally eaten. This phenomenon, known as 'pica', tends to be dismissed by physicians as a sort of hysteria, but may well be hunger for specific bioactive substances for which the woman or her unborn child has a special need.

Given this, and if the hunger for nutrients evident in animals is also present – albeit muted – in humans, it follows that sedentary people who consume typical industrialized diets will remain hungry after they have eaten enough to keep them in energy balance.

Our need for various nutrients including some vitamins and minerals is certainly independent of our need for dietary energy. This means that the less physically active we are, the greater our need for foods that are good sources of these nutrients. Highly processed foods are typically high in sugars and fats that are poor sources of most nutrients – other than energy. In turn this means that sedentary people in energy balance will often be malnourished – short of various nutrients while not being clinically deficient in them.

People who remain sedentary, and who do not change their diets, in effect have two choices: to remain somewhat undernourished or, by consuming adequate nutrients from their food and drink, to increase in weight and to become overweight. The startling conclusion is that sedentary people who consume typical industrialized diets may be better off being overweight.

Cravings, which often cause compulsive eating and what amounts to addiction to particular foods and drinks or even food in general, are experienced as an intense and even uncontrollable hunger. Some foods and drinks may be compulsively consumed – alcoholic drinks are the obvious example. So may processed foods and drinks formulated to make them tempting or 'more-ish'. There are a number of packaged foods I have learned not to open because I know my initial desire will be magnified once I have taken my first bite, and that then I am liable to scoff the lot. The scientists who concoct convenience foods and drinks are clever people. The main cause of general craving for food and drink is semi-starvation, including the time during and also after dieting regimes. (There is more on craving and addiction later in this chapter and in the notes.)

The bottom line here is, again, to prefer fresh and lightly processed foods. These are nourishing, are most likely to satisfy a healthy appetite, and are least likely to cause cravings and compulsive consumption.

DO OBESE PEOPLE OVEREAT?

The fifth mistake is that obesity is caused by greed. In days gone by when obesity was not common and not connected with major diseases, and before the glittering prospect of obesity drugs beckoned, physicians and other health professionals were irritated by fat people. Obesity was then thought usually to be caused by self-indulgence. If patients were brave enough to ask what to do about being obese, the physician might dole out a 'diet sheet' including advice to eat less, or count calories, or cut carbohydrates – like the one Tibor Csato gave me in the mid-1970s. Or, later, cut fats. And maybe get some exercise. Or ask the receptionist on the way out for the telephone number of the local TOPS ('take off pounds sensibly') or Weight Watchers branch.

Obese people are rarely greedy

Yes, some people do get and stay fat because they are always eating and drinking. In his confessional book on obesity and dieting, William Leith describes an encounter on a train with three grossly obese people – a mother and her son and daughter. 'The guy inhales two large bags of crisps in three or four minutes. The girl kills a Mars bar in a couple of gulps. Then . . . she eats the Pringles in 2-inch stacks. When she runs out of food . . . she tries to snatch her brother's food bag . . . The mother bops the girl on the head, and gives her another Mars bar.' You may have seen very fat people who behave like this in public.

Also, some people are fat because they are gourmands – they choose to indulge in delicious, high-quality, 'rich' meals, and pay the price. Among British monarchs Henry VIII comes to mind – the legend says that after his active days were over he flaunted his wealth with great feasts, in which he guzzled sack, flung gnawed haunches of beef over his shoulder for his hounds, and gorged on plum puddings. Edward VII is said to have gobbled breakfasts of partridge pie, cold mutton, truffles, half a dozen plover's eggs, and kedgeree, washed down with a pint of claret, and ended his days with seven-course dinners. Such people, in the current unlovely phrase, are making personal lifestyle choices.

Behaviour like that of the family on the train, or that of kings of old, is conspicuous but unusual. Some people do eat and drink constantly and compulsively and become and stay very fat, or control their weight by vomiting and purging. 'Greed' does not characterize such eating disorders. Overall in the US adult population a figure of 3 per cent has been suggested, with maybe much higher percentages for young women. But in his clinical manual on obesity John Garrow, writing from much experience as director of a UK Medical Research Council obesity centre, says: 'Most (but not all) obese patients have eating patterns which are indistinguishable from those of normal-weight people.'

Heavy people may eat less than light people

Short of compulsion and greed, practically everybody assumes that fat people consume more energy from food and drink than slim people, even though many fat people complain that they don't eat or drink much, and say they know there are slim people who eat more than they do. Most thinking and writing here remains muddled. Part of the problem is terminology.

A number of studies have reported that fat people do consume less energy from food than slim people. But what exactly does this mean? If the only significant difference between the two groups of people is that one is heavier than the other, this cannot be true. On average the heavier group must be consuming more energy from food and drink than the lighter group, otherwise the laws of thermodynamics would be broken.

Some studies can be discounted, because relying on what people say they consume when asked to fill in forms or when interviewed. John Garrow points out that these results are contradicted by those of other studies in which people are confined and their diets controlled. When asked in the context of weight control, people tend to underestimate the food and drink they have consumed; and fat people are more likely to forget or to fail to record all that they have consumed. Also, fat people may be following a dieting regime at the time the question is asked.

This said, fat people often do consume less dietary energy than slim people, when the fat people are inactive, and the slim people are better described as lean, because of being fit and physically active. Constantly used, muscle is far more metabolically active than body fat, lean tissue weighs more than fat, and physical activity uses energy.

At the same weight, lean active fit people are bound to be in energy balance at levels higher than fat out-of-shape sedentary people. This difference can be up to 500 calories (about 2,100 kilojoules) a day, or more. For example, a sedentary fat woman weighing 196 pounds (89 kilograms) needs only about 450 calories (about 1,900 kilojoules) a day more than a sedentary fat woman weighing 133 pounds (60½ kilograms); but if the lighter woman becomes physically active, fit and lean, she may well turn over at least an additional 450 calories a day and therefore be consuming at least as much as the fat woman who is 63 pounds (29 kilograms) heavier. At less extreme contrasts of body weight, relatively light, lean fit people can stay the same weight while consuming more – even a lot more – energy from food and drink than relatively heavy, overweight sedentary people. Correspondingly, sedentary fat people can increase weight while eating less than fit lean people whose weight is stable.

Another point is historical. In general, people now are consuming a lot less energy from food than did people of the same height and weight in previous decades, and much less than in the early 20th century, when most people were physically active. Compared with those times, the difference is roughly between 400–600 calories (about 1,675–2,500 kilojoules) a day, depending mostly on size, gender and age. It follows that in general, fat people now are consuming less energy from food and drink than fat people did a generation or two ago. Indeed, many fat people now are consuming less than lean and lighter people did even as recently as the 1970s.

The bottom line here, if you are sedentary and overweight, is that you may well be consuming less energy from food and drink than people who are lean and fit. The answer is to become more physically active.

PRIMAL HUNGER

The points made so far are a necessary prelude to what follows. The method I use from now on is conventional in any scientific investigation. I start by noting stories suggesting that dieting may cause the problem it is meant to cure. I then summarize some human experiments and surveys of the relevant scientific literature. Then I outline the biology explaining why dieting makes you fat. Finally, I set out the general theory based on the most reliable foundation, which is human evolution and adaptation.

How to fatten a pig

We all know now that eating fish is good for us. Popular magazines say correctly that oily fish are rich in types of fat that nourish our cardiovascular and nervous systems. We owe our knowledge of the value of these essential fats to a network of researchers, many of whom have been inspired by the nutrition scientist Hugh Sinclair, a friend of mine in the last decade of his life.

I gave Hugh a copy of the first version of this book and asked him what he thought. He told me that when young he bred pigs, and that every stockbreeder knows that the most effective way to fatten pigs for market is first to starve them. This knowledge goes back at least 2,500 years. Aristotle, in his *History of Animals*, says: 'Before the fattening process begins, the creatures must be starved for three days ... after these three days of starvation, pig breeders feed the animals lavishly.' He also says: 'Animals in general will take on fat if subjected previously to a course of starvation.' This phenomenon is now known as 'overcompensation' in animals, and 'overshoot' in humans.

Researchers who work with animals are careful to say that what is true of a mouse, rat or other experimental mammal may well not be true of humans. Pigs are not humans. But nor are they rats or mice. Of all domesticated animals, the digestive and other body systems of pigs are closest to those of humans. Hugh thought that pig breeders know something we need to know. His experience, and that reported by Aristotle, was confirmed in 1951 by Isabella Leitch of the Rowett Research Institute, then the leading animal nutrition research centre in Britain.

How to fatten a child

Twenty years later in Brazil, I mentioned the idea that dieting makes you fat to my wife Raquel. She told me that the phenomenon of *fome histórica* (historic hunger) is well known to health workers in Brazil responsible for impoverished and undernourished small children who, once they get their hands on unlimited food, gorge and become fat.

This is confirmed in the literature. For example, a team from the Federal University of São Paulo and Tufts University in Boston, reporting in the *British Journal of Nutrition* in 2004, found that Brazilian children who are unusually short – stunted – because they were undernourished before and after birth 'have a preference to accumulate or spare body fat to the detriment of lean body mass' once they have access to plenty of food. The conclusion was: 'These findings may contribute to the understanding of why there is an increased prevalence of overweight and obesity among poor populations.'

Reporting in the *British Medical Journal* in 2000, a team from the UK noted the effect in small children of accelerated growth induced by extra feeding, usually with formula feeds and then energy-dense foods, so that the children 'catch up' with what were then the approved growth standards. The conclusion was: 'Children who showed catch-up growth between zero and two years were fatter and had more central fat distribution at five years than other children.'

Such results are now confirmed by those of studies in many countries. All over the world, children who begin life short of food will preferentially store food as body fat once they can eat as much as they want – especially if the food they are given is energy-dense. In 2002 and 2006 reviews published in the *International Journal of Obesity*, Abdul Dulloo of the University of Fribourg, Switzerland, and colleagues comment on this literature. They state: 'Body fat is recovered at a disproportionately faster rate than that of lean tissue.' They also state: 'Studies from South Africa, Brazil, Russia, China and India suggest that stunted children have a 2 – 8 times greater risk of becoming overweight.'

ENERGY RESTRICTION: THE CLASSIC EXPERIMENTS

Animals are not humans, children are not adults, and being short of food before and after birth is not the same as dieting. So the next stage in the investigation is to see what happens in a controlled environment to human adults when they restrict their energy intake from food and drink, and then what happens afterwards.

Dr Benedict's ravenous volunteers

A meticulous experiment was conducted almost a hundred years ago in the USA by Francis (F G) Benedict, director of the Nutrition Laboratory in Boston. He was given the task of finding out what would happen to volunteers prepared to reduce their weight in controlled laboratory conditions. The purpose of the study was to see how people could best survive the rigours of wartime. The results of what became known as the Carnegie Experiment were published in 1919 in a 700-page report, *Human Vitality and Efficiency Under Prolonged Restricted Diet*.

Two dozen male students of normal weight, divided into two groups, agreed to restrict their daily energy intake from their usual 3,000-plus calories to 1,800 or fewer (roughly from 12,500 to 7,500 or fewer kilojoules). They consumed the same food as other students, but a lot less of it. By the time they had reduced their weight by the specified 10 per cent, their basal metabolic rates – the rate at which the body turns over energy at complete rest – had decreased twice as much, by around 20 per cent.

Other associated vital signs such as blood pressure and pulse rates also dropped remarkably. The volunteers found it hard to keep warm, and became lethargic. They became ravenous. Towards the end of their period of weight reduction, if they ate more than around 2,100 calories (about 8,500 kilojoules) a day – almost 1,000 calories (about 4,250 kilojoules) fewer than their normal intake – they started to put on weight.

Once they had reached their target weight, one group was left free to eat and drink whatever they liked. Their consumption and its effects were observed and measured. All the men gorged, up to and above 5,000 calories (about 21,000 kilojoules) a day – 'there was an excessive consumption of cakes, candies and pies'. After the end of the experiment everybody gorged. Their weight 'overshot': three months after the period of energy restriction had ended the average weight of the group had increased by 3 kilograms (6½ pounds), and they were fatter.

Overshoot with Dr Keys

Francis Benedict was a pioneer. He did not expect that dietary energy restriction would have such an impact. In those days obesity was uncommon, as was dieting, and the relevance of the Carnegie Experiment results to the impact and effect of dieting was not recognized at the time.

A convention in science is to treat the results of any one study, however well conducted, with reserve, and to be impressed only when its results are confirmed by another study using comparable methods carried out by a separate team. The circumstances in which a second study was mounted were those of the Second World War.

Ancel Keys of the University of Minnesota in Minneapolis, who died aged 100 in 2004, was already influential in the 1940s: the K rations used by US paratroops in the war were devised by and probably named after him. Like Francis Benedict, he determined to investigate and understand the physiological and psychological effects of semi-starvation. The purpose was to support the rehabilitation of displaced and other undernourished people in mainland Europe.

The methods he and his team used were similar to those of Francis Benedict, but much more ambitious and even more meticulous. He recruited 36 healthy average-weight male conscientious objectors. The whole programme took almost two years, from November 1944 to October 1945 with follow-ups until September 1946. After three months of assessments and measurements, Dr Keys dropped the energy intake of the volunteers from their then normal 3,200 calories (about 13,500 kilojoules) a day to 1,570 calories (about 6,600 kilojoules).

The experimental diet consisted mostly of wholegrain bread, other cereals (grains), cabbage and root vegetables, with small amounts of meat and other animal foods. It was a simple version of current standard low-fat dieting regimes. Nutritionally the main difference from their normal diet was that this contained less than a quarter of the amount of fat measured as weight – around 17 per cent of total energy – and less than half the weight of protein. Dr Keys required them to walk for 22 miles a week, and kept them on the regime for 24 weeks. The results of this Minnesota Experiment were published in 1950 as *The Biology of Human Starvation*, a two-volume 1,385-page report.

At first the volunteers' body weight dropped very quickly, then weight reduction slowed, and after 20 weeks was negligible. By the end of the 24 weeks, the total average weight reduction was 24 per cent, dropping from an average of 69.4 kilograms (152½ pounds or just under 11 stone) to 54 kilograms (119 pounds or 8½ stone). This translates as about 15 kilograms or 33 pounds.

As with the Carnegie Experiment, the basal metabolic rate of the volunteers dropped more precipitately – half as much again, by 39 per cent. Again, the signs were evident in much slower pulse rates, very low blood pressure, low body temperature, feeling cold all the time, loss of strength and endurance, lethargy, apathy, irritability, mood swings, and depression. The volunteers abandoned sports and recreation, lost interest in social life and sex, and had problems with girlfriends. In his account one volunteer wrote: 'My body flame is burning as low as possible to conserve precious fuel and still maintain life processes.'

All became obsessed with food. They licked their plates clean. Some drank vast amounts of coffee and tea until limited to nine cups a day. Some started to smoke, or smoked more heavily. Four cracked, binged, and were taken off the programme. While working in the grocery store one of these 'suffered a sudden "complete loss of will power" and ate several cookies, a sack of popcorn, and two overripe bananas before he could "regain control" of himself. He immediately suffered a severe emotional upset, with nausea . . . and promptly made a complete confession to the Staff, trying at first to save face by referring to his loss of control as a "mental blackout".' Another chewed up to 40 packets of gum a day, ate garbage, and stole another person's lunch.

Ancel Keys and his team paid special attention to what happened after the 32 remaining volunteers ended the regime. After the 24 weeks the volunteers were put on a gradual re-feeding programme for 12 weeks, restricted to around 2,500–3,000 calories (10,500–12,500 kilojoules) a day. The men remained ravenous. After that they were then able to eat whatever they wanted, and were measured for eight weeks. A smaller group of 12 volunteered to be followed up 20, 33 and 58 weeks later.

They gorged, consuming an average of 5,200 calories (21,750 kilojoules) a day, and some up to 7,000–10,000 calories (29,250–42,000 kilojoules) a day. Some became ill from overeating. They snacked incessantly. They felt hungry even during and after vast meals: one comment was of 'an odd sensation of being full yet still hungry'. After 20 weeks those measured had regained and overshot their original weights. Their average body weight was 5 per cent above what it had been originally, and their body fat was 52 per cent higher. The report commented: 'The recovery of adipose tissue was more rapid than that of the muscles.'

This colossal increase in body fat then subsided. After 33 weeks average body fat was 39 per cent higher. At the final follow-up, over 18 months after the experiment started, the men measured were only 2 per cent heavier than before the experiment started. But they had on average put on 1.25 kilograms (2¾ pounds) or 10 per cent more body fat, mostly where it is most readily stored and available, on the abdomen and backside. Their body composition had changed.

Of the volunteers at the final follow-up the report said: 'The "overweight" is fully accounted for on the basis of increased fat storage.' The men started slim and ended somewhat flabby, with more body fat. Dr Keys called this phenomenon 'post-starvation obesity'. Eight months after the period of restriction the volunteer quoted above wrote: 'I am fat and healthy although my muscles have not yet returned to their former tone.' The foreword to the report stated: 'The presence of undernutrition makes a special kind of person, different morphologically, chemically, physiologically, and psychologically, from his well-fed counterpart.'

As a general statement, Dr Keys and his colleague said: 'In re-feeding, especially when the caloric intake is high, fat deposits tend to increase at a faster rate than the "active" tissues.' Is all this generally true? Writing three decades later John Garrow said: 'When normal subjects, who have been on a restricted diet, are given access to *ad libitum* food [eating all they want] they tend to increase in weight beyond the original baseline value.'

DIETING: THE MODERN EVIDENCE

The human studies so far mentioned remain the most meticulously conducted investigations of their kind. The researchers had no special professional interest in the results of their studies, except to observe and record what happened. The conditions were almost as close as humanly possible to those of an experimental laboratory in which animals are studied. But the studies happened a long time ago in a different world, the participants were men who on average were slim in the first place, and the circumstances of the studies may feel different from dieting. So, what about modern studies of people who restrict energy intake by dieting?

Since the second half of the 20th century, many hundreds of studies on the effects of dieting on overweight and obese people have been published, at an accelerating rate. The increased interest is not just academic. As overweight and obesity has become more common, and identified as a public health emergency in the USA and other materially rich countries, more researchers have moved into the field. Public funds are increasingly available for studies of methods designed to control and reduce weight. Also, commercial slimming organizations hire scientists to advise them and to refine and validate their dieting programmes, and also fund investigations published in scientific journals.

So how is it possible to make sense of the mountains of studies on the effects of dieting regimes? The best resource is methodical reviews of the relevant scientific literature undertaken by independent researchers without special interest in the results of their work. Some have now been published.

Dieting predicts weight increase

In 2004, the *British Journal of Nutrition* published a review and commentary by Andrew Hill, a behavioural scientist from the University of Leeds. He collected nine prospective studies by seven separate research groups in which the effects of energy-restrictive dieting regimes were followed up and checked for periods between 1 and 15 years after they had ended (with one exception that checked weight gain over a holiday period). He then compared the results with those for comparable groups who did not go on a diet. In all but one study, dieting predicted greater weight increase. Dr Hill observed: 'On the face of it, this provides the clearest empirical evidence that dieting facilitates weight gain.'

The review was compiled in response to the first version of this book, and Dr Hill apparently did not want to believe its thesis, for he said that 'a great deal of effort is required to counter Cannon's paradox'. His conclusion was that being fat makes you diet. This is true, but does not explain the rather impressive results of his review and in particular the consistent conclusion that dieting predicts greater weight increase.

Piling the weight back on

Much more was to come. In the spring of 2007 I was working in London. On 10 April the headline in the *Independent* was: 'Most dieters "end up heavier".' Its story said: 'Though many [dieters] succeed in shedding pounds while dieting, they pile the weight back on as soon as they stop, with most ending up heavier than they did to start with.' The *Daily Telegraph* headline was: 'Health warning: all diets make you fat.' Its story said: 'When you diet, something funny happens to your metabolism – it gets better. Better, that is, at making you fat.' Other major newspapers in the UK and in the USA ran similar stories.

When I returned to Brazil the headline in the weekly news magazine *Veja* was: '*Fazer regime engorda*', Portuguese for 'dieting makes you fat'. Janet Tomiyama, a researcher from the University of California, Los Angeles (UCLA), was quoted as confirming the finding of Andrew Hill's small review: 'Dieting consistently predicts additional increase in weight.'

The futility of dieting

These headlines were all about the results of a comprehensive review published in the *American Psychologist*. This had been undertaken by Traci Mann of the department of psychology at UCLA, with Janet Tomiyama and other colleagues. They had systematically collated and analysed the results of all the studies they could find that both examined the effects of dieting regimes and included follow-up checks carried out two or more years after dieting had ended. They located a total of 31 studies.

Seven studies were found whose design compared the effect of dieting in a group of obese people with the weights of a 'control' group who were not dieting, and that also included follow-ups for at least four years after dieting had ended. Many other studies with this design were rejected because they included no long-term follow-up.

Taken together, the results of the seven studies were that on follow-up the dieters had put back on almost all the weight reduced on the various regimes. At that point they were 1.1 kilograms (2.4 pounds) lighter. 'Clearly, these participants remain obese,' the UCLA team observed, and: 'It is important for policy-makers to remember that weight regain does not necessarily end when researchers stop following study participants.' Of these studies the one whose results showed the greatest weight reduction on follow-up also included 'large amounts of physical activity . . . this may be the potent factor'.

A total of 14 studies were found whose design did not include a control group, where dieters were followed up for at least four years. Of the 14 studies taken together, followed-up results were that the participants reduced an average of 14 kilograms (just over 30 pounds) on the regimes, then became obese again, and at the final follow-up were recorded as being an average of 3 kilograms (6.6 pounds) lighter.

That sounds like modest success. The UCLA team said that the net weight reduction could well have been caused by exercise. Many studies specified that participants be more physically active. A clue was found in one study that controlled for the effects of physical activity. This divided participants into two sub-groups: dieting only, and dieting plus physical activity. In this study, all participants on average had reduced about the same amount of weight at the end of the dieting regimes. Follow-up results were that the dieting plus activity people were a net 2.5 kilograms (5.5 pounds) lighter, whereas the dieting-only people were 0.9 kilograms (2 pounds) heavier than when they started the regimes.

The third type of study, of which ten were reviewed and analysed, identified people who did, or who did not, go on dieting regimes, and followed them up. Most of these prospective studies had been reviewed by Andrew Hill, and the UCLA team's analysis confirmed his. The results of one study were that four years later, dieters had reduced some weight. Two studies found no relationship between dieting and weight. The remaining seven studies found that dieting predicted a net weight increase.

The UCLA team also noted the results of three previous reviews published in 1991, 1995 and 2001, one of which concluded: 'It is only the rate of weight regain, not the fact of weight regain, that appears open to debate.' In 2007 Traci Mann commented: 'We found that the majority of people regained all the weight, plus more . . . We concluded that most of them would have been better off not going on the diet at all.' She added: 'My mother has been on diets and says what we are saying is obvious.'

The false hopes of scientists

The results of the UCLA review could be interpreted simply as showing that dieting does not work. This is indeed one of the conclusions reached by Traci Mann and her colleagues, but they go further. They state that epidemiological studies of free-living people designed to check the efficacy of dieting regimes are systematically biased in the direction of showing that energy-restrictive dieting regimes are effective, in at least seven different ways.

First, since the 1980s the vital importance of sustained regular physical activity has become generally recognized, so much so that it can be considered unethical to design a weight-control programme that excludes additional exercise. As mentioned, most of the studies specified increased physical activity as well as dieting. Any sustained drop in weight may well be because of increased exercise. The findings of the US National Weight Control Registry – mentioned above – support this interpretation.

Second, most participants in the dieting programmes were actually not followed up. They did not turn up, did not return forms, or could not be found. People prepared to be followed up are more likely to be pleased with their results. Those who put back all the weight reduced by dieting and so feel they have failed, and so will be a disappointment to the investigators, are less likely to be available.

Third, researchers excluded participants from follow-up for failure to reduce enough weight, bariatric surgery, failure to return telephone calls, refusal to attend earlier follow-ups, and other reasons. The UCLA team commented: 'Although studies find numerous reasons to exclude participants who might make the diet look ineffective, it does not appear that any studies exclude participants who might inappropriately make the diet look effective.'

Fourth, more than half of the participants followed up in the 14 non-controlled studies were not weighed, and instead reported their weight by mail or telephone. Some studies allowed for weight under-reporting, usual in these circumstances, by adding on 2.3 kilograms (5 pounds). Two studies have found that dieters under-report their weights by an average of 3.7 kilograms (over 8 pounds).

Fifth, between a fifth and two-thirds of the dieters continued to go on dieting regimes – after completing the one specified – during the follow-up period. One study found that participants had reduced an average of 11.8 more kilograms (26 pounds) on other dieting regimes before follow-up. In such cases follow-up records will not show long-term results but short-term weight reduction on the other regimes.

Sixth, the dieters wanted the regimes to work. That is why they enrolled in the studies in the first place. They may also have wanted to please the investigators. In such circumstances it is inevitable that people will under-record their weights or, if they feel they have failed, either start on another dieting regime or else drop out.

Seventh, the investigators wanted the regimes to work. A rule in science is that investigators should be disinterested. But many researchers responsible for dieting regime studies believe in the efficacy of dieting. Also – the UCLA team did not say this, perhaps being too polite – many leading researchers in the field are directors of their own obesity clinics, or may be consultants to, or funded by, slimming businesses – or both.

Also, the results measured and analysed were of body weight. Measures of body fat before and after the regimes, and at follow-up, would have been more illuminating. Taken all together, the results of epidemiological studies of free-living dieters, however conscientiously undertaken, have to be examined carefully, as Traci Mann and her team did. They concluded: 'Dieters who gain back more weight than they lost may very well be the norm.'

The biospherians

The lines of evidence so far – anecdotal observations, the experience of animal breeders, the results of re-feeding after energy restriction in undernourished children and in normal-weight men, and followed-up studies of free-living obese adult dieters – point in the same direction. All the same though, my own training has taught me that the clinching studies are of humans in experimental conditions. But would a controlled human experiment ever be carried out again? The limiting factor is not so much cost, as practicality and ethics. Who would ever commit months of their lives to undergo such an arduous study?

New Agers, is the answer. In 2000, half a century after the Minnesota Experiment, the results of the Biosphere 2 Experiment were published in the *American Journal of Clinical Nutrition*. Medical officer for this project was the physician, gerontologist and nutritionist Roy Walford of UCLA.

Biosphere 2 was built between 1987 and 1991 at a cost of $US200 million in Oracle, Arizona. One of its purposes was to see what life might be like for humans who colonized space. With a structure inspired by the visionary engineer Buckminster Fuller, and an inside area of 3.15 acres (1.27 hectares) it remains the largest closed ecosystem ever. Inside were areas of rainforest, coral reef, mangrove, desert and cultivated fields, and buildings. The eight biospherians, including Roy Walford, had to grow their own food. They remained inside for two full years from 1991 to 1993, in touch with colleagues outside by radio, telephone and computers, but otherwise sealed off from Biosphere 1 – the Earth.

The dieting experiment came about because of a mistake: the biospherians were unable to grow enough food to keep them in energy balance. Roy Walford proposed that they accept this dietary energy restriction, which they did for the two years.

The biospherians were four women and four men aged between 29 and 67. Six were slim or of normal weight, two were somewhat overweight. For the first six months, and for a total of 21 months of the two years, they consumed a daily average of around 1,800 calories (7,500 kilojoules) of highly nutrient-dense food from the produce they grew, plus supplements. After six months their weights had dropped by an average of 9.1 kilograms (20 pounds). After that more food was sometimes available, and their weights stabilized for the remaining 18 months. They stayed physically active. The study as published did not report on their levels of hunger or their behaviour.

After they left the biosphere and were eating whatever they wanted, five of the group agreed to be monitored for six months. At the end of that time their lean tissue was not recovered, but their fat had overshot. They had put on 8.8 kilograms, practically all the weight reduced in the previous two years, and almost all of it was fat. They had become fatter.

You can say with some confidence that anybody who restricts energy from food by going on a dieting regime is likely to overshoot – the reduced weight will go back on, and the proportion and amount of body fat will increase. Thirteen years before Traci Mann's review was published, a commentary in the *British Medical Journal* said: 'It is no longer a mystery why diets have such a poor record of long-term success.' It added: 'The failure of fat people to achieve a goal they seem to want – and to want almost above all else – must now be admitted for what it is: a failure not of those people, but of the methods of treatment that are used.' But the juggernaut dieting industry rumbles on.

WHAT HAPPENS WHEN YOU GO ON A DIET?

But how and why does dieting make you fat? There have been some clues so far, in the epidemiological studies and the human and animal experiments. In this and the next sections I give a brief account of the biological processes involved when you go on a diet, when you come off a diet, and when afterwards your body adapts to being fatter. It's a story involving physiology, biochemistry, metabolism, and other disciplines including one that may hold the key to why dieting makes you fat – microbiology.

A long and winding road

The story is also of a journey that has included false turnings and wrong paths taken. Even now, many researchers in the territory, most promoters of dieting regimes, and therefore no doubt hundreds of millions of people who try to reduce body weight and fat, are confused. Much of the most reliable information now is coming from both older and younger generations of scientists who have remained open-minded or else have never been committed to an attitude based on ideas that are a mismatch with experience.

Many of these researchers are specialists in energy metabolism and energy balance. Others work in infant and childhood development, exercise physiology, microbial ecology, natural history, and systems theory, and other disciplines requiring broad minds. And as with other topics of intense public interest, some of the most illuminating insights are being posted on the internet by people without academic qualifications, usually dieters or ex-dieters themselves, who have decided to find out what goes on.

The fundamental fallacies

First though, you need to be well aware of another series of mistakes. Until recently dieting regimes – especially those that 'count calories' – have been based on the idea that if you restrict dietary energy, the weight you reduce will be body fat, and also that the weight you reduce simply depends on how many calories you cut. Some regimes still claim or imply as much. This is wrong.

Thus in the previous chapter I mentioned *The F-Plan Diet*, a smash-hit bestseller in the early 1980s. This assumes that the female reader is in energy balance on 2,000 calories a day – higher than usual even then – and says: 'If we were to put you on a slimming diet providing you with 1,500 calories a day, you would be 500 calories short of your requirement and these would have to be taken from your body fat. It has been scientifically estimated that a pound of your own body fat provides approximately 3,500 calories. So during a week you would be likely to shed one pound of surplus fat.'

Even until the late 1980s, people who devised dieting regimes could hardly be criticized for saying that steady body weight and fat reduction is just a matter of cutting calories. They were simply repeating what was said by scientists with the status of world authorities on energy balance, obesity, and weight control.

For example, Jean Mayer, who became President of Tufts University in Boston, was with Ancel Keys the most influential nutrition scientist specializing in obesity in the USA in the third quarter of the 20th century. In a paper published in book form in 1971 he wrote: 'A loss of 2lb per week (corresponding roughly to a deficit of 1,000 calories per day) seems to be reasonable for most adult patients; a loss of 1lb a week (corresponding to a deficit of 500 calories a day) would still lead to a weight loss of 50lb in a year.' Reg Passmore of the University of Edinburgh was at that time comparably prominent in the UK. In a standard textbook co-edited by him and published in 1986 he wrote: 'Treatment is simple in principle. If a patient eats a diet providing 500–1,000 kcal (1–4 MJ) less than is needed for the activities of daily life, then and only then will the excess reserves of energy in adipose tissue be drawn upon and weight lost at a rate of 0.5–1.0 kg (1–2lb) each week.'

As you can see, these statements make or imply three inter-related points, taken to be true by many dieting regimes. First, that the amount of weight reduced is simply a function of body fat having an energy value of 3,500 calories (about 14,700 kilojoules) per pound (roughly half a kilogram). Second, that with dietary energy restriction, weight reduction will be steady. Third, that weight reduced is - or can be assumed to be - just body fat. This is all wrong.

You do not just reduce body fat

Once any regime of dietary restriction is well under way, most of the weight reduced will normally be body fat. But at no stage, on any regime, will it be only body fat. That's just wishful thinking. It's what you want, but it's not what happens.

Depending on the nature, severity and length of the regime, you will also lose lean tissue from muscles, and eventually from other organs of the body. As a rough and ready calculation, for sedentary people after the first week or two the proportions of weight reduced are about 75 per cent body fat and 25 per cent lean tissue, mostly muscle. That's why dieters usually get to feel weak. The proportion is a rough approximation: it varies depending on the nature of the regime and the state of the person.

There is a saying, 'use it or lose it'. At any time of food shortage or of famine, the body protects its tissues that are most needed, such as that of the brain, the heart, and other vital organs. It releases energy from its stores to compensate for what is not being supplied from food and drink.

The bodies of physically fit and active people will tend to spare muscle tissue from being used as fuel, because it is in use all the time and is therefore needed. By analogy, if you are short of wood to make a fire to keep you warm, you use what is in store first, together with any unused and least valuable furniture. This does not imply that there is a little person inside your body checking you out and saying 'need that, keep that, don't need that, sling that'. It is the result of how we have trained our bodies, a process of physical training of which we are normally not conscious.

You dehydrate

Any weight-reduction programme claiming to reduce 4½–7 kilograms (about 10–15 pounds) a week and implying that this is of body fat is making a false and misleading claim. A simple calculation proves the point. Suppose you are in energy balance at 2,500 calories a day (a lot higher than most basically sedentary women). Assume the energy value of body fat is 3,000 calories a pound (which it is, the 3,500 calorie figure is inaccurate – see the notes to this chapter). Then if you consumed zero calories a day on a water-only fast you could not possibly reduce more than around 6 pounds (under 3 kilograms) of body fat in a week.

The calculation goes like this. First take 2,500 (daily calories needed to stay in energy balance, which, because consumption is zero, all come from the body's stores). Second there are seven days in the week; 2,500 multiplied by 7 is 17,500 calories. Third, this 17,500 divides by 3,000 (calories per pound of body fat). That all makes 5.8 pounds (about 2½ kilograms). This is the absolute maximum of body fat that theoretically could be burned in a week.

Suppose instead that the regime supplied around 1,500 calories a day, which many do. When you use the same calculation, but with 1,000 calories a day as the difference, the result comes to a maximum of 2.3 pounds (1 kilogram) of fat a week – as indicated by Reg Passmore.

The folks who mastermind dieting regimes also know how to use a pocket calculator. They tend to evade the arithmetic by claiming that the foods and drinks on their system have special fat-burning powers. Even were this so, nothing could account for body-fat loss of 5–7 kilograms (about 10–15 pounds) a week.

Only a small amount of any initial impressive weight reduction is of body fat. It is mostly water. This comes from two sources. One is contained in all your tissues – you become drier generally. The other is the body's immediately available source of energy. This is glycogen, a form of glucose stored in the muscles and liver. By analogy with money, you can think of glycogen as your current account, and body fat as savings.

Glycogen is stored bound up with water at the ratio of roughly 1 part glycogen and 3 parts water. Overall the body contains roughly 700 grams (roughly 1½ pounds) of 'solid' glycogen, bound up with roughly 2 kilograms (4½ pounds) of water. Glycogen is a type of carbohydrate with an energy value of roughly 400 calories per 100 grams. Water in cells needs little energy to be released. It only takes around 400 calories to burn off a pound of glycogen and the water that comes with it.

This, plus the release of water from other parts of the body, explains how dieting regimes can deliver on their promise of a drop in weight of 4½ kilograms (10 pounds) or more in the first week. All you need to know is that little of this is body fat, and that once you are off the regime, this weight will all go back on again. To use the money analogy again, your current account will be back in balance.

You slow down

On any typical dieting regime, your body slows down. The process may be conscious, and is also unconscious. Dieters notice that suddenly the programmes on television are more interesting, that they don't have time to go for a brisk walk, and that it's nice to have a nap in the afternoon and lie-in during weekend mornings. Your body adapts to inadequate energy from food by making you less physically active. This partly frustrates your purpose in dieting.

Also your metabolic rate – the level at which your body is in energy balance – drops. Other things being equal, the metabolic rate of a lighter person is lower than that of a heavier person. But an invariable feature of dieting is that your metabolic rate drops lower still. In his textbook John Garrow states: 'People who are on a restricted diet show a decrease in metabolic rate which is greater than would be expected from tissue loss. The literature has been reviewed . . . and there is no investigator who has looked for this effect and has failed to find it.'

This 'undershoot' drop in metabolic rate also partly frustrates the intentions of dieters. The body of a dieter becomes more inactive, externally by less physical activity of all sorts – from fidgeting to running – and internally by turning over more slowly. This is as close as we get to a state of hibernation.

These processes explain why after the first period of fast weight reduction, which is mostly water, for a while weight reduces at a fairly steady rate – the speed mostly depending on how severe is the dietary restriction – and then slows right down, and eventually, unless you are almost literally starving yourself, will stop. Your body has adapted to its new circumstances. You are thinking about reducing your weight and fat. Your body is responding to a situation of food shortage, and has been evolved and adapted to do so since the emergence of the human species. Indeed, after a while on a dieting regime, your body will respond in ways that conserve its fat. To use the analogy with money again, it is as if your body has got the message that you are rapidly running out of readies, and is prudently holding on to the savings account to stop you becoming bankrupt – or, in the situation of dieting, to which the body reacts as if famine or starving, dead.

WHAT HAPPENS WHEN YOU COME OFF A DIET

So at some point you come off the diet. This may be because you have reached your target of weight reduction. Or it may be because you have become bored with or tired of the regime, or feel tired or depressed, or because you have been thinking about food all the time, or have become frustrated. What happens then?

Your body stores fat

What happens, if you are sedentary, is that you put on weight more or less to the level it was before the diet started, and you become fatter. When you come off a dieting regime, and start to eat and drink 'normally', you may not feel hungry immediately. But as soon as you have consumed your first meals, your body is likely to respond by making you feel very hungry. It reacts like the body of a person who has been starved – which describes a dieting regime.

This hunger may be intense and compulsive. In the first chapter I mentioned the experience of going with my colleague Russell Twisk for a celebration blow-out immediately after the weigh-in that culminated our lose-weight contest. On another occasion, during the regime I had been thinking about pickles, and my first 'meal' after I finished dieting was a big jar of pickled onions, with half a loaf of bread. During and after both binges I felt sick – especially after the onions – and yet for a few weeks afterwards I did not – could not – stop myself eating. (There is more on compulsive eating later in this chapter.) The hunger after a regime has ended drives us to put on the weight reduced by dieting. And it also enables our bodies to accumulate extra fat, the better to survive the next time when food is short.

It may well be that this effect of body fat overshoot is more pronounced and more difficult to control when dieters are sedentary and unfit – as most dieters are. The idea is that if you are physically out of shape, on a dieting regime your body will shed more lean tissue than it would were you active and fit, simply because you have unintentionally trained your body to discard under-used lean tissue. Likewise, when you stop dieting your body will preferentially put on fat essentially for the same reason – the regime has trained your body to conserve fat. Anecdotal evidence that supports this idea is that active people like boxers, jockeys, dancers and actors seem to find it comparatively easy to reduce and to regain weight when they need to do so for their work, without losing body tone.

Do you stay slowed down?

After dieting regimes does your metabolic rate remain depressed? After successive regimes does it become gradually lower, as your body gets the message that food will go on being short? Animal experiments show this, and from the evolutionary perspective it makes sense that the body will respond to situations of regular famine by progressively slowing down its functions. But relatively short-term studies with usually sedentary and obese humans checked before, during and after dieting regimes do not show this – evidently after a regime has ended, their metabolic rates eventually return to the previous level.

This makes sense when body composition and overall level of physical activity remain constant before and then eventually after dieting regimes. If, however, people become gradually less and less active, and their lean tissue becomes gradually wasted, then at the same weight resting and overall metabolic rate must drop. The reverse must also apply. When instead of dieting people become regularly physically active, and become lean, at the same and even lower body weights their bodies will turn over more dietary energy.

Bugs may explain everything

When you go on a dieting regime you train your body to hold on to its fat, and when you come off the regime and your weight increases again, your body composition usually changes so that you are fatter. The evolutionary explanation is given later in this chapter – briefly though, the dieting process triggers responses designed to enable us to survive food shortages and famine. But how is this done within our bodies?

At the time of writing in mid-2008 the following hypothesis is being investigated by scientists in the USA and Europe. My colleague and friend Tore Midvedt of the Karolinska Institute in Stockholm indicates that the answer is likely to be known with some confidence around 2010. It is to do with bugs – the 500 or more species of bacteria inside our guts that altogether make up over 90 per cent of the cells of the human organism. We are evolved in association with bacteria, and among many other functions depend on them for the metabolism, digestion and excretion of our food. Much of faeces is bacteria.

The bacteria in our colons are made up from two classes, the bacteroidetes and the firmicutes, each of which include many species. Experiments on laboratory animals were reported in *Nature* at the end of 2006. These show for sure that firmicutes 'harvest' energy from food far more efficiently than bacteroidetes, that firmicutes are dominant in the guts of obese animals, that this dominance is increased when the animals are subjected to energy restriction, and is sustained after they are given normal rations.

Is this also true in humans? So far it looks like the answer is yes. Work so far is showing that firmicutes are also dominant in the guts of obese humans, and that this dominance is increased by dieting. If so this means that dieting breeds the type of bacteria inside us best able to extract energy from food, and best able to store this as body fat. If this turns out to be true, the leading scientists in this field, who include Jeffrey Gordon of Washington University in St Louis, Missouri, and his colleagues, are likely to be nominated for Nobel prizes.

ADAPTING TO FATNESS

Some time after any dieting regime has ended – maybe months, maybe years – your weight will almost certainly increase to more or less what it was before you started the regime, and then usually more or less level off.

But not necessarily. You might stabilize at a lower level. One way to achieve this is in effect to go on a diet after the diet has ended – to keep restricting your dietary energy, allowing for your body both needing less energy at a lower weight, and needing to become adapted to a lower energy balance. Some people of iron willpower may be able to do this. The other way is to be physically active. But with depleted lean tissue and extra body fat, this is also very hard to do – unless you become a lot more physically active while you are on the diet, in which case the activity will be using and thus protecting your muscles. Better, is to skip the dieting regime in the first place and simply become a lot more physically active – on this, see below, and chapter 6.

If, however, you are and remain basically sedentary, you may well eventually stabilize at a somewhat heavier weight. You will almost certainly be fatter, because you have trained your body to build up its fat reserves.

Body fat is metabolically active, but needs less energy for maintenance than vital organs and active muscle, so at this higher level of body fat – and maybe also body weight – your energy turnover could well be lower. This creates a vicious cycle in which you gradually continue to become fatter; the more so if you follow one dieting regime with others.

Also, levels of energy balance drop as people get older. Even with sustained levels of physical activity, the bodies of older people at a constant weight turn over less energy; another reason why weight tends to drift upwards.

The moving set-point

If you read articles and books on dieting you will be aware of 'set-point theory'. The general idea is that the body contains a weight regulator, maybe in the hypothalamus, like thermostats that keep rooms at constant temperatures. This theory has some charm. It suggests that some people are bound to be slim and other people are bound to be fat, and that's that. It also has some plausibility. Studies both of under- and overeating always show that decrease or increase of body weight, in humans as well as animals, is slower than it would be if weight was just a function of amount of energy consumed.

But set-point theory as usually proposed is obvious nonsense. It cannot explain the fluctuations in body weight and fat historically, or as between different countries, or within countries. Also, it is not true that individual people usually stay the same weight over time, nor is there evidence that this has ever been so.

Breaking our appetite controls

My conclusion is that the human body does contain some sort of 'appestat' that 'buffers' body weight reduction or increase, like a thermostat, but with a crucial difference. Suppose a room thermostat is set at 25° Celsius or just under 80° Fahrenheit. As long as the machine is working, this is the temperature at which it will turn on or off, keeping the room at the same temperature. But the human body is not a machine; it adapts. When people increase in weight – the equivalent of the room being too hot – their 'appestat' will adapt and drift upwards to the equivalent of a new setting.

The mechanisms the body uses to control appetite and thus body weight and fat are not static, but dynamic. Therefore while the 'appestat' does 'defend' body weight and body fat, it does so around a constant weight only if the person stays at a stable weight and in energy balance more or less at the same levels of energy intake and expenditure. But when people gradually increase body weight, the point to which the 'appestat' is set is raised to accommodate these circumstances. After any dieting regime the 'appestat' will signal hunger – typically intense hunger – until body weight returns to the level that it was before the regime began. But the difference, for a basically sedentary dieter, is that each regime has the effect of reducing lean tissue and increasing body fat. The new amount of body fat, and maybe weight also, which the body will then 'defend' will be higher.

Also, the constant stress of continued dieting might derange – in effect break – the body's weight-control mechanisms. This would explain why some people who frequently go on diets – weight cyclers, also known as 'yo-yo dieters', suffer body weight and fat increases that spiral out of control, and can be treated only by surgery. There is more on weight cycling later in this chapter.

The conclusion? The 'moving set-point' theory is the best working hypothesis. It helps to explain why dieting is counterproductive – and possibly risky.

WHY PHYSICAL ACTIVITY IS CRUCIAL

The message that shines out of the methodical survey of Traci Mann and her colleagues is that it is regular sustained physical activity, not dieting, that controls body weight and body fat. Activity can be of any type. It can be travel (cycling or walking to work), occupational (outside or inside, in the workplace or in the home), or any form of recreational activity (walking, running, cycling, dancing, swimming, tennis, football, fitness-centre work, and so on). What matters most is that to make us fit and healthy, much – and preferably most – physical activity should be as vigorous as we can make it.

Here is the good news

Another key message of this book is that sedentary people are in artificially low energy balance. Humans are designed to turn over something like 400–600 calories (roughly 1,675–2,500 kilojoules) a day more than is now usual. This higher level was usual three generations ago, and has been normal for the 200,000 or so years of *Homo sapiens*. The range is approximate and allows for size, age and gender. At this higher level our bodies work well. When it is easy to get plenty of nourishment from food and drink, our system are more tolerant of pleasures like snacks, desserts or alcoholic drinks.

When we use and train our muscles, our bodies preferentially convert dietary energy into building and maintaining lean tissue. Regular sustained physical activity nourishes all the body's systems – brain and nerves, heart and blood vessels, immune system, lungs, stomach, liver, kidneys, and other vital organs, as well as those of consumption, digestion, metabolism, and excretion. Activity makes us healthy as well as fit.

The uses of energy

Now I will show just how valuable sustained physical activity is. This I have done by setting out the amount of energy needed every day by people of different weights, body compositions, and levels of physical activity. The table on the next page page is adapted and developed from the classic textbook *Energy, Work and Leisure*, and follows discussions with John Durnin of Glasgow University, one of its co-authors.

Most of the energy our bodies need is used when we are at rest. An athlete in training or a miner may use as much as or even a bit more energy in activity as at rest, but you and I do not. At rest, our vital organs do most work. Our brains use roughly 20 per cent of the energy we take in from food and drink, and our other metabolically most active vital organs – liver, heart and kidneys – about 45 per cent. Of the remainder, for an average sedentary person almost 20 per cent is used by muscle; and almost 20 per cent is used by all our other organs – including body fat, which is metabolically active. Also, about 10 per cent of the energy in our diets is used in the process of digestion and absorption of food.

The one very variable number here is the percentage of energy used by muscle. During physical activity muscles use anything up to 20 or 50 or even more times the energy they do when at rest, depending on how vigorous the activity is, and also depending on the condition of the muscles – that is, how fit you are.

Now look at the table. The first two columns on the left show categories of body composition. Thus 'lean' does not mean 'thin' or 'light'. It refers to people with a high proportion of lean tissue – muscle in particular – and not much body fat. By definition, lean – as distinct

Energy used at rest (basal metabolic rate) in women and men of different body compositions and weights

Figures within the table are approximate and illustrative only, for people aged 16-60.
Values for those older than 60 are lower. For kilojoules multiply by 4.18

Women	Men	51kg 112lb	60.5kg 133lb	70kg 154lb	79.5kg 175lb	89kg 196lb
Body composition	Body composition	BMR calories	BMR calories	BMR calories	BMR calories	BMR calories
	Lean¹	1450	1550	1650	1750	1850
Lean¹	Medium²	1300	1400	1500	1600	1700
Medium²	Fat³	1150	1250	1350	1450	1550
Fat³	Very Fat³	1000	1100	1200	1300	1400
Very Fat³		850	950	1050	1150	1250

1   Lean because physically fit from regular activity, exercise
2   Medium for early 21st century. Intermediate body composition, basically sedentary
3   Fat (flabby) or very fat, and also sedentary

from slim – people are physically fit. They may be light (see the next column) or they may be heavy. Likewise 'fat' and also 'very fat' does not mean 'heavy'. Here it refers to inactive people with a high proportion of body fat to lean tissue. They may be heavy (see the columns to the right) or they may be flabby or very flabby but not particularly heavy, or even relatively light.

Thus if you are a basically sedentary woman of medium body composition and you weigh 60.5 kilograms (133 pounds) your body will turn over around 1,250 calories (about 5,250 kilojoules) every day at rest. If you have the same proportion of body fat and lean tissue and weigh 70 kilograms (154 pounds) you will turn over around 1,350 calories (about 5,700 kilojoules) every day at rest. (The reason why a 'medium' woman corresponds to a 'fat' man is that women have more body fat than men.)

To take another case, a woman whose lean tissue is wasted, because she is sedentary and repeatedly goes on diets, will be flabby – fat – and may also weigh 60.5 kilograms (133 pounds), or less if she is short. She will turn over something like 1,100 calories (about 4,600 kilojoules) every day at rest. But if she is lean she will turn over around 1,400 calories (5,900 kilojoules) every day at rest. That is 300 calories (about 1,250 kilojoules) a day *at the same weight*. There is no magic here. If you are lean you are physically active. If you are flabby you are physically inactive.

What the table indicates is that if you are relatively lean, your body uses more energy all the time, not only when you are being active. Measurements made of the energy value of physical activity only during the activity itself – on a treadmill, for example – underestimate the energy value of physical activity. Any sustained physical activity uses more energy after as well as during the time of activity. As people become physically fitter and leaner, they are training their bodies to work at a higher level of energy turnover all the time.

People who have changed their ways of life and become physically fit and relatively lean, know this. They feel warmer all the time. They wear lighter clothes and are less likely to 'wrap up' when it is cool outside. They prefer rooms at lower temperatures, and open windows. This all means that their bodies are turning over more energy, all the time, waking and sleeping.

The news gets better

People are not relatively lean by chance, but because they are physically active and fit. Here is where the story becomes more remarkable.

Given that energy turnover at complete rest (what is known as basal or resting metabolic rate – the two rates are similar) is given a value of 1.0, sedentary people will use something like an additional 0.4–0.5 in all their physical activity and also for the digestion of food. This is known as a physical activity level (PAL) of 1.40–1.50. So the inactive 'medium' woman who weighs 60.5 kilograms (133 pounds) whose basal metabolic rate (BMR) is 1,250 calories will have a total energy turnover of something like 1,750–1,875 calories (about 7,350–7,875 kilojoules) a day. An inactive woman of the same weight who is fat and whose BMR is 1,100 calories a day will have a total energy turnover of something like 1,550–1,650 calories (about 6,500–6,950 kilojoules) a day. Metabolism slows down with age, and such a woman aged around 65 could well increase her body fat on a dieting regime designed to supply 1,500 calories a day. This shows why a relatively fat inactive (albeit relatively light) woman – or man – may 'eat like a bird' and yet put on more fat.

By contrast, a physically active, fit and lean person will be at a PAL around 1.70–1.80. So the lean woman of 133 pounds whose BMR is 1,400 calories a day could be turning over a total of 2,380–2,520 calories (about 10,000–10,575 kilojoules) a day – something like 600 calories (roughly 2,500 kilojoules) a day more than the 'medium' woman

This closely corresponds with the average energy requirements calculated for United Nations agencies for women of that weight in the mid-20th century. This explains why a relatively lean active (albeit heavy) man – or woman – may 'eat like a horse' and yet remain at the same weight.

Fit active lean people can eat almost the equivalent of a whole meal a day more than unfit sedentary fat people and stay lean, while in-active people get fatter.

WHY DIETING MAKES YOU FAT

Expressed in so many words, 'dieting makes you fat' is a paradox. The word 'paradox' has two meanings. One is an idea that is contrary to reason. The other is an idea that seems contrary to reason but which turns out to be true. This is the sense in which 'dieting makes you fat' is a paradox. Here now is the general theory stating why as a rule it is true. This theory is the best fit with the facts.

The fundamental reason why dieting makes you fat concerns our origins and nature as a species, and how and why humans have evolved, adapted, survived, and multiplied. Once knowledge of human biology is seen in the light of human evolution and history, what at first seems absurd becomes obvious.

200,000 years of adaptation

You were born in the 20th century, and live in the 21st century. You are also a member of a species evolved and adapted over the last 200,000 years. If you periodically restrict your energy intake with the intention of becoming less heavy – and less fat – what you do unintentionally is activate, develop and strengthen a series of inbuilt processes. These conserve and increase your body fat, whose purpose is to keep you alive and functioning in times of food shortage and famine.

History helps explain why. For most if not all readers of this book, food and drink are abundant. If you live in a materially rich country, you are surrounded by shops stocked with what seems endless variety. You probably can eat and drink as much as you like, and more, any time. But for most humans, what is your daily food and drink has been consumed only at feasts and other special occasions.

You may never meet somebody who has experienced starvation or famine. But in terms of human evolution, always having plenty to eat and drink is a rare experience. Food insecurity has been the main single threat to human survival since *Homo sapiens* emerged.

The gatherer-hunter and pastoral communities that went forth and multiplied most successfully were those who survived epic migrations over vast distances of land and ocean. They were dependent on what they could carry – on and in their bodies – as within the last 100,000 years they found and populated Asia, Australia, the Pacific, Europe, and the Americas. They became increasingly well adapted at surviving long periods of semi-starvation. Less well-adapted migrant communities died out or stayed put.

We are the descendants of the successful survivors. Their ability to withstand starvation is bred into us. We humans are born to conserve the fuel we carry within us, which is our body fat. Without this special quality *Homo sapiens* might well have never moved out of Africa, or else have become extinct.

Within the last 10,000 years, communities in the Middle East, Europe, Asia, Africa, the Americas and the Pacific islands developed food systems driven by the need to make supplies more secure. Grains and other plant foods were bred, sowed, cropped and stored. Animals became domesticated and were bred as additional sources of food. But peasant agriculturalists still needed the special human ability to conserve body fat. Even in times of peace most people subsisted on frugal diets. Famines caused by war, flood, plague and infestation wiped out those least adapted to withstand starvation, and their bloodlines therefore ended.

Body fat as treasure

In pre-industrial societies, people whose food was most secure were most liable to accumulate excess weight. Fat people were obviously powerful. Some rulers and elders were obese, and in some societies women were fattened to show the prosperity of their husbands. In food-secure societies, rich women may wear their visible wealth outside in the form of jewellery. In food-insecure societies, rich women often wear their visible wealth inside in the form of fat. Fatness remains esteemed as a sign of wealth and health in many countries and cultures.

Before industrialization, most people lived and worked on small quantities of food, and so were small and lean. If they had no food stocks they suffered the consequences of severe food shortage and famine, including the infectious diseases most liable to kill babies and young children. Again, survival of the fittest meant survival of those bloodlines most adapted to food shortages.

All this remained true until after food supplies in some and then many countries became secure following industrialization. This began around eight generations ago. Only then could most people in Europe, and then in North America and other materially rich countries, be sure of enough food almost all the time. It was then that being slim began to be seen as a sign of good health.

People in industrialized countries often remained short of food until well into the 20th century. Conditions for working-class families in cities throughout Europe were generally abominable. Many millions of 21st-century US citizens are descendants of families who escaped starvation by emigrating from Europe a few generations ago, or whose antecedents were slaves until the mid-19th century.

The rate of increase in obesity, especially since the 1980s, has been very rapid in countries whose populations are either mostly descended from impoverished rural communities, such as India and China, or from impoverished urban communities or recent immigrants, such as in the UK, the USA and associated countries. Populations with a history of frugal ways of life become overweight and obese very quickly when they suddenly become sedentary and have unlimited access to energy-dense food and drink. Saudi Arabia is a striking example.

Training to survive famine

The evolution and survival of the human species gives us the context that explains why restricting energy intake by dieting has an effect on our bodies that otherwise seems inexplicable. The reason is biological in its fundamental sense.

Every time you go on an energy-restrictive dieting regime you turn on processes in your body that explain how the human species has survived and developed. Once you start eating normally again, these processes increase your store of body fat as a safeguard against the next time of deprivation.

The extent to which dieters' bodies become trained in this way varies. Age and genetics are factors. So is gender. Nature favours women because they give birth to and nurture children. Women carry a greater proportion of body fat, withstand semi-starvation better than men, and generally put on more body fat than men when by dieting they provoke their bodies to respond as if to famine.

The most important factors are the severity, length, and frequency of dieting. Sedentary people are in artificially low energy balance all the time. People who restrict their energy intake by around 10 per cent – by say 200 calories (around 820 kilojoules) a day – are less likely to trigger the mechanisms that protect the body against famine. People who restrict their intake by around 30 per cent – by say 600 calories (around 2,500 kilojoules) a day, to around 1,200–1,800 calories (5,000–7,500 kilojoules) a day, roughly what many dieting books 'prescribe', are training their bodies to adapt to an environment of regular food shortages. Those who regularly endure lower energy dieting regimes, of say 1,000 calories (4,200 kilojoules) a day or fewer, are 'telling' their bodies to react so as to survive regular famines.

Much of what our bodies do is beyond the control of our minds, which, if you think about digestion, heartbeat and breathing, is just as well. You know the differences between dieting or fasting on the one hand, and starvation and famine on the other hand. But if you speak nicely to your body, and say: 'Listen body, this is not a famine, this is a dieting regime,' your body does not hear you.

At times of food shortage your body slows down its vital physical functions, to keep going as long as possible and to conserve its fat stores. Then when plenty of food becomes available and is consumed, these processes preferentially convert the food into body fat. As an analogy from conscious life, when prudent people are suddenly short of income they spend less cash, and then when plenty of money becomes available again, they remember the bad times and put any surplus cash into savings.

The more often this happens, and the more severe the restriction, the more efficient the body becomes at conserving its own fat stores. Adipose tissue is the built-in larder essential at times of privation when the body sustains itself and stays alive by consuming its own internal energy stores. Camels, evolved to survive in deserts, store body fat in humps. Humans, adapted to survive through severe winters and during epic migrations, store body fat elsewhere – as you know.

Babies, children and adults are all liable to become overweight and obese when they always have plenty of readily available food, especially when it is energy-dense. This is particularly so within sedentary populations, whose energy balance is unnaturally low. Children frugally fed when in the womb are most vulnerable to becoming obese whenfed artificial formula feeds and then energy-dense diets.

Historically, and until eight generations ago or fewer, food security, energy-dense food and drink, and sedentary ways of life, were unusual and very rarely found all together. But now they all are typical in many if not most parts of the world. In these circumstances, the very worst thing you can do is provoke the human drive to store excess fat by restricting dietary energy intake.

We are not adapted to plenty. We are adapted to famine. We are evolved to be slow to shed body fat, and quick to put on body fat. That's the fundamental reason why dieting makes you fat.

IS DIETING DANGEROUS?

But this is not the end of the story. Any cause of increased body fatness must, for this reason alone, be a cause of disorders or diseases the risks of which are increased by being fat. How serious is this? Also, dieting itself affects how our bodies work. Is this damaging?

Common sense suggests that isolated dieting is not a problem. When people reduce substantial amounts of their body weight and fat once or maybe even a few times in their lives, at any speed, and by any methods other than drugs or surgery, it seems unlikely that they will harm themselves – although as you will see below, this may well be an optimistic view. Occasional or even regular dietary restraint is in itself likely to be salutary. Indeed, I recommend fasting in chapter 6 as an enlightening discipline – but not as a way to reduce weight.

But people who restrict dietary energy often – maybe usually – do so regularly. They try one regime after another. This regular or even constant process of dieting is known as weight cycling, or 'yo-yo dieting'. The point at which dieting becomes weight cycling is a matter of judgement, but anybody who goes on diets regularly can be defined as a yo-yo dieter. In his 2002 review, Abdul Dulloo and his colleagues observed: 'A large section of the human population is predisposed to . . . accelerated fat recovery or catch-up fat. This includes . . . tens of millions of "yo-yo" dieters.' But apart from – or as well as – this, is weight cycling dangerous?

An official line

The National Institutes of Health, a federal US government agency, have a weight control information service, known as WIN. Their current official position on weight cycling is: 'Experts are not sure if weight cycling leads to health problems. However, some studies suggest a link to high blood pressure, high cholesterol, gallbladder disease, and other problems . . . Weight cycling may affect your mental health too.'

Is staying overweight healthier than weight cycling? 'That is a hard question to answer . . . However, experts are sure that if you are overweight, losing weight is a good thing.' For overweight and obese people, reducing 10 per cent of body weight is suggested: 'Try to eat a healthy diet and get plenty of physical activity.'

The first position on weight cycling made by the US National Institutes of Health was published in 1994. This was based on a review of studies, some of which showed associations between weight cycling and increased risk of various diseases and of death. It concluded: 'The currently available evidence is not sufficiently compelling to override the potential benefits of moderate weight loss . . . Obese individuals should not allow concerns about hazards of weight cycling to deter them from efforts to control their body weight.'

Both these position statements sound rather ominous. And no question, there are problems caused by weight cycling – the only serious debate is about their importance, extent and severity.

The feeling of failure

Nobody practices yo-yo dieting for fun. Every cycle admits that the previous regime failed. Continual futile attempts to reduce body weight and body fat on dieting regimes are depressing and make people feel they are failures. Most women, a sizeable proportion of men and now significant numbers of children in the USA, UK and other high-income countries find that dieting does not work. As a result, they are often left feeling that if they can't control their own weight, they can't trust themselves.

The conclusion? Weight cycling is a cause of depression, rates of which have greatly increased in many high-income countries in recent decades.

Craving and its consequences

Weight cycling deranges the natural senses of desire for food, and of appetite, hunger and satiety. Hunger is a primal drive, built into us to keep us alive. The compelling felt need for food after the end of a dieting regime is as powerful as the craving for tobacco or 'hard' recreational drugs – many people would say even more overwhelming. To say that weight cycling can cause appetite disorders misunderstands what typically happens after dieting has ended: this *is* an appetite disorder.

The sense of hunger, appetite and satiety is also liable to be disordered during the period of dietary energy restriction. Depending on its nature, quality and severity, dieters may feel fine. Or they may feel raging hunger liable to cause bingeing. Or they may lose all sense of hunger, which may lead to self-starvation. These also *are* appetite disorders, and put dieters at risk of anorexia 'nervosa' and bulimia – compulsive self-starvation, and gorging followed by vomiting, both now common, particularly among young women in many high-income countries.

The conclusion? Seen in this light, weight cycling is a cause – maybe the most common cause – of anorexia and bulimia. Indeed, the anorexia-bulimia syndrome can be seen as an extreme version of weight cycling.

Is weight cycling addictive?

This point is more conjectural. People who are heavy drinkers of alcohol, or smoke cigarettes, or use 'hard' recreational drugs, do not aim to get addicted. But that's the risk. After a time they are liable to find that they are hooked. Weight cycling can be seen as a comparable process. It can become a habit that is very hard to break. It does change the biochemistry of the body and its metabolic processes, as well as depressing mood and deranging appetite. This pathological process is similar to that of physical addiction.

The conclusion? The process by which weight cycling keeps your body in training to focus on staying alive during times of famine can be seen as addictive.

What happens to yo-yo animals?

The WIN statement mentions depression and appetite disorders, but its main focus is on chronic physical diseases. This is a controversial topic – probably more so than it should be, as you will see.

One line of evidence is from experiments on animals. As we know, rats are not people. But dogs and pigs as well as mice and rats, when subjected to the equivalent of yo-yo dieting, show yo-yo hypertension – their blood pressure overshoots.

Paul Ernsberger and Richard Koletsky of Western Case Reserve University in Cleveland, Ohio, and colleagues elsewhere, have carried out and also reviewed many animal studies. Their results, published in the *Journal of the American Medical Association* and elsewhere, also find that weight-cycled animals have enlarged hearts, higher levels of adrenalin, kidney damage, and more abdominal fat. Animals naturally liable to become fat when fed freely, become progressively fatter as a result of weight cycling, especially when this takes the form of fast weight reduction followed by slow weight increase. These results partly explain the cautionary tone of the WIN position.

What happens to yo-yo humans?

What about humans? A number of studies have shown that blood cholesterol as well as blood pressure overshoots in weight cyclers. For example, a US study published in 1989 found that large weight fluctuations in men were associated with higher blood pressure and blood cholesterol, and double the deaths from coronary heart disease. Another large study using US data published in 1991 found that women and men whose weight varied a lot were more likely to die from heart disease and also from all causes. The extra risk relative to people with stable weights was between 1.27 and 1.93, which averages out at 60 per cent additional risk of death. In the USA, a million people die from heart disease every year, and many millions of people in the USA are weight cyclers. More generally, the evidence suggests that weight cycling increases the risk of metabolic syndrome. This is the associated cluster of obesity, diabetes, high blood pressure and stroke, and deranged blood chemistry and heart disease.

Most studies of large populations evidently show that weight cycling is risky, but some have been criticized because of not allowing for the possibility that fluctuations of weight could be caused by illness. This was allowed for in a large study published in 2005. This divided a representative sample of the US population into five groups: stable non-obese, stable obese, people gaining weight, people losing weight, and people whose weight fluctuated, and adjusted (screened) for poor health and pre-existing disease. Its conclusion for both obese and non-obese people was: 'Weight fluctuation is associated with higher risk of all-cause and cardiovascular disease mortality in the US population.'

Association does not prove cause. But the biological reason why weight cycling increases the risk of death from heart disease is obvious. Our blood biochemistry is affected by what we consume. Typical industrialized diets are high in processed sugars, saturated fats and trans-fatty acids, mostly from processed foods. These all increase the types of fatty substances in the bloodstream that increase the risk of heart disease. The nature of adipose tissue (body fat) is also, naturally enough, affected by the nature of dietary fat. So when people who consume industrialized diets restrict their dietary energy, their unhealthy body fat floods back into the bloodstream again. There is evidence that heart attacks are provoked not so much by slow and gradual silting of the arterial walls, but by sudden rushes of such pathogenic blood fats. Given this, it would be odd if weight cycling did not increase deaths from heart attacks.

The WIN position is that 'experts need to learn more about weight cycling'. Paul Ernsberger says: 'Recognition of the hazards of repeated loss and regain of weight is a serious threat to the weight loss industry . . . as they depend on repeat business . . . If only persons who had never dieted before were encouraged to join weight loss programs, the industry would collapse overnight.'

The conclusion? Taken together, the evidence shows that dieting, in the form of weight cycling, is not only futile, but dangerous.

WHAT'S WRONG WITH BEING FAT

So far this book may seem to imply that it is bad to be fat. Is this so? Most people now would say 'yes'. The better answer as far as personal health is concerned is what most people probably would have said until recently: 'It depends'. Meaning that you may be fat and ill, or you may be fat and well. Much depends on your age, your attitude, how fat you are, and – crucially – not necessarily fatness itself, but the causes of fatness.

The definition of 'fat'

The senior classics master at my school, Derrick Macnutt, a man of vast intellect (he set the *Observer* 'Ximenes' crossword) was also a man of vast girth. We unfeeling boys used to stick pillows under our coats and mimic something he said about himself: 'I'm not fat. I'm comfortable.' We thought this was funny.

But what is 'fat'? Being fat is now usually equated with being overweight or obese, and these terms are defined – for adults, not for children – by using the body mass index (BMI) system which measures weight as a proxy for fatness. You can calculate your own BMI by dividing your weight in kilograms by the square of your height in metres. (If you use pounds and inches, the calculation is more complicated – see the notes to the Introduction.)

Take a person who weighs 75 kilograms (165 pounds) who is 1.70 metres (5ft 7in) tall. The BMI of this person is 75 (weight) divided by 2.89 (square of height), which is 25. The range of BMIs between 18.5 and 25 is defined as 'healthy' or 'acceptable'. BMIs between 25 and 30 are defined as 'overweight' or sometimes 'pre-obese', BMIs over 30 as 'obese', and over 40 as 'severely' or 'morbidly' obese. Anything under BMI 18.5 is 'underweight'. When you have a general health check-up, the professional you consult will probably calculate your BMI.

The good advice you hear from almost all sides now is to stay between BMI 18.5 and 25. The 1.70-metre-tall person would be underweight at 53.5 kilograms (118 pounds) and below, obese at 86 kilograms (189 pounds) and above, and severely obese at 100 kilograms (220 pounds) and above. For this person anything in the broad range above 53.5 and below 75 kilograms (115–165 pounds) is 'healthy' or 'acceptable'.

It is as certain as anything in biological science can be, that obese people are more likely to suffer from various serious chronic physical diseases. Obesity is itself now usually – but not always – identified as a disease, and as such suitable for treatment. This starts with attempted weight control usually by some form of dieting regime, or also exercise, or maybe drugs, if the physician is compliant or enthusiastic. Then, at BMIs of 35 or 40 and above, surgery is on offer.

Stopping being fat before it starts

So, what about being fat? The most effective approach is to stop overweight and obesity before it starts. At the beginning of life, a 'bonny bouncing' overweight baby fed cow's milk-based formula and then energy-dense food, who becomes a fat child, is pretty likely to become an overweight or obese adult. So for infants and children, what's best is exclusive breastfeeding for up to six months, lots of opportunities for and encouragement of physical activity, lots of fresh wholefoods and drinks, and avoidance of processed sugary, fatty, energy-dense diets. There is more on this in the next chapters.

How do you feel about being fat?

It is one thing to prevent fatness in the first place. It is quite another thing to control and to reduce body fatness when you are already overweight or obese. If you are fat and hate this, then being fat is a bad thing for you; but forget dieting. The right way to gain and maintain health and wellbeing, and also in due course to reduce body fat, is shown in chapter 6.

Fatness and health

Now for a topic that is the subject of furious debate. As you know, since the 1980s the incidence of overweight and obesity has greatly increased all over the world. Also, since around the mid-1990s it has become generally accepted that being fat causes a vast number of deaths every year. This position is now accepted by relevant United Nations agencies and many governments.

Thus in 2001 David Satcher, then US Surgeon-General, issued a Call to Action, stating: 'Overweight and obesity may soon cause as much preventable disease and death as cigarette smoking.' This position was backed by the findings of a 1999 study by the Centers for Disease Control and Prevention (CDC), a US government agency. This concluded that in the USA the annual number of adult deaths 'attributable to obesity' is around 300,000. This translates to around one in every eight deaths. Even bigger numbers, corresponding to one in every five deaths, have been published in leading US journals, have also been massively publicized, and are emphasized by commercial weight-loss organizations.

What is the basis of these claims? In the previous chapter I quoted the 2006 European Charter stating that 'more than one million deaths . . . annually are due to *diseases related to excess body weight*.' The key phrase I have put in italics. The assumption is that deaths from diseases usually, but not always, agreed to have obesity as a cause – rarely if ever the only cause – are caused by obesity. This is a big jump. Likewise, in their conclusion the US Surgeon-General and the CDC have assumed that deaths *with* obesity are deaths *from* obesity. This is not the same thing.

The obesity wars

Debates on fatness and physical health and disease have become known as 'the obesity wars'. There is overwhelming evidence that being fat, in the sense not only of being obese but also overweight as defined by the BMI method, is indeed risky. Sometimes even BMIs within the 'healthy' or 'acceptable' range are also identified as in themselves risky.

Targeting obesity – and also overweight – as the biggest cause with smoking of premature death implies that fatness itself must be treated, and accepting that fatness (obesity and even overweight) is itself a major cause of heart disease, various cancers, and other serious diseases, then it sounds like good sense to reduce weight – if this can be done. This argues for surgery, drugs, and also energy-restrictive dieting regimes – if they work, which as you now know, as a rule they do not.

This approach is medical or quasi-medical. Treating obesity, and also overweight, keeps the wheels of commerce turning. This is good for the pharmaceutical industry, the medical profession, the research community, and the dieting industry. It distracts attention away from the basic causes of serious diseases and of fatness, and so makes life easier for politicians and the food manufacturing industry. It stops tough questions being asked and tough actions being taken that would involve economic, social and environmental reform, and new thinking about what being healthy really means.

That's on the one side. On the other side, a number of academics specializing in nutrition, physiology and other disciplines, and also some non-academic writers, have a different view. They say that the official edifice agreed by United Nations agencies and national governments, and organizations in the dieting business, has no sound foundation. They say that fatness is a sign or symptom rather than a cause of chronic diseases. They are not impressed by the evidence that overweight, and even obesity below BMI in the mid-30s, is itself a major direct cause of chronic diseases or of death. They point to evidence that from later middle age, moderate obesity may prolong life.

They are not isolated contrarians. In 1998 the *New England Journal of Medicine* published an editorial stating: 'The data linking overweight and death, as well as the data showing the beneficial effects of weight loss, are limited, fragmentary, and often ambiguous.' Further, estimates of deaths a year caused by obesity are 'derived from weak or incomplete data'.

The true crisis

So what's the answer? This is a crucial issue, for international and national governments, industry, the health professions, schools and other institutions, civil society organizations, the media – and no doubt for you or your family or friends. If you are fat, and don't want to be fat, what should you do, right now?

Those who say that obesity is safe are wrong, and if they persuade obese people not to be concerned, they have done wrong. That said, the true global public health crisis here, which affects your country, your community, and very likely your family, is premature suffering and death from disabling and deadly diseases such as diabetes, heart disease and various cancers. All of these physical diseases have causes that are in common with the causes of overweight and obesity.

What this means is that the right approach is to focus on these causes rather than to treat overweight and obesity in isolation. And even if fatness in itself is a major cause of these diseases, the expense and risks of drugs and surgery, and the general futility of dieting regimes, also show that the right way is to work towards eliminating the causes of fatness.

This approach involves the family and the community. It puts fatness into its general biological and also economic, social and environmental context. It needs time and care and love rather than money, is safe, and if followed should be effective.

The common-sense view

So much depends on why people are fat. Diseased processes within the bodies of fat people are generally not so much a function of body fat itself, as of what is making them fat. Would you say that an inactive overweight person whose diet is mostly snacks of highly processed food is likely to be as healthy, happy and protected against disease as a physically fit overweight person whose high level of energy balance comes from regularly consuming meals of whole fresh food? I would not. Such an idea makes no sense.

The same point applies the other way round. Take a sedentary woman whose continual weight cycling has devastated her lean tissue, who is in energy balance maybe at 1,500 calories (about 6,300 kilojoules) a day or fewer, and who is flabby and shapeless while being light in weight with a BMI below 25. Would you say that she is likely to be better nourished, healthier, and better protected against disease than a considerably heavier woman who walks a lot, enjoys her food, has either never dieted or has stopped dieting, who is in energy balance maybe at 2,250 calories (9,400 kilojoules) a day or more, whose BMI is a few points higher, and somewhat above 25? I think you would not. This also makes no sense.

Women all over the world – and men too – are now assailed with advice on weight control, and are pushed to reduce weight. Good advice for fat people is to forget energy-restrictive dieting regimes, which as you now know are risky as well as counterproductive. Instead, they can enhance their lives by becoming a lot more physically active, and in this way raise the level of their energy balance while eating delicious high-quality meals. Authoritative recommendations are given in the 2007 World Cancer Research Fund/American Institute for Cancer Research report, referenced in the notes to this chapter. If they want, they can also eventually reduce a substantial amount of body fat, and some weight too. This may mean you.

The bottom line here is that there is nothing necessarily wrong with being fat. If you are a bit overweight while not being obese, are physically active, eat well, like the way you are, feel fine, and have no symptoms of disease, then enjoy yourself the way you are. If you prefer to reduce your body fat – and there are very good reasons to do so, to prevent serious diseases and enhance your wellbeing – turn to chapter 6.

PART 2
CONSCIOUS WELLBEING

The word 'health' in English is based on an Anglo-Saxon word 'hale' meaning 'whole'; that is, to be healthy is to be whole . . . Likewise, the English 'holy' is based on the same root as 'whole'. All of this indicates that humans have sensed always that wholeness or integrity is an absolute necessity to make life worth living.

David Bohm

Food is . . . crucial . . . for the whole problem of the pollution and exhaustion of our environment, with the danger that man may make this planet uninhabitable within a short century or so. If food is grown in strict relationship to the needs of those who will eat it, if every effort is made to reduce the costs of transportation, to improve storage, to conserve the land, and there, where it is needed, by recycling wastes and water, we will go a long way toward solving many of our environmental problems also.

Margaret Mead

4. EVERYTHING ELSE THAT MAKES YOU FAT

Fast food has joined Hollywood movies, blue jeans, and pop music as one of America's most prominent cultural exports. Unlike other commodities, however, food isn't viewed, read, played, or worn. It enters the body and becomes part of the consumer . . . By eating like Americans, people all over the world are beginning to look more like Americans.

Eric Schlosser

Epidemics are great warning signs against which the progress of civilizations can be judged.

Rudolf Virchow

It is not just dieting that makes you fat, of course. There are four types of reason driving our choices, with roots in human evolution, history and ideology. These basic causes are biological, economic, social, and environmental.

Usually it is not food that makes us fat, but what is done to food, in its production, preservation, processing, and promotion. Obesity makes money. There is no big official, commercial, or medical business interest in wellbeing.

Dieting is a mistake. So what is the right thing to do? This depends what you want, for yourself, for the people in your life, and for the future. A theme of the second part of this book is that enjoyment of good food and drink, meals and feasts, is a central part of well-led, convivial and rewarding personal and social lives. Getting out of the dieting trap and on the path to an active and truly healthy way of life will make you feel and look better. Being able – maybe for the first time in your adult life – to eat and drink all you like, without ever again worrying about your weight, may be a vital freedom. This will also be one part of your general fulfilment as a human being.

Food is not and never has been just a matter of what people purchase and consume. The quality of food systems, which begin with growers and farmers near us and also all over the world, affects our physical health. But that's not all. Conscious wellbeing involves living in the right relationship with the people in our lives, with society in general, and with the living and physical world.

In this 21st century we know that our food choices affect the way other people live. They also affect the way in which animals live, and have an impact on natural resources such as soil, water, energy, and climate. Conscious wellbeing begins with what we habitually put into our mouths in order to sustain ourselves. Much follows from these acts.

The previous chapters focus on the immediate reasons for weight increase, overweight, and obesity, and explain why dieting is a trap. But these are only one part of the story. This chapter outlines the reasons why more and more people became fat in Europe, the USA and other materially rich countries after industrialization, and then why rates of obesity have increased very rapidly all over the world since the 1980s. You need to see this big picture in order to make the right decisions in your own life: for yourself, your family, and for everybody touched by your choices.

THE MEDICAL MODEL

So what – apart from dieting – makes you fat? Like priests who cast bones and read runes, when specialist scientists are asked questions like this they tend to give enigmatic answers. Papers in journals that publish academic research use phrases like 'obesity is a pathology of complex multi-factorial aetiology and multi-disciplinary nature', and may add that more research is needed. Such statements are also sometimes used in accounts of obesity for the general reader. You can read many meanings into them. They don't amount to much more than 'aha!' or 'we don't know' or 'wait and see'.

There are as many technical accounts of obesity as there are relevant or interested professional disciplines. When physicians and other medical professionals who think of us mainly in terms of our physiology, biochemistry or pathology are asked what causes obesity, they will say something like this: 'The human body is nourished with energy from foods and drinks, which is used for the body's natural processes when awake and asleep, and for physical activity. Balance is achieved when energy input equals energy output over time. People decrease in weight if they take in less energy than they use, and increase in weight if they take in more energy than they use. Excess energy is mostly stored as body fat. It follows that an excess of energy input over energy output will, over time, lead to increase in body weight and fat, and eventually to obesity. The speed of this process largely depends on the degree of excess energy input.'

Well, yes indeed. You can find statements like this in any textbook or report on obesity. They are accurate, but describe rather than explain. They are based on the medical model, which positions people as individual patients or clients. They isolate us, almost as if we are laboratory animals. They respond to questions of 'what?' and 'how?' but not to 'why?' or 'when?' They refer to the immediate physical cause of obesity. But inasmuch as they imply that dietary energy restriction is suitable treatment for overweight and obesity – the advice usually given by physicians – they are not much help. (There is more on the medical model, in the notes to this chapter.)

In a case of murder a jury would not be impressed by expert testimony that death was caused by the bullet penetrating the brain. Detached statements like this are objective but unhelpful. What judges and juries want to know are the answers to other types of question, such as who bought the gun, who fired it, and why. These are the most relevant and important types of question to ask, in order to find out what makes you fat.

IT'S NOT ALL IN THE GENES

So what are the significant causes of obesity? High-powered and well-resourced research scientists are now most interested in one biological cause: genes. This is where the big research money is and the drug bonanzas are. Media stories with headlines like 'obesity – new breakthrough' are usually reporting the claim of some research team that some 'obesity gene' has been identified. Thus in April 2007 front-page news in the UK was 'Scientists find the gene that makes you fat'. This was about 'the discovery of an "alphabet soup" of genes that influence obesity'. In January 2008 another headline was 'Gene map will lift lid on diseases'. This heralded the $US50 million '1,000 genes project', designed to 'allow scientists to pinpoint the genetic causes of common disorders swiftly and help tailor medical treatment to individual patients'. That's to say, if such claims stand up, patented drugs can then be formulated, designed to zero in on the gene, maybe with the researchers and their institutions cut in on the action.

Once approved by regulatory authorities, the drugs will be promoted to physicians to prescribe to fat individuals with lots of disposable income or with unusually comprehensive health insurance, as well as to desperate people without much money. Some research scientists foresee the possibility of genetic modification of infants to stop them getting fat. The genetic approach to obesity attracts scientists and industry and is also valued by governments, whose tasks include the promotion of science, business and trade. Any such procedures are unlikely to be available in my or your lifetime, and are likely to be risky.

REASONS WHY WE GET FAT

In any case, genetics does not explain why throughout history obesity has been generally rare except in materially rich people, why it becomes more common with industrialization and urbanization, and why since around 1980 global rates of overweight and obesity have accelerated. As said in a 2000 World Health Organization (WHO) report on obesity: 'The rapid increases in obesity rates in recent years have occurred in too short a time for there to have been any significant genetic changes within populations.'

Humans now are not genetically different from humans in 1980 or 1950, or for that matter 1800. We are all born different in some ways, more or less protected against and more or less vulnerable to all sorts of disorders and diseases. Some people are more likely to become fat than others. Fatness does indeed 'run in families'. But susceptibility is not inevitablity. The effective causes of obesity are those that trigger our susceptibility to increase in weight or, as the WHO obesity report says, 'have overwhelmed the physiological regulatory processes that operate to keep weight stable'.

In this chapter, four types of cause are identified, all of which have historical origins. These are biological, and in particular how we are evolved and adapted as humans; economic, including prices and food industry practices; social, including access to food and also the impact of official policies and practices; and environmental, including the state of the built, living, and physical world.

The Long Island revelation

Experience of different countries, even just on visits, can be illuminating. I was impressed in the mid-1970s by what was for me as an Englishman the exotic culture of US suburbia when I stayed for a while with a family living on Long Island in the state of New York. While I had visited the USA a number of times previously, these were quick visits to mid-town New York City and down-town San Francisco, cosmopolitan enclaves that in some ways have more in common with Left Bank Paris and West End London than with the country as a whole.

The everyday contrasts with life in Britain as I knew it amazed me. The Long Island way of life felt to me more like science fiction. Supermarkets were vast and stocked hundreds of packaged ready-to-eat and ready-to-heat dishes bought and piled in vast home freezers and refrigerators. There were television sets in the eating area and bedrooms. Everybody drove everywhere on roads often without sidewalks. The father of the house was putting on weight and was close to obese, but he didn't know why; he didn't connect what was happening to him with the nature of his world, or with his night-time raids on quart tubs of fudge sundae ice creams. He played golf at the local country club where his Cadillac was valet-parked, and he drove a cart from clubhouse to tee to hole to tee. He asked my advice – I was in a slim phase at the time – and said that a lot of his colleagues and neighbours had a 'weight problem'. Apart from suggesting that he emigrate I didn't know what to say, so I changed the subject.

This was a glimpse of international things to come. Such ways of life, then uncommon outside the USA, have now become usual in Britain and in many other high-income countries, where rates of overweight and obesity have increased three- or fourfold since the 1980s.

Brazilian cellos and double basses

In middle-income countries ways of life have now also changed. Physically active people who eat to live are lean. But the homes of prosperous middle-class Brazilians now have garages with two or more cars, kitchens with more than one refrigerator, and several television sets – some turned on much of the time.

In the 2000s, upper-middle-class suburban Brazilian ways of life have a lot in common with those of suburban Long Island in the 1970s. As reported in chapter 2, there are now a lot of fat people in Brazil. For Brazilians the ideal female shape as seen in the magazines is that of a violin. But the streets and beaches now also include a lot of cellos and some double basses.

What the experts say

We can all think of reasons why people get fat. Children get rewarded for good behaviour with chocolate, ice cream, candies, and other fatty or sugary foods. Many young people rarely eat home-prepared meals, because their parents work and rely on convenience food such as pre-prepared supermarket dishes. Office workers may buy lunch at shops and bars selling fast food and snacks, not having found alternatives. Parents may want their children to play active games out of doors, but may feel that the streets are unsafe, and so keep them indoors where they watch television or play video games.

What do the experts say? The 2000 World Health Organization obesity report mentions big international economic issues such as structural readjustment and economic globalization, official subsidies for and dumping of fatty and other energy-dense food, and a series of related industry practices such as concentration within the food industry, and increased production and promotion of cheap foods, fatty or sugary convenience foods and fast foods, energy-dense foods, large food-portion sizes, and sugared drinks. Social factors mentioned include inadequate government regulation of food, and the selling of school and other sports and recreation grounds. (For more on fast, convenience and junk foods, see the notes to this chapter.)

The WHO report also lists 'possible strategies'. These include family approaches like limitation of children's television viewing time, economic policies like subsidies for growers of vegetables and fruits, social strategies like improved food labelling, restriction of food advertising to children, and environmental practices like city and building design that emphasizes pedestrian precincts, cycle paths and stairs, and reclaiming of land in cities to grow vegetables.

Contributors to the UK government Foresight report on obesity published in late 2007 also identify what they believe to be some economic and social causes. These include the IBM personal computer introduced in 1981; daytime television, which began in the UK in 1986; the drop as from the 1980s in the relative price of food; and more chilled ready-to-heat meals in supermarkets and correspondingly more home freezers and microwave ovens.

The 2007 World Cancer Research Fund/American Institute for Cancer Research report on prevention of cancer includes a chapter on personal causes of weight increase, overweight and obesity. Those emphasized are sedentary living, consumption of energy-dense foods, sugary drinks and fast foods, and television viewing. Protective factors are identified as regular physical activity, consumption of foods low in energy density, and being breastfed. One recommendation is: 'Avoid weight gain and increases in waist circumference throughout adulthood.' Another is: 'Consume "fast foods" sparingly, if at all.'

IN DEFENCE OF INDUSTRY

Now for an interjection. If you are getting the impression that this book is hostile to industry in general, or to food science, technology and processing, or to food manufacturers, distributors, retailers and caterers as such, I am misleading you. While all sectors of industry are responsible for their policies and actions, and should expect to be held to account in the public interest, the notion that 'the food industry' has malicious intentions is absurd.

The food industry as a whole includes family and community farmers and growers all over the world. Assuming a narrower definition, of highly capitalized businesses, the networks of industries directly and indirectly responsible for global and national food systems generally do not operate like the tobacco industry. It is specific sectors of the big food and drink and allied industries, albeit very resourceful and powerful, whose products tend to make you fat and to increase your risk of various diseases; and only some of these actively seek to conceal or subvert reliable evidence on hard fats, say, or sugar, or convenience and fast food.

Technology has been used to modify food since the first deliberate use of fire. The food industry as a whole continues to ensure security of food supplies in most parts of the world. Just as correct responses to climate change now need collaboration with and indeed leadership from the energy industry, leaders in the food and drink industry must now become partners in the necessary shift to healthy global, national and local food and drink supplies. Some big manufacturers, caterers and retailers are now beginning to respond to the issues set out below and in the next chapter. All this needs to be said.

BASIC REASONS WHY WE GET FAT

The stories, analyses and recommendations mentioned so far point the same way. You may think you have a lot of freedom of personal choice. Compared with most people in the world you probably do. People as individuals and as family and community members are getting fat because they have become more sedentary and are consuming more energy-dense foods and drinks. But the economic, social and environmental circumstances of our lives influence and constrain our choices. So does history. So do prevailing beliefs. So has the technology that shapes the food systems that generate food supplies – what's in the shops.

The general increase in overweight and obesity since food systems have become industrialized has one fundamental cause. This is our biological built-in desire for sugar and fat, together with its commercial exploitation by food manufacturers. There are three other associated and inter-related economic and social causes. These are the chemicalization of food, the degradation of food, and malign food processes.

These factors drive patterns of food supply and consumption that are altogether different from those with which humans evolved, and to which we are not adapted. Some of these tend to be neglected in expert and popular accounts of obesity. Why, is indicated by the naturalist E B Ford, who says, 'evolution is the key-note of biological study and research', and who goes on to say: 'The historical setting of a subject has a value which, so it seems to me, is somewhat underestimated, at least in science.'

HUNGER FOR SUGAR AND FAT

We who live now have not escaped our identity. Who we are and what we do is influenced by our evolution and adaptation, in the long period of the development of *Homo sapiens* when people were usually active all their lives and probably rarely survived after their children were self-supporting.

In the previous chapter I explained why we are – as the phrase is – hard-wired to protect and conserve body fat. It is our evolution that explains why dieting makes you fat. In common with animals, we humans are also evolved to seek out sugar and fat. As the 2000 World Health Organization report on obesity says: 'Inherent demand for sugary, salty and fatty foods . . . seems to stem from the evolutionary need to benefit from small amounts of these formerly scarce resources.'

We desire sweetness because this taste tells us that fruits and other plant foods are ripe and safe to eat. Fruits are evolved to become sweet so that birds and animals – and humans – will eat them and then excrete and propagate their seeds. In nature wild honey is raided by humans – and apes and bears – despite the fury of the bees. For thousands of years fruits have been dried to preserve them and concentrate their sugars. Ancient writing is a witness. The Song of Solomon, the Old Testament erotic poem, compares the body of the beloved to dates, figs, and sweetness. People now may call their partners 'honey', 'sugar', 'sweetie', and so on.

We desire succulence because fat is the most concentrated source of energy, readily stored as body fat. In all societies whose supplies of food are insecure and unpredictable, people are literally insulated against hard times by their hunger for fat that is consumed in easy times and stored as body fat. For people without access to processed food – and for carnivorous animals – gorging on the fattier parts of animals is the most efficient way to lay down personal fat stores. The Bible's New Testament says that the return of the prodigal son was celebrated by the killing of a fatted calf.

When food is insecure or scarce, seeking out sweetness and succulence protects against deficiency of dietary energy and specific nutrients, as well as infections. It also encourages mutually useful relationships between humans and the rest of the living world.

These desires are the basic biological reason why, given an abundant supply, humans have an appetite – including when we are not hungry – for food or drink that is sugary and fatty. As soon as food systems became industrialized, and sugar and fat became cheap, manufacturers inevitably devised and developed more and more sugary, fatty, processed foods and drink, and say quite correctly that they are responding to what consumers want. So do restaurateurs and caterers. So for that matter do parents, confronted with what children demand. Hard-wired human appetites make sugary and fatty products more attractive and more profitable.

Sweet nothings

Sugar was traded internationally centuries before food systems became industrialized. Sugar is a wonderful commodity. It is uniform, stable, compact, does not rot, and packs and travels well: it is as close as anything edible can be to metal. It has been the foundation of many mansions in the Americas, and a fuel for the 'industrial revolution' and the British Empire.

As derived from cane, and originally cheapened because grown, cut, crushed and processed by slaves, sugar – also derived from beet, and now as high-fructose syrup from corn – has been the most profitable legal edible mass cash crop for centuries. It is also a preservative and 'bulking aid', and makes fat palatable in very many energy-dense processed foods and drinks.

When 'refined', sugar is a source of energy but no nutrients, and so is sometimes called 'empty calories'. Britain was the first country to have a 'sweet tooth', induced by mass importation of increasingly cheap sugar and mass-produced sweetened foods and drinks. In the early 19th century, the relatively active population of Britain on average consumed around 5–10 kilograms (around 10–20 pounds) per head of 'refined' sugars a year, mostly added in home cooking and at the table. World sugar production increased from around 8 million tonnes in 1900 to about 50 million tonnes in 1950. Writing in the mid-1970s, Wallace Aykroyd, former head of nutrition at the Food and Agriculture Organization of the United Nations, observed of sugar: 'No other human food has shown an increase in production of this order.'

By the mid-20th century, sugar in the form of sucrose supplied annually to the increasingly sedentary populations of the USA, Britain, and other industrialized countries amounted to around 45–50 kilograms (around 100–110 pounds) a head. In around six generations, sugar consumption in these countries increased between five- and tenfold, from around 2–4 per cent to around 15–20 per cent of total dietary energy, which is reckoned by industry to be about the saturation point for any country. In 2008 world sugar production is projected at 157 million tonnes. Given that about a tenth is wasted, this amounts to an average for everybody on earth of around 22 kilograms or just under 50 pounds a year. This roughly corresponds to a consumption of 450 grams (a pound) every week.

Big differences between the mid-20th century and now are the increase of sugars added to processed foods and drinks, and the use of US-government subsidized high-fructose syrups, especially in cola and other soft drinks. The strategic goal of Big Sugar – the associated transnational and national companies whose products depend on sugar, as well as sugar 'refiners' – is to achieve world production and consumption of sugars at the current levels of fully industrialized countries.

Hard facts

Animals have been domesticated to supply milk, cheese, butter and other dairy products, and fattened to produce succulent meat, for thousands of years. Animal husbandry, together with the growing and breeding of cereals (grains), characterize peasant agriculture and enable people to live in towns and cities, where they become dependent on food and drink brought in from outside. Traditional diets of societies all over the world are usually plant-based, with relatively small amounts of animal products, and substantial amounts of meat eaten only occasionally. Chronic overweight and obesity is rare except among rich people, and those who are inactive because they are infirm or elderly. With some exceptions, fats and oils traditionally have on average supplied around 15-20 per cent of total dietary energy.

In Europe, the USA and their dependent and associated countries, these dietary patterns were replaced from the mid-19th century onwards. Meat became an everyday food as a result of the raising of cattle and sheep in the wide-opened spaces of the USA, Argentina and Australia, and development of technology including the mechanization of slaughter, refrigerated train and ship containers, and faster processing techniques. In countries with dairy surpluses, milk from cows became identified as an ideal food, especially for children. The hydrogenation process made hard 'brick' margarine a mass product, and also enabled industry to transform all edible soft fats and liquid oils into uniform 'purified' hard fats. These are now used, often together with sugars, as a main ingredient of many if not most lead line products on sale in supermarkets.

Within industrialized countries, the supply of fats and oils roughly doubles, up to around 35-40 per cent of total dietary energy. Overall around half and often more of the energy consumed by sedentary people in these countries comes from sugars and fats. As food supplies become industrialized, their sugar content increases to and beyond 15 per cent of total energy and their fat content increases to and beyond 35 per cent of total energy.

Physically active populations whose sugars mostly come from fruits and other naturally sweet foods, and whose dietary fat comes mostly from free-ranging and wild animals, birds and fish, dairy products, and relatively unrefined oils, rarely become overweight. The issue is not sugar and fat as such, it is added sugars and fats. These, in the amounts contained in industrialized food supplies – now mostly in the form of energy-dense processed foods and drinks – make you fat. The problem is in the processing.

Desire for sweetness and succulence is not just a matter of personal taste and choice that can be changed at will, with suitable information and education. If we think this we are mistaken. The desires are fundamental. They are a reason why our species has survived. They are hard-wired into us.

THE CHEMICALIZATION OF FOOD

We also have not escaped our history. Since the mid-19th century, food has been identified with its chemical constituents, in reference books, expert reports, popular accounts, and on processed food and drink labels. The chemicalization of food enables products to be formulated from cheap, attractive natural and artificial ingredients.

Rocket fuel

Parents worry about processed foods and drinks whose main ingredient is added sugar. Kids love them. As just one example, sweetened cocoa drinks are popular. The label of an international leading line, a hot seller in Brazilian supermarkets, says it is rich in vitamins and is a source of calcium and iron. The ingredients list sugar, cocoa powder, maltodextrin, minerals and vitamins, and innocuous preservatives. The nutrition label lists calcium and iron, magnesium, and thiamin, riboflavin, niacin, vitamin B_6, vitamin B_{12}, pantothenate, and biotin. The labels do not say how much sugar the product contains, but in every 20-gram serving there are 17 grams of carbohydrate. It tastes like cocoa-flavoured sugar. My taste buds tell me that it's more than 80 per cent sugar. A 400-gram (14-ounce) tin retails at the equivalent of a bit over $US2 or £1. The tin, useful for storing small toys, may cost the manufacturer as much as its contents.

Sugar flavoured with cocoa is essentially no different from hundreds of other products made by national and transnational companies. These are all rocket fuels, in the form of sugar plus other ingredients. They are sold as 'fortified' breakfast cereals, biscuits, 'energy bars', sweetened yoghurts, and many other products, as well as sweetened drinks marketed as if they are yummy vitamin and mineral pills. (See also the note to this chapter on glycaemic indices.)

Look at the labels

An expert committee reporting to the British prime minister in the early 1980s stated: 'The ability to fractionate and recombine food components will create more opportunity for the fashioning of food products in novel ways.' So it has proved. Look at the ingredients and nutrition labels of processed foods. Many if not most of these are made out of 'macronutrients' – fats, carbohydrates, and proteins – stripped out of foods, 'purified', 'refined', and 'modified' into uniform raw material using techniques such as hydrogenation and hydrolysation.

They are then put together again with bits of foods such as nuts, seeds and herbs, often 'fortified' with analogues of micronutrients, and made more attractive with cosmetic chemical additives – colours and flavours – and other chemicals such as stabilizers, firming agents, aerating agents, anti-caking agents, bulking aids, texture improvers, thickeners, thinners, binders, buffers. They also contain water, which may be declared, and air, which is not declared. These are not foods as celebrated in song and commemorated in culture and cuisine and everyday meals. They are edible chemistry sets.

Addictive additives?

A pizza parlour in Washington DC advertises its products with a charming notice: 'Warning: may cause cravings.' As many parents know, and as you may know for yourself, cravings for types or specific brands of food and drink are no joke. Some of these are or may be addictive, alcoholic drinks being an obvious example. For many years I depended on coffee. Quitting was as difficult as stopping smoking, and the physical effects of withdrawal, including throbbing headaches and 'the shakes', made me feel worse than when I was kicking my nicotine habit.

Is craving – even to the point of addiction – a reason why some energy-dense processed products make you fat? The sugar industry does not like to hear that processed sugars as contained in some sweet products can be addictive, but the impact of sugary foods and drinks on the blood chemistry of vulnerable people is well known. What about additives? Could some of these, individually, or as part of a chemical 'cocktail', or in combination with other ingredients, have an addictive effect?

Consider this. Competition between manufacturers of sugary or fatty energy-dense convenience and fast foods, snacks, and drinks, is intense. The race is always on to formulate new products that more consumers most want to go on and on buying, eating or drinking. Food engineers and technicians hired by manufacturers have great scope to combine and permute attractive chemicals.

When people crave a food or drink product, and feel bad if they can't consume it, and go out of their way to buy and consume it, and talk in terms of 'hit' and 'rush' and not being able to stop consuming it, that's more than ordinary desire. Can chemical additives have such an effect? We don't know. Experiments that test for toxicity of additives focus mostly on cancer and other diseases, rather than on the eating patterns of rats and other laboratory animals. Very many flavours and fragrances added to processed foods are not declared on the label. Of course responsible food manufacturers do not want consumers to become addicted to their products, and would not market any product they believed was addictive. But intention is one thing and effect is another. There may never be 'hard' evidence that any combination or permutation of chemicals in any sugary or fatty processed foods and drinks cause cravings, let alone addiction.

Where did the sugar go?

The identification of food with its chemical constituents is evident on all nutrition labels of processed products. Take a look. These usually list amounts of protein, carbohydrate, fat, saturated fat, dietary fibre, and maybe some vitamins and minerals, contained in the products. It is practically impossible to make sense or use of most of the information about food on nutrition labels.

Here is one example: carbohydrates. The Atkins Diet and other dieting regimes are based on the idea that carbohydrates make you fat. As indicated in chapter 2, Robert Atkins later sort-of retracted this idea in favour of saying that processed products high in 'refined' starches and sugars make you fat.

Carbohydrates – like fats and ethanol (alcohol) – are combinations of oxygen, carbon and hydrogen, hence their name. They were identified as such in the 1820s. Chemically all carbohydrates are similar, but biochemically they are different. What fresh foods high in carbohydrates – like wholegrain cereals, pulses (legumes), starchy roots and tubers, and fruits – do to you is different from the effect of starches and sugars stripped out of these foods and combined as main ingredients of processed foods. The notion that carbohydrates as such make you fat or are harmful to human health in any other way is nonsense.

Why are carbohydrates listed on nutrition labels? This is useless information. Manufacturers are not obliged to state what proportions of the carbohydrates in their products are from starch and what from sugars, unless they choose to make associated health claims. So they don't. This is because companies whose profits and share prices depend on adding sugars to their products have combined their forces, and made sure in their dealings with regulators that the volume of added sugars in processed foods and drinks generally remains a mystery.

Human humvees

The most audacious and catastrophic example of food chemicalization is artificial milk formulated for babies. In the mid-19th century enthusiastic food chemists invented feeds they claimed to be improvements on human milk. Then, with more prudent formulations, Henri Nestlé of Vevey in Switzerland founded the fortune of what is now the biggest food manufacturer in the world.

The key chemical constituent in formula feeds was and is protein. Cow's milk contains over three times as much protein as human milk. Protein pushes growth. Babies are evolved to grow slowly, calves to grow fast. The reasons to promote artificial formulas and condensed, dried and fresh cows' milk for babies and young children as from the late 19th century were both social and economic. European governments and industry wanted to raise big strong generations of young people. Formula feeds gave them this opportunity. Those who wanted to make money had an interest in replacing breastmilk with priced products, and those who sought power wanted a strapping working class to endure work in factories and to fight land wars. Scientists and philanthropists supported these reasons of state and business.

Thus was born the paediatric principle that accelerated growth in early life is the measure of good child health, and thus was bred the 'bonny bouncing baby', meaning the overweight and even obese baby. This view persisted. In 1985 the World Health Organization published guidelines for optimum infant and young child growth and health. These were based on measurements mostly made between 1960 and 1975 of the average increase in heights and weights of children of middle-class parents in the USA, almost all of whom were fed artificial formula feeds.

These guidelines, which show how to make babies all over the world the same size and shape as formula-fed babies born in the USA, were the official measure of infant and young child growth and health by governments and by health professionals at national, regional, municipal and local levels throughout the world, until they were finally replaced in 2006. When the growth of babies has not matched that of babies in the USA fed obsolete formulations of artificial milk, mothers have been told that their babies are 'failing to thrive' and advised to switch to artificial formulas. According to the US Institute of Medicine, in 2006 around one in ten babies in the USA were obese.

The new United Nations standards are based on studies of exclusively breastfed babies and young children. They are part of a new global strategy approved by all member states. This includes the recommendation that infants and young children be exclusively breastfed for six months. The standards confirm that the natural rates of human growth are slow. What are now the agreed UN energy requirements for breastfed babies up to 3 months are 17 per cent less than for formula-fed babies, and 20 per cent less between 3 and 9 months. These are big differences.

Formula feeding causes overweight and obesity early in life, probably because this breaks the bond between mother and child and confuses the child's natural sense of satiety. Also the nature of breast-milk changes during feeding, which may prompt breastfed babies to feel satisfied towards the end of the feed. Artificial baby feeds followed by energy-dense diets have bred human humvees. (There is more on the new global strategy on infant and young child feeding in the next chapter.)

THE DEGRADATION OF FOOD

Various techniques to preserve food and to extend its 'shelf life' were developed on an industrial scale between the 19th and the early 20th century. Some, like bottling, canning, and refrigeration, have made seasonal and other perishable food more available, and do not in themselves greatly affect its quality. Other techniques such as the mass 'refining' of wheat grain to make white flour that is used to make bread and baked goods, degrade food and make it less satisfying. Industrial meat and poultry production make meat fattier and more energy-dense, and deplete it of those fats which, like vitamins, are essential for health and life itself.

Store food

Store food stores well. In the 19th century it was the main stock of shops in the rapidly expanding cities of Britain, the USA and associated and dependent countries, and in frontier general stores, and it is still stocked in small shops and supermarkets. Store food includes dried foods like grains and beans, drinks like tea and coffee, tinned and often concentrated products such as condensed milk, and white flour, 'refined' sugar, hard fats, salt, smoked, pickled or salted meats and other animal products, baked goods like biscuits and candies, and liquor.

Other than what is dried, most store food is degraded. The most nourishing food is perishable; it decays or becomes rancid. Good food goes bad. Perishable nutrients in long shelf-life products are usually depleted or destroyed. This is why store food has a long 'shelf-life'.

At first in Britain, 'company stores' were set up by factory owners who paid employees partly in coupons redeemable for food only at these stores. Factory conditions made it impossible for mothers to breastfeed their babies. Much of the working-class population suffered deficiency diseases. Multiple-deficiency states and also obesity are now common among populations, communities and families who subsist on old-fashioned types of store food. These include native peoples throughout the Americas, the Australian aboriginal people, and Pacific islanders.

Impoverished people in rural as well as urban areas all over the world may rely on modern types of store food, which now also includes dried pasta and noodles, sugared soft drinks, ultra-heat treated (UHT) milk and its products, together with many branded biscuits and cakes, other baked goods, chocolate and confectionery. These supply 'cheap calories' to people who remain short of nourishment, while often consuming more than enough energy from such sugary, fatty and degraded products. In middle- and low-income countries, deficiency states and obesity co-exist within the same communities and families – and even within the same individuals.

Distressful bread

White bread and confections such as cakes and pastries made with white wheaten flour were luxuries until the second half of the 19th century. Until then the common bread was coarse or wholegrain, made from wheat or rye, and bread was practically unknown where cereals such as rice, corn or oats, or roots or tubers were the staple crops. As from the 1870s steel roller mills replaced traditional milling of wheat, efficiently separating the bran and the germ of the whole grain and making flour from the endosperm, the part of the grain that supplies energy in the form of starch.

White flour and white bread were preferred by the milling and baking industry because the essential fats in the germ of wholegrains become rancid. Stripped of germ, flour and bread has a longer shelf life. Also, bran and germ have separate markets, as animal feed, and as a human nutrition supplement and health food. Dorothy L Sayers, who once worked in an advertising agency, explains in her 1933 detective novel *Murder Must Advertise*. 'By forcing the damn-fool public to pay twice over, once to have its food emasculated and once to have the vitality put back again, we keep the wheels of commerce turning, and give employment to thousands – including you and me.'

Like processed sugars, processed starchy foods are unsatisfying: they lack the natural bulk of the whole food, and also are assimilated unaturally fast. What gives you the buzz also makes you fat. Minerals and vitamins in whole grain are also depleted in the 'refining' of white flour. White bread is usually 'enriched' with versions of a few of these nutrients. This degradation is insignificant for active populations and people whose diets are generally nutritious and who don't eat much white bread. It is a different story for sedentary people who consume a lot of degraded food including white bread.

Abused animals

Production and thus consumption of red meat – beef and pork especially – of processed meat, and other animal products, rocketed after the development of industrial-scale methods of rearing, slaughter, freezing and transport in the late 19th century. Before the middle of the 20th century meat and other animal foods became the centre of daily main meals not just of relatively rich people in industrialized countries, but also middle-class and better-off working-class families. Food culture epitomised by meat took various forms in different countries: in the USA steaks, in the UK roasts, in Germany sausages.

Animals bred in factory conditions are fed concentrates to make them as heavy and fat as quickly as possible. Meat itself does not make you fat. Wild animals are lean. What does make you fat is meat from industrially produced animals that are unnaturally fat, and whose fat has been hardened and made more saturated by concentrated feeds. By the 1970s, many foods of animal origin became identified as problematic because of their high fat and saturated fat content, and for this reason were agreed to be a cause of heart disease, and also of overweight and obesity.

MALIGN FOOD PROCESSES

Benign food processes preserve or improve the qualities of foods and drinks that protect against disease and enhance wellbeing, directly or in effect. Malign processes have the opposite effect. Directly or in their effects, they cause disorders and diseases.

Time to abolish hydrogenation

Most food preservation techniques, such as drying, fermenting, pickling, salting, and smoking, and refrigeration by use of ice, have ancient origins. On a mass scale, freezing and cooling followed bottling and canning as features of industrialization, and domestic refrigeration was not widespread even in the USA until the mid-20th century.

The 'refinement' that creates sugar and white flour is malign in its effect because it enables production of energy-dense processed foods. The technology that is most malign – directly as well as indirectly – is hydrogenation, the process that hardens all sorts of oils into uniform solid fat.

Before refrigeration, oils were not much use to food manufacturers. They are liquid, volatile, various, become rancid, and, in packaged products, seep. A standard fat is solid, uniform, and long-lasting – almost like sugar. All packaged products with long shelf lives that include fat, such as biscuits and cakes, are made possible by hydrogenation. This process also creates *trans*-fatty acids, also mostly an artefact of food chemistry, which Walter Willett of Harvard Medical School, the highest-profile nutrition scientist in the USA, believes may well be the main single nutritional cause of cardiovascular disease.

Together with the industrialization of meat production, and now the supply of cheap plant oils, hydrogenation has done most to increase the supply of fat, saturated fats and *trans*-fats in the world's food supplies since its invention at the beginning of the 20th century. Refrigeration and in-store cold-chilling has now made it largely obsolete, and some manufacturers and retailers are now eliminating it from the products they make and sell. You can encourage its extinction by not buying any product containing fat marked 'best by' more than a week ahead, or that lists 'hydrogenation' in its ingredients lists, and by telling your supermarket manager this is what you are doing – and why.

WHY WE ARE GETTING FATTER

Here follow the main reasons why obesity has become so much more common than it was as recently as the 1970s, in materially rich countries and throughout the world. They are arranged into six 'master' reasons. The first three all have economic, social and environmental aspects. These are the illusion of comfort, the cheapening of food, and food as an energy bomb. The second three reasons also have political and ideological aspects. These are economic and cultural globalization, the dogma of individual supremacy, and the confusion of wealth with money.

All six reasons pre-date 1980, but have become much more widespread and powerful in their effect on body fatness since around that time. Their power is in their combination. What's here, together with the notes to this chapter, is brief and illustrative, and is meant to guide you in your decisions and choices as a community and family member, as a customer and consumer, and as a citizen.

THE ILLUSION OF COMFORT

An environment of machines and cities tends to make humans inactive. This tendency has accelerated from the 1980s onwards. You know why. Many hundreds of millions more people now are driving cars, sitting at work, watching television, and using computers. The biggest recent change is that so many more children now are inactive. There is no sign of an end to any of these trends.

The shift to inertia

The quantity of food we can consume before we start to become fat dropped in the second half of the 20th century, and started to drop faster towards the close of the century. The energy balance of basically sedentary people is now artificially low, well below the level to which humans are adapted. Our need for nutrients is largely independent of our need for energy from food. This means that if you are basically sedentary you will either become short of vital nutrients or increase your body fat, unless you ensure that your diet is unusually nutrient-dense.

Reliable estimates of human food energy requirements have been made for centuries in Britain and Europe. In the USA in the first half of the 20th century, Francis Benedict and Ancel Keys, whose studies on the effects of energy restriction are summarized in the previous chapter, made exact measurements of normal energy requirements. Reports published around the mid-20th century consistently show that in general, adult men of average size and weight were then in energy balance at round about 3,000 calories (12,500 kilojoules) a day, and most average size and weight adult women at round about 2,300 calories (9,500 kilojoules) a day.

Now these averages have dropped by around 20 per cent or 500 calories (about 2,000 kilojoules) a day, to around 2,500 and 1,800 calories (10,500 and 7,500 kilojoules). In the USA and other countries the figure for the 'reference person' (men and women combined) is taken to be 2,000 kcal/day (8,374 kilojoules), for the purpose of nutrition food labelling.

The reason for this sudden drop in human energy requirements is because physical activity in the home, at work, and for moving from place to place, has been taken over by machines that do our work and supply entertainment for us. This shift towards physical inertia, which has economic and social drivers, gives us an illusion of comfort. But being obese is uncomfortable.

Watching the box

There are a number of reasons to single out television viewing as a cause of obesity. A 2008 UK survey states that children aged between five and 16 watch television on average for more than five hours a day, and four out of five have television sets in their bedrooms. Many homes in many countries have television sets in most main rooms, including bedrooms. People commonly watch television sitting or sprawling on easy chairs or sofas or lying in bed. Watching television takes the place of doing something more active.

People often snack on energy-dense foods and drinks or eat ready-to-heat meals while watching television. Children watch programmes whose breaks are saturated with advertisements for energy-dense fatty, sugary or salty foods and drinks marketed for children.

THE CHEAPENING OF FOOD

How we spend our money and time affects our happiness, health – and also shape. Mass-manufactured foods and drinks have become transformed since the 1970s and 1980s. The ready-to-eat and ready-to-heat products dominating the high-rent central aisles of supermarkets, and also sold in fast-food outlets and now in shops of all types including automobile and human filling stations, are prodigiously advertised as good because they are convenient and cheap. This economic factor is also ideological. When we consume cheapened food the cost to us and also to society is higher than the price of the products in the shops.

The increase in the volume of sugars, fats and oils in European, North American and other industrialized food supplies since the 19th century has largely been because of the artificial cheapness of these commodities. Now history is being repeated as sugary, fatty energy-dense products are flooding markets in Asia, Africa and Latin America.

'Good food costs less'

Most manufacturers of computers, cars, carpets, clothes and all sorts of other commodities spend their biggest advertising and promotion budgets on up-market models and styles. Food and drink is the one major commodity still mainly promoted as good because of being cheap.

Once I took a chance to say my piece on this topic. In 1990, at a meeting at the headquarters of the then leading UK supermarket chain, held to charm members of the UK Guild of Food Writers, I literally cornered the then boss of bosses, Lord Sainsbury. I told him that the 'classic' slogan, 'Good food costs less at Sainsbury's', was pernicious and foolish. First, any such claim was false. Second, if consumers had been bludgeoned into believing this absurdity, it would make them care less, and spend even less on food, which would ruin Sainsbury's, and the nation's health. The good food Lord was obviously not used to being spoken to like this, so I kept it pithy. A perspiring public affairs director interposed himself.

In the 1990s Sainsbury's market share plummeted, and in 2005 its slogan was 'Try something new today'. However, as you can see by looking at advertisements, flyers and displays, retailers continue to promote cheapened and discounted foods and drinks.

Less spend on food

Shoppers in materially rich countries are spending less and less on food. In the USA in 1930, people on average spent about one quarter of their available income on food and drink, almost all of which went on food prepared and eaten at home. By 1980, when obesity in the USA had become widespread, the figure had almost halved, to just over one eighth. By 2000, total spending on food and drink consumed in and out of the home in the USA was under one tenth of available income, of which close to half was – and is – spent out of the home.

In the USA the total proportion of disposable income spent on food consumed in the home has been under 6 per cent since 2000. After the USA, the country recorded as spending least on food consumed in the home is the UK, at just over 8 per cent. The proportion of total spending on food and drink consumed out of the home is higher in the USA and the UK than in other countries.

By contrast, the average spend in and out of the home in France and Italy, two European countries whose average personal available income is similar to the UK, and where the tradition of fresh food and shared meals is preserved, is respectively over 30 and over 50 per cent higher than in the UK. Rates of obesity in the UK are a lot higher than in France and Italy.

An inconvenience truth

We are also spending less and less time on food. Manufacture and sale of fast food has rocketed since the 1970s and 1980s. These ready-to-eat or quickly available energy-dense fatty, sugary or salty meals, snacks, foods and drinks, often super-sized and usually relatively low in nutrients, are served in transnational franchised 'restaurants' and their national and local equivalents, and also stocked in supermarkets, convenience stores, vending machines, sandwich shops, takeaways, bars and petrol stations. Typical meals and dishes served in transnational 'burger bars', such as those franchised by McDonald's or Yum! Brands, are fast foods. Most foods and drinks offered in sandwich and snack bars are fast foods.

'Convenience' ready-to-eat or ready-to-heat foods, drinks and dishes are a form of fast food. Many of these products are made from rock-bottom priced ingredients – highly processed starches, sugars or fats, as well as the even cheaper air or water, sophisticated with cosmetic additives, attractive packaging, and glamorous brand-imagery. These may not be cheap to buy, but they are cheapened.

This is not what manufacturers want you to think: their advertisements typically feature slim, smiling, attractive, athletic young people playing sport and having fun while enjoying their products. The reality is otherwise, as you can see in the streets of any city.

The end of the meal

European visitors to New York a century or so ago were amazed by the speed of meals. The Frenchman Paul de Rousiers reported in 1892: 'Nobody goes home in the middle of the day. They eat wherever they happen to be: in the office, while working in clubs, and in cafeterias . . . In blue-collar restaurants thousands of people eat standing up, with their hats on, all in a line, like horses in a stable . . . While lines of men dig in to plates brimming with meatballs, others wait to take their place.'

Even in the USA this fast food style remained a feature only of big cities until the second half of the 20th century, and the gradual and then accelerated rise of fast-food 'restaurant' and takeaway chains, at first on highways. Hanging out at drug stores that served soda, and then driving around and browsing and grazing at fast-food joints, became embedded in 1960s rock'n'roll themes. Convenience food took off in a big way throughout cities in the USA in the 1970s, and domestic penetration was enabled by the mass use of industrial and domestic freezers.

Until the 1970s, the fast food style was exotic in Europe, and in some parts is still unusual. Many families in German, Italian and French cities still have lunch together at home. Where the habit of eating together at home – if not at lunch then in the evening – remains normal, this celebrates the family and the meal as well as food and drink, the quality of which is part of the conversation. In much of the world now the family meal, and with it the family, is disintegrating. People eat while they do something else.

The French writer Claude Fischler says that spies could have told Saddam Hussein when Baghdad was about to be bombed in 1991, by infiltrating the Washington food-takeaway delivery system. On 16 January Domino's biked 55 pizzas to the White House, rather than the usual 5, and 101 pizzas to the Pentagon, rather than the usual 3. It's a safe guess that the US president and the joint chiefs of staff did not discuss the pizzas.

The business of business is to deliver profit. In the food industry, the best business is branded products whose ingredients are stable, safe, and cheap. In high-income countries, the less money and time people spend on food and drink, the more likely they are to become fat.

Thus for most people living in industrialized and urbanized societies, food and drink mean less than ever before in history. Lots of cheap foods and drinks are available all the time. So food is not valued, and people tend to overlook and ignore the ill-effects of habitual consumption of bad foods and drinks on health and wellbeing, until they are suitable cases for medical or surgical treatment at late stages in disease processes. This gives us added value as customers and consumers.

FOOD AS AN ENERGY BOMB

Fast and convenience food characteristically delivers more calories for any given amount of weight or volume than fresh food, and is manufactured and promoted in ever bigger sizes. This double whammy means that the most immediately available and attractive products are those that are most likely to be overeaten. Energy-dense foods and drinks are piled high in supermarkets and are on sale everywhere.

Snack attack

People who are worried about their excess body fat often imagine that if they avoid meals in favour of snacks, they will reduce weight. Wrong! This tactic won't work, because our sense of satiety comes from a feeling of fullness as well as from energy delivered. Most processed snacks are energy-dense. Suppose, for example, you have a cup or two of black coffee for breakfast, a couple of chocolate biscuits (cookies) in the morning, that you take away some no-cal soft drinks at lunchtime with two packets of crisps (chips), have a slice of carrot cake in the afternoon, eat nothing except a slice of pizza with a salad in the evening, together with more no-cal soft drinks, and reward yourself for being so disciplined with a confectionery bar and more black coffee before bed.

Here come the first and only calorie-counting sums in this book, in my report from supermarket sleuths in the USA, the UK, and Brazil. A couple of chocolate biscuits contain around 125 calories. Two 50-gram/2-ounce packets of crisps (chips) contain around 525 calories. A 100-gram/3½-ounce slice of cake may be 400 calories, a 150-gram/5-ounce slice of pizza may be 450 calories; and a 75-gram/3-ounce bar of confectionery may be 375 calories. This, plus say 25 calories from the salad, and nothing from the coffee and 'diet' soft drinks, adds up to 1,900 calories (8,150 kilojoules), which is around the amount of energy you may think that an average-size sedentary woman uses in a day.

So, you might think, that's all right. Wrong! For a start, this is somewhat more than many if not most sedentary women can take on board without gaining weight. Energy balance would be more likely without the biscuits, or even without one of the packets of crisps. The basic point though is that all such foods are very concentrated in processed starches, sugars, fats and salt. There is no way that a total of around 500 grams of food a day, roughly the weight of four apples or oranges, will satisfy you. Our bodies are designed to digest around 2 kilograms (4½ pounds) of food a day, more or less according to our gender, size and age. Snackers are ravenous much of the time, and tend to eat extra snacks that they don't mention, or even notice. All this is great for the snack trade, whose products are formulated and engineered to be more and more moreish.

Wallerstein's Bane

Super-sizing first began in 1955, when company boss Robert Woodruff agreed to market Coca-Cola in 10- and 12-ounce 'king size' and 26-ounce 'family size' bottles, as well as the traditional 6½-ounce size. The same principle was applied to fast food by David Wallerstein, who until the late 1960s managed a chain of movie houses in Texas. People would not buy more than one bag of popcorn because, he reckoned, going for seconds would seem to be greedy. So he made the containers bigger. This worked. In 1968 he was hired by McDonald's, and persuaded Ray Kroc, who by then owned the business, to sell bigger servings at a discount. This also worked. The Big Mac was born. Mostly starting in the 1980s other fast-food chains followed, with discounted Thickburgers, Colossal Burgers, Megabreakfasts, Triple Whoppers, Biggies, Meat 'Normouses, BK Stackers, Big Gulps, Triple Deckers, Great Americans, and Monsters. In Brazil Porção, a chain of *churrascarias* in and around Rio de Janeiro, has the face of a grinning pig as its trademark, and its name is a pun on *porcão* (pig) and *porção* (big portion). In *churrascarias* you pay a set price and then eat as much meat as you want.

Liquid candy

The manufacture and consumption of soft drinks, sometimes known as 'liquid candy', and in particular carbonated cola drinks, increased tenfold in the USA between 1942 and 2002. Between 1970 and 1997, production of sugared cola and soda drinks in the USA increased from 22 to 41 gallons per person a year, well over a 12-ounce bottle or can a person a day. Big Gulps, also known as the large Coke, are now 32 ounces or 2 pints (roughly a litre). What was more than king size in the 1950s is now the 16-ounce small Coke. By the turn of the millennium, people in the USA were drinking 13.15 billion gallons of carbonated drinks a year.

In the USA, boys aged between 13 and 18 on average drink the equivalent of two 12-ounce (350 millilitre) cans of soft drinks a day, which if sugared deliver around 300 calories (1,250 kilojoules) a day. The average for girls of the same age is the equivalent of 1½ 12-ounce cans or around 200 calories (850 kilojoules) a day. Average adult consumption of soft drinks in the USA also delivers around 200 calories a day. As you can see simply by walking the streets and noticing shop fascia, cola and other soft drinks are mammoth business all over the world.

Between 1975 and 2000, production and consumption in Brazil of *refrigerantes* (sugared cola and other soft drinks) increased by almost 400 per cent. Two-litre plastic bottles of Coke each deliver 850 calories (3,570 kilojoules), or 85 calories per 200-millilitre serving, as suggested in small print on the label. Do people usually drink a glass of a fizzy drink and then replace the cap for tomorrow? I suggest not. The 2003 World Health Organization report on prevention of chronic diseases states: 'It has been estimated that each additional can or glass of sugar-sweetened drink that [children habitually] consume every day, increases the risk of becoming obese by 60 per cent.'

There is also the matter of advertising and marketing. Consuming a cheeseburger and a cola drink is highly predictive of consuming a lot more cheeseburgers and cola drinks. But of course! Advertising and marketing budgets amounting to billions of dollars a year that press all available primeval buttons – including desire for fun and sex as well as sugar and fat – are not for nothing.

ECONOMIC AND CULTURAL GLOBALIZATION

The food systems determining what is supplied to shops do not just reflect consumer preference. They are shaped by the decisions and practices of the transnational and national food and drink and associated industries. They are also shaped by the policies of powerful national governments, working through international agencies such as the World Trade Organization, the World Bank and the International Monetary Fund. As economists say, what we eat and drink is not so much demand-driven as supply-driven.

The phenomenal acceleration of international communication, business, trade, and money flow since the 1980s known as 'globalization' has many aspects. Economic globalization is supposed to promote the free flow of capital and goods. In its present form it tends to enrich high-income countries and further impoverish low-income countries. It causes obesity in middle- and low-income countries by displacing low energy-dense traditional food systems with high energy-dense industrialized food systems. Cultural globalization is creating a homogenized food culture throughout the world.

From sugar and spice to burgers and brownies

Globalized trade is not new. The spice routes from the East helped to make Venice immensely rich. The triangular trade of which slaves from Africa to the Americas was one side, and sugar and then tobacco and coffee from the Americas was another, enriched the European powers and changed the food supplies of Britain, France, the Netherlands and other countries. At primary school in the mid-20th century my teacher taught the class geography by getting us to arrange food labels on a map of the world – oranges from South Africa and Palestine, lamb from New Zealand, butter from Australia, bananas from Jamaica, dates from Egypt, corned beef from Argentina.

Now the scale of global food trade has vastly increased. Evolved agriculture systems based on local foods that require mainly human inputs are ripped up and replaced by capitalized systems producing cheapened milky, meaty, sugary, fatty, processed foods usually of foreign origin. In Brazil, unsustainable cattle ranches and farms producing soya, mostly for animal feed, are replacing great tracts of the Amazon rainforest and the *cerrado* (savannah) region.

Big differences between the mid-20th century and now are the relative and absolute cheapness of meat, processed meat, and fats and oils, the further drop in physical activity throughout the world, and industrialization of the food systems of Asia, Africa and Latin America. In China, the traditional meat is pork, but its beef supply was up to 20 kilograms per person a year (55 grams a day) in 1985, and 50 kilograms per person a year (136 grams a day) in 2008. In Chinese cities, use of edible oils increased 440 per cent between 1979 and 1999. Global meat production is projected to increase from 229 million tonnes in 2000 to 465 million tonnes in 2050.

Subsidies and dumping

Trade remains unfair. For example, since the 1980s soft drinks in the USA have been sweetened with high-fructose syrup made from corn. The price of corn is kept artificially low by US government subsidies of around $US10 billion a year to Midwestern farmers, whose corn used as animal feed has accelerated the factory farming of cattle and poultry. The vast profits of the giant soft-drinks industry in the USA come in part from these subsidies. Economies of scale have almost eliminated family farming, and are exhausting the land of its water resources.

Export of subsidized crops and foods, and dumping of staple foods in the name of trade and aid, is contributing to destitution of farmers in impoverished countries where the price of farm produce is not protected. These policies make the rhetoric of 'free trade' very different from its reality. Powerful countries have always protected their own industries, and forced open the markets of weaker countries.

These forces may seem nebulous to those of us who lead comfortable lives. Not so to the makers of food. Many types of food, not only those that make you fat, are unfairly traded. Hector Chavez, a smallholder in Chiapas, Mexico, has said: 'I don't know how American farmers can sell corn to this country at such low prices. I have heard that their government gives their money. What I know is that we cannot compete with their prices. Imports are killing our markets and our communities.' Exports of massively subsidized milk powder from Europe in the mid-1990s devastated the livelihoods of family farmers of milk and dairy produce in Jamaica.

With sugared soft drinks, federal political and economic policies are a cause of overweight and obesity. Consumption of soft drinks sweetened with high-fructose corn syrup peaked in the USA in the early 2000s. Coca-Cola, PepsiCo and other giant manufacturers are now preparing for business in a new world.

The global food system

Transnational food and drink manufacturing companies, such as Nestlé, Unilever, Coca-Cola and Kellogg's, established their brands globally in the first half of the 20th century. Even more influential than these conspicuous signs has been the general adoption of industrial methods of farming and growing, food technology, and distribution and marketing throughout the world, to produce food for internal consumption and also for export. In the late 20th century, international trade in various basic food commodities became increasingly concentrated and controlled by a small number of gigantic US-based enterprises such as Cargill, ConAgra and Archer Daniels Midland.

An increasingly global food system means increasing approximation to the food system of the USA and other materially rich countries. In turn, this means the replacement of traditional food produced by rural farmers by industrialized products to feed urban workers. Accelerated in many countries by 'structural adjustment', under which the World Bank and the International Monetary Fund insist on indebted and impoverished countries opening their markets wider to imports, this phenomenon is changing the shape of the human world in the most literal sense.

With India, China is the biggest prize. India and China together contain roughly one-third of the world's population, and already there are more people with cardiovascular heart disease in India and China than in all high-income countries put together. China is now 'developing' very fast. A Red Cross report published in 2004 stated that 70 per cent of the people of Beijing, Shanghai and Guangzhou said they were tired, unfit or ill. The Chinese Academy of Sciences has reported sharp decreases in life expectancy, most of all among the educated and professional classes – intellectuals are dying at an average age of 58 years, 10 years below the national average. The life expectancy of managers and programmers in China's 'silicon valley' is 53 years, of Shanghai journalists 45 years.

The global food culture

Given the richness and variety of their culinary and other traditions, why do Indians and Chinese want to become part of a homogenized convenience-food culture? One answer is Mickey Mouse. In China, burgers and brownies are not positioned as cheap convenient fuel but as chic eats, part of the Good Life beckoning from the West.

Transnational food and drink companies are in China for the long haul, and they have multi-billion-dollar budgets. As an example, 1.8 million people a day visited McDonald's 770 joints in mainland China in 2007. The company's goal that year was to have 1,000 'restaurants' in place in time for the 2008 Beijing Olympics, of which McDonald's – along with Coca-Cola – is a sponsor. McDonald's has also signed a deal with Sinopec, the state-owned oil company, for first refusal on human fuelling stations within its 30,000 automobile fuelling stations across China. The company's middle-term target is to make China its second biggest market after the USA – an ambition it shares with Starbucks.

On holiday in the Sri Lankan forest in the mid-1980s, we stopped by a metal Coke advertisement, underneath which was a boy selling the local refreshment. While I took photographs, he sliced the tops off two coconuts with his machete, and offered them to us. He gestured at the sign, grinned and said: 'No good. Chemical.' Maybe now he is the big boss of the Sri Lankan refreshment industry. Maybe.

THE DOGMA OF INDIVIDUAL SUPREMACY

Treating people as individuals is another reason why we get fat. The idea that humans as individuals are separate from and transcend humans as members of families and communities and as part of society is now so generally accepted in North America, much of Europe, and other materially rich and powerful countries, as to be almost taken for granted. Historically this ideology is recent, and is still not assimilated into the culture of most civilizations.

The vision of Tony Blair

Let me illustrate what this has to do with weight increase and obesity. In July 2006 the then UK prime minister gave a speech on public health. This was in part prompted by a populist campaign fronted by the 'celebrity chef' Jamie Oliver, whose purpose was to raise the nutritional standards of British state-school meals.

Tony Blair began by saying: 'Our public health problems are not, strictly speaking, public health problems at all. They are questions of individual lifestyle – obesity, smoking, alcohol abuse, diabetes, sexually transmitted diseases. These are not epidemics in the epidemiological sense. They are the result of millions of individual decisions, at millions of points in time.' In the entire lecture the word 'family' occurred just three times, once with reference to dysfunctional families. Rather like Margaret Thatcher, who when prime minister declared 'there is no such thing as society', he emphasized five times, in different phrases, that 'all of us' are 'individuals, companies, and government'. In the 1980s Margaret Thatcher was pioneering an ideology. In 2006, Tony Blair, in his tenth year as prime minister, was confirming the separate supremacy of the individual.

'Individual lifestyle choice'

Obesity is now positioned as being the result of individual 'lifestyle choices'. This notion has little to do with the realities of obesity – or of diabetes, smoking, alcoholism, or of various common diseases. Abandonment of the concepts of society and of public health is a consequence of the dogma of individual supremacy. This first originated in Europe in the form of Protestantism and its belief in salvation not through good works but through faith. It took root as a political and social ideology in the USA in the 19th century, mainly perhaps because of the frontier spirit and the vision – represented by presidents like Andrew Jackson, Abraham Lincoln and Ulysses Grant, all commemorated on banknotes – that everybody, however humble their beginnings, can make good.

The idea of individual 'lifestyle choice' is very new. It was developed at first in the USA in the 1970s. It underpins the ideology of the 'free market', the new version of *laisser faire* ideology that, since the accessions of Ronald Reagan and Margaret Thatcher, has now been accepted by most if not all main political parties in most high-income countries.

Governments justify demolishing regulations and giving industry a free hand by stating that the results of industry policies and practices, such as those so far summarized in this chapter, are a matter for individual choice. If you are fat and this bothers you, join a fitness centre, or eat more vegetables, or go easy on fatty foods, and if you don't make choices like these, well hey, that's your choice and it's not the job of government to interfere.

This notion resonates with politicians and policy-makers in materially rich countries, because as very privileged people they personally have extraordinary freedom of choice. It is also politically handy, because it implies that industry has no responsibility for the consequences of its actions. The limits of responsibility that free-market governments will accept is identification of the best evidence on personally healthy and unhealthy foods and drinks, and publication of guidelines summarizing what the experts say. Here's the pamphlet, now you choose. That's the idea.

This approach may seem to make sense to you. After all, you, the reader of this book, don't have to consume fast food or sugared soft drinks – although you may find it hard to discourage your children from doing so. People who buy books generally do have a lot of freedom of choice. Indeed, the final chapter of this book is all about making personal choices that will enhance your health and wellbeing. But for many families and communities in your country, wherever you are, and for most families and communities throughout the world, it's a different story.

The meaning of people

To say that obesity is a 'lifestyle disease' implies that individuals are free to choose whether or not to be fat, which in turn implies that prevention is only about education and information – or drugs or surgery. The more privileged people are, the more scope they have. But it makes little sense to say that consumption of foods and drinks that are craved, let alone those to which people can become addicted in a real sense, is a matter of 'lifestyle'. Also, babies and young children do not become overweight and obese because of their 'lifestyle'.

Dietary guidelines addressed to individuals are not part of the solution but part of the problem. They are part of a world where people browse and graze in fast-food joints, in the streets, and at home. Without intending to do so, they undermine shopping and cooking for others, the family meal, the identity of the family itself, and its communal fabric.

We value our selves. We are also members of families, communities and societies. As a simple example, within any family often one person makes most of the decisions on what food to buy, prepare and serve. The family table and meal is fundamental to the fabric of the family, the community, and society. The dogma of the supremacy of the individual, applied to food, is destructive of society, the family, and of ourselves. It also makes us fat.

THE CONFUSION OF WEALTH WITH MONEY

Money makes the world go round. It is the measure of material things, and is used to gauge the wealth and development of nations. This being so, the rocketing cost of obesity is excellent news for governments as well as for industry, the medical profession and pharmaceutical industry, and all who service fat people, including the dieting industry. In becoming fat we embody added value.

Adam Smith wrote *The Wealth of Nations* to advocate his theories of effective use of capital and trade as a means to the end of human health, welfare and happiness, which was roughly what 'wealth' meant in the 18th century – hence the word 'commonwealth'. Since then 'wealthy' has come to mean 'having and using a lot of money'. The means has become the end.

Obesity as development

Governments and government agencies in high-income countries are now proclaiming the cost of obesity. Remember that scene in *Crocodile Dundee* where our hero scoffs at the switchblade of a would-be mugger and whips out his massive weapon, saying: 'Call that a knife? *That's* a knife'? In 2004, a UK House of Commons Committee estimated the then national cost of obesity at around £3.5 billion a year. In late 2007, the UK government's advisory Foresight group – like a poker player pushing a pile of chips into a big pot, leaning back and saying 'double, and triple double' – came up with a projected £45.5 billion for 2050. *That's* a statistic. If the UK is taken to be sort-of average, this figure could be conjured into a heroic global 2050 figure of $US10 trillion. Now *that's* a statistic: even higher than the US national debt. United Nations agencies and organizations that study obesity identify ever-increasing percentages of international and national treasure spent on obesity: 1 per cent, 3 per cent, 5 per cent – who knows?

Suppose such extrapolations and percentages are officially accepted. Do jumbo numbers, once taken on board and recited by politicians, mean that at last governments will act to reduce obesity? No, they do not. Obesity is good for business. More than that, it is a sign and a cause of national success as now measured.

'Development' is a money measure. To 'develop' means to unfold, mature, evolve. But as now applied to countries, the word has a technical meaning. The gauge for degree of development is money, expressed as GNP (gross national product), averaged as per head per year irrespective of the distribution of money within the country. 'Development' is not of freedoms and entitlements, as the Indian Nobel prize-winning economist Amartya Sen advocates, or of safe water, protected forests, families, beauty, biodiversity, culture, intelligence, serenity, security, or any other indicators of wealth that are hard to measure or are immeasurable. It means more cash being turned over and spent.

Subsistence farmers are 'undeveloped' – more so if they do not use agrochemicals – whereas consumers are 'developed'. A rainforest is 'undeveloped', whereas the strip-mines and cattle farms that replace the forest are 'developed'. Countries in which more people spend more money on food and drink, on medicine and surgery, and on treatments for body fatness, are increasingly well 'developed'. Obesity and chronic diseases that show early in life and are medicated for half a century or more are characteristic of 'highly developed' countries.

Money makes the world get round

Health professionals say that the soaring cost of obesity is a bad thing. You might think that governments would be appalled, and would institute legal and fiscal measures such as those that require motorists to wear seatbelts and that restrict guns and tax liquor and tobacco.

To the contrary. Politicians say that rates of obesity are appalling and that something urgent really must be done. And? In January 2008, the UK government rolled out its 'Healthy Weight, Healthy Lives' education package, while deciding not, after all, to regulate advertising of junk food on television before 9 p.m., explaining that this would cost over £200 million a year in advertising revenue.

The more money obesity turns over, the better the shape of finance, industry, agriculture, food and trade ministries, the more glittering the bottom line of the industries these ministries sponsor, and therefore the more 'developed' the nation. True, obese people are more likely to be out of work and thus a drag on social security. But this will only be a big deal in full-employment economies with social welfare systems that include publicly funded health services, and these are now becoming phased out, except in Canada, Scandinavia and a few other countries. Civil servants are trained to be hard-headed and, as they see things, unemployed zeppelin helots knocking back junk food and drink while watching television and playing computer games are cheaper for the state to maintain than muscular *hoi polloi* who get into trouble and spend much of their lives working out in the gym in the slammer at the taxpayers' expense.

This is not to say that your head of state positively *wants* you to be fat, simply that if you and half the population get fat on gut-busting food, your elected representatives are not going to bust a gut to stop the trend. Besides, what you do and what happens to you is your responsibility, remember?

Consider some of the effects of populations steadily gaining weight. Makers of airline seats have jobs for life. Dieters double or quadruple sales of suits and dresses. There is a bariatric surgeon's yacht in every marina. Academics are replenished with multimillion-pound grants from government agencies and the drug industry. Obesity conferences supported by convenience food and designer drug companies are hot academic tickets. The sugar industry endows university professorships of human nutrition. Students continue to fund their studies with money from casual work in burger bars. Fat people take drugs for diseases thought to be caused by obesity, all their adult lives. Fast food, pharmacy and fitness high street chains boom and consider synergistic mergers.

Hospital administrators demand more hospitals. Television series showing obese children on trekking trips are a primetime novelty success. Forests are cut down to produce guidelines and pamphlets, which is good for the woodcutting and printing trades, and tape-measures are placed in every schoolchild's lunchbox, which cheers up the haberdashery accessory manufacturers. Activity! The bottom lines showing the profits of transnational drug and snack companies continue to be healthy, and their share prices rise. Ching, ching!

Obesity is fuelling national 'development' all over the world because 'developed' countries are those that turn over most cash. Money is the measure of progress and success. If you look after yourself you are bad for business. There is no added value in wellbeing. This ideology is mad, and it can't last, but it's the way the world works now. The business of all 'market economies' is business. Obesity makes money. Obese and diseased people are good for business. All over the world, policies and practices sponsored and promoted by governments are making us fat.

5. THE PLACE OF FOOD
IN OUR WORLD

*It seems to me that our three basic needs, for food and security and love,
are so mixed and mingled and entwined that we cannot straightly think
of one without the others. So it happens that when I write of hunger, I
am really writing about love and the hunger for it . . . and warmth and
richness and the fine reality of hunger satisfied . . . and it is all one.*

M F K Fisher

*How and what we eat determines to a great extent the use we make of
the world – and what is to become of it.*

Michael Pollan

In which I tell some stories of the value of food and drink, as personal and shared pleasure and a centre of family and social life, as well as protection of our health and enhancement of our wellbeing. We can act on this knowledge now.

In this 21st century it is time to revive the value of food as a precious resource, thinking and acting as customers, consumers and citizens, and as members of one species with special responsibilities within the whole living and physical world.

Practically all readers of this book are materially rich in many ways beyond the dreams of bygone emperors. We can travel to other continents within the same day, listen to great music at the touch of a button, communicate immediately all round the world, and use drugs to assuage many symptoms of illness.

An adverse effect of these wonderful privileges is that we tend to forget or neglect what is most fundamentally valuable in our lives, and most of all that which we share with all humanity, such as family, friendship, conviviality and wellbeing – and also, our daily food and drink.

It's good to be the size and shape you want to be, to be comfortable within your skin, to feel in control of yourself, to enjoy the sun and the sea, to run for fun, to climb hills joyfully, and to wake up and live in the day and go to sleep with a sense of wellbeing you have earned and gained. Time spent in cycles of becoming overweight and then dieting and then becoming overweight again is a miserable experience, if only because this diminishes the joy of living.

What to eat and drink from day to day? The question is bound up with larger questions. What to do? How to live? How to be? How much choice and how many freedoms do we really have? What most matters? How can we support the makers of food most effectively? What about the size and shape and wellbeing of our children? What will become of us? We are also becoming more aware of the impact of world food systems on resources such as soil, water and energy. What sort of a world will we leave? One way to sense answers to such big questions is to become more conscious of what we eat and drink and why, and what this does to us.

This chapter indicates the right way with food. If you started reading this book to find out what's wrong with dieting, why else we are liable to become fat, and how to reduce body fat and weight, I hope that by now you are also looking forward to enjoying delicious food and celebrating its value. This and the following chapter will encourage you to forget about dieting regimes and instead to celebrate food and drink and meals that are a pleasure to consume, and that are altogether good for you.

THE REAL VALUE OF FOOD

The enjoyment of food and drink is part of the good life well led. Food is also part of the story of the ascent of humanity. Great civilizations are defined partly by the quality of their food systems and food culture. How land is used for the cultivation of food shapes the environment for which we have a responsibility. The preparation of food – for everyday meals and for special occasions with family and friends – contributes to human fellowship.

When food systems are not industrialized, people know where their food comes from. They are bound to know, and to appreciate and understand the value of food, because much of their life is devoted to finding, growing, preserving, storing, making and preparing food. Privileged people – like me and, no doubt, you – are released from such obligations by industrialization. We can spend most of our time paying no special attention to food. As a result we are liable to lose the sense of its value – or never gain such a sense.

As shown in the previous chapter, this makes trouble for us. For most people in materially rich countries, cooking remains as a remnant of old skills with food, and often not even that. These days, when supermarkets are stacked with ready-to-heat food, when shops of all kinds stock snacks, fast foods and other ready-to-consume goods, and when more and more meals are eaten in bars, diners, canteens, cafés and restaurants, the nature, origin and meaning of food is gradually becoming a mystery.

We want our food and drink to be available, affordable, safe, varied, delicious and healthy. So do the many millions of communities and families who remain short of food and whose water supplies are often contaminated. We have the better chance of getting what we want, and our gain is often their loss. We can learn from the fact that food is more fundamentally important to impoverished people than it is for us. It will become more valuable whether we like this or not, as the world's natural resources dwindle.

THE BEST THINGS IN LIFE

While preparing this book and discussing its scope with friends and colleagues, I was asked a couple of times – why this chapter? The question went something like this. 'You encourage readers not to go on dieting regimes, you explain what else makes them fat, and you outline a path to better health. OK. But now you are also encouraging readers to buy fair-traded food, be concerned about animal welfare, do their bit to slow down climate change, and support Oxfam and Friends of the Earth. Is this a health book or a save the world book?'

It's both. Here is why. In one of his plays Johann Wolfgang von Goethe writes: 'You owe to others what you are.' This refers for example to what children gain from their mothers. Writers may reflect on all those who have taught them. And by the necessary acts of eating and drinking, we owe to animals and plants what we are, and also plants owe their being to soil, water, air and light. This awareness of our co-existence with the living and physical world may be more effective in moving us to eat and drink well, than preoccupation with our individual selves.

Conversely, Mahatma Gandhi speaks to our concerns about the prospects for planet earth in his saying: 'Be the change you wish to see in the world.' Eating and drinking in awareness of and with respect for the makers and sources of our food is a basic act of solidarity with real meaning and value, for the world out there, and also for the world in here – literally, inside ourselves.

Separating the sensual, culinary and nutritional aspects of what we eat and drink from its biological, economic, social, political and environmental dimensions, is a mistake, and also unrealistic and increasingly unwise. Whether we want to reduce body fat and weight, or to reduce our risk of diseases of which industrialized diets are a cause, or to nourish our families, it is best to think of food and drink as a whole, and also as part of a bigger picture – which it is.

If your main personal interest is to find out how to control your body fat and weight, this may seem all too much. Trust me. Eating, drinking and living well in all ways involves time, care and respect. We can all begin by being prepared to spend more time on food and drink, and when better quality means a higher price – sometimes it does, but often it need not – also to spend more of our money on what we and our families eat and drink and maybe less on other things.

That's enough generality. Here as illustrations are three stories of the value of good food, of which one is a classic, and the other two are from my own experience. They are about omelettes in France, salmon in Scotland, and snacks in China. They are also about what food means, and can mean.

Sure that eggs are eggs?

The first story is about quality and simplicity. In an essay written in 1959, the cook and writer Elizabeth David tells of the omelettes made half a century earlier by Annette Poulard, owner of the Hôtel de la Tête d'Or on Mont-St-Michel in Normandy, for her devoted customers who came from all over France and indeed Europe. What was Madame Poulard's secret? All sorts of rumours circulated. She mixed water with the eggs? No, the secret was cream. She had designed her own pan. She had added foie gras to the omelettes. She had reared her own breed of hens. Rival recipes of increasing elaboration for *omelette de la mère Poulard* appeared in French magazines and cookery books.

Long after retirement Madame Poulard told her secret. She said: 'I break some good eggs in a bowl, I beat them well, I put a good piece of butter in the pan, I throw the eggs into it, and I shake it constantly. I am happy, *monsieur*, if this recipe pleases you.' Elizabeth David tells the story gleefully. But the days when it truly could be said 'sure as eggs is eggs' are long gone. In those days anybody – well, anybody in northern France who cared about food – knew a good egg and a good piece of butter, and half a century ago Mrs David paid her readers the compliment of assuming that they also knew.

The hens that produced the eggs for Madame Poulard's omelettes lived in much the same way as hens had lived for the previous thousand years and more, in backyards or genuine free-ranging flocks of a few hundred at most. Eggs look roughly the same as they always have, and their chemical composition seems to be roughly the same. But they have changed.

The degradation of chickens by modern methods of agriculture into living machines, units in an industrial process involving tens and even hundreds of thousands of caged birds, results in poultry that is flabby, and eggs that cannot be cooked and enjoyed as were those of Madame Poulard. Once you have savoured real free-range eggs, the experience of eating battery eggs becomes distasteful. Most shoppers who make sure they buy genuine free-range eggs do so because they are disgusted by the factory farming of chickens. Some do so because they know that eggs laid by chickens treated with respect are delicious.

At home in Brazil, once again touched by this story and its messages, I make supper. I break two *ovos caipira* – eggs from hens reared in a local backyard – in a bowl, and beat them. Compared with the eggs I used to cook when I lived in England they are small and their shells are thick; the mixed yolk and white is like custard. I heat the iron pan I bought in London in the 1970s and keep oiled, and toss in a knob of butter made in Lima Duarte, a local country town. Fizz. Then I add the eggs and do the shaking, and turn the omelette with a two-handed toss of the pan. Serve on thick slices of wholegrain toast. Mm. *Pas mal.*

The nature and quality of any animal food is affected by what the animal eats and the conditions in which it lives, just as the nature and quality of any plant food is affected by the quality of the soil in which it grows. The only issues are by how much, and the significance of the difference. People who appreciate food are sensitive to these things. Elizabeth David, writing of what she called 'the art or the discipline, call it what you like, of leaving well alone', says that 'it's a capacity that would make meals a lot cheaper and cooking a great deal easier'.

What goes round, comes round

On 21 April 1987 I was taught a lesson about the value of food at the Holly Tree restaurant at Kentallen by Appin in the Highlands of Scotland. This is the second story, also about quality, and respect. At dinner overlooking Loch Linnhe, thinking to be knowledgeable, I explained to my companion that of course the salmon we had been served was farmed. Alasdair Robertson, then the owner, overheard me, and came to our table, polite but seething. 'I serve real fish here,' he said, and thrust me a book with photographs showing the differences between wild and farmed fish: the texture and colour of the flesh, the amount and nature of the fat between and within the muscles, the condition of the skin, fins and tail, and the whole look of the fish. He kindly did not say that if I couldn't taste the difference, what was I doing in his restaurant?

The intensive farming of animals for human food has profound public health implications. Michael Crawford, an authority on brain chemistry, points out that much of the essential fat in animals, birds and fish is lost when they are produced by factory methods and is in effect replaced by saturated fats. This, he says, is a threat to the functioning of our brains and nervous systems. Maybe eating too much dead food at that time was why I could not immediately taste the difference between wild and farmed salmon. In Appin was I on the way to losing my marbles? Ever since then I have preferred to eat the meat of creatures that when alive were physically fit hunters and foragers and lived a real life.

Ecologists say that the abuse of nature by humans has a karmic effect. Treat living creatures bred as human food well, and they will treat you well. Abused, their meat and their products will in time make you ill. What is true of salmon is true of cattle, sheep, pigs, turkeys, geese, chickens, other fish and – see below – seafood. The Brazilian philosopher Leonardo Boff writes of 'the ecological culture that respects plants, animals, soil, and humans – all living things that are part of the fabric of life . . . in solidarity with future generations'.

The alley of snacks

The third story takes place in Hangzhou, capital of the province of Zhejiang, not far from Shanghai, and is about food traditions and culture. In the midst of the Alley of Snacks off Hefang Street are tables for eight, which on the day of my visit towards the end of 2006 were crammed with couples, often with their one child, concentrating on their meals. The Alley of Snacks is serious business. Two facing rows of stalls offer endless possibilities, for each has its owner and cook preparing crabs, prawns, clams, scallops, jellyfish, pork ribs and jointed chicken in their own styles, and also many mysterious – to me – seafoods and organ meats, endless varieties of succulent greens, and the sticky black rice for which Zhejiang is famous. I chose one of the many seafood congees which, together with a whole round crisp loaf fresh from the oven and shaped like a great fat coin, set me back 5 yuan (about 70 US cents or 35 UK pence) and was plenty for lunch.

The people of Zhejiang are renowned for their good health and long lives, and their diets meet the current World Health Organization recommendations for vegetables and fruits and for dietary constituents. This is not because communities and families in Hangzhou are examining expert reports. They know anyway. Love of food in Zhejiang has a very long history. Towards the end of the 13th century at the time of the Mongol emperor Qubilai Qan (Kubla Khan), Hangzhou, then the capital of the empire of southern China, was said by Marco Polo to be 'the finest and noblest in the world', and may also have been the richest and most populous city on earth. Green tea has been roasted or fermented in Zhejiang for 4,000 years, and prepared and drunk as an art, a stimulant, a remedy, a ceremony, and a centre of food culture, like wine in France.

Chinese natural philosophers at and before the time of Qubilai Qan did not distinguish between food and medicine, and their scholarship included celebrations of cuisine and compilation of cookbooks, many of which have survived. Nearly a thousand years ago the people of Hangzhou by day shopped in markets that sold fish, meat, poultry, vegetables, fruits, fungi and herbs in wonderful variety and abundance, and by night dined out with their families in tea houses, the first restaurants.

There is balance here between what's ancient and what's new, and an informal system involving food, activity, livelihoods, and personal and public health, in a social, economic, environmental as well as personal context. In addition to choosing what's best from other places, may the people of Hangzhou preserve what they have.

OUR PRIVILEGES AND CHOICES

Stories of respect for our food, and for its origins and makers, speak to us now. They do not imply that the world would be a better place, or that we would be better off, if we all lived as if we were gatherer-hunters or peasant-agriculturists. This is a fantasy, because it isn't going to happen, and a fallacy, because pre-industrial populations did not have it all good.

Most people who live in nature and whose tools give them only simple advantages lead arduous and often debilitating lives, and in many parts of the world are vulnerable not only to the weather but also to human predators such as rival tribes, landlords, warlords and invaders. The splendours of pre-industrial empires such as those of the Egyptians, Greeks, Romans, Franks, Venetians, Mongols, Aztecs, Spanish and Russians, involved constant oppression, slavery and massacre of civilians. One aspect of such general insecurity is that for many communities food supplies were, and still are, often uncertain, monotonous and depleted.

What a contrast with our ways of life, if we live in peace, and are relatively affluent. Where I live now in Brazil, my family's food comes from our garden, from local farmers, from makers of speciality produce, from small shops and the municipal market, from the Brazilian supermarket chain Bahamas, and also from the international French-owned chain Carrefour, whose supermarkets are very big business here. When I am travelling, in London I shop at Waitrose and in Washington at Whole Foods, both astonishing emporiums with spectacular choices of vegetables, salads, fruits, and other fresh and benignly processed foods, some locally sourced, some supporting family farmers and farmers' co-operatives, and also many shipped, flown and driven in from all over the world.

If we act on the knowledge of what is good for us, our health will be improved and our wellbeing enhanced. But of course many people do not know what is good for them, and many people in almost all countries do not have access to adequate good food or the means to buy or grow it. Dietary advice is of little value to an African mother who has to use her small allotment plot to grow cash crops for money to feed her family, who has access only to small shops selling processed basic foods and drinks, and whose produce and home are threatened by drought or civil war. Much the same is so for unemployed or otherwise impoverished families living in city slums in the UK and the USA, as well as in the slums and shantytowns of Asia, Africa and Latin America.

You probably have scope, if you choose, to buy, eat and drink well. If you are wise, you will do so in practical sympathy with the makers and producers, wherever they are. (Some of the ethical aspects of shopping at supermarkets are outlined below, and also see the notes to this chapter.)

THE BIGGER PICTURE

What we eat, where our food and drink comes from, and what determines the shape and nature of food systems, are all related. It's best that we dissolve the distinction between ourselves as consumers and as citizens. Jean Anthelme Brillat-Savarin had the right attitude. Nearly 200 years ago he said: 'The destiny of nations is determined by what and how they eat,' and also: 'If you tell me what you eat, I will tell you who you are.'

Here are two more stories about the value of food in our lives. The first is dark, the second is optimistic. Both illustrate the nature, scale and power of the forces that shape food systems and food supplies. Events and decisions that take place far away from us can and do affect the food that we – and babies and young children – consume. More than this, they may be matters of life and death for us.

The price and the cost of prawns

Here is what can happen when the price of food in the shops does not take its true cost into account. It is a story about traditional ways of life being destroyed by local producers and entrepreneurs, by international 'development', and by the drive to supply cheapened food to supermarkets. The deaths of the 250,000 and more people swept away by the Asian tsunami at the end of 2004 – one third of them children – were not as generally supposed solely a natural catastrophe. Here is why.

Your local supermarket may stock jumbo bags of frozen prawns and shrimps: easy to cook, tasty and nutritious (unless you worry about dietary cholesterol), and at a remarkably low price. Since the 1970s and 1980s, the main dietary message in the USA and other countries has been to consume less fat. Sales of low-fat food of animal origin have boomed. Dieting regimes have encouraged these new markets: prawns and other seafood are part of the high-protein and also the low-fat dieting messages.

In the mid-1980s the World Bank loaned and granted money to businesses in Asia to boost industrial-scale prawn and shrimp farming. National governments gave further support in the form of loans and tax breaks. One purpose of these enterprises is to earn foreign exchange and to pay off debts to international moneylenders. In 2000, Thailand exported 300,000 tonnes of prawns and shrimps, Indonesia plus India another 150,000 tonnes. Close to half the annual Asian total of over half a million tonnes is imported by the USA, with a market valued in 2000 at around $US10 billion.

So exactly where do these prawns and shrimps come from? Mangroves, anchored in mud in estuarine ecosystems, once made up almost a quarter of the littoral of Southeast Asia. Fishers in Brazil call mangroves *berçários do mar*, 'sea cradles' that protect hatchlings from predators and provide safe mooring for boats. Husbanded mangrove ecosystems provide stocks of fish for local consumption and for a wider market; part of traditional food systems and a source of communal livelihoods.

Like estuarine fish, prawns and shrimps mature in a mixture of fresh and salt water. Asia's coastal wetlands have been and are being destroyed for shrimp 'farming' for the export and tourist trade, and also for new ports and resorts for tourists. Throughout Asia, reefs and mangroves continue to be dynamited and bulldozed. More than half these natural commons are now gone for ever. Thus Thailand once had 380,000 hectares of mangroves; by 2000 two-thirds, a total of 253,000 hectares, had been destroyed.

Some people gain; most lose. Fishing communities are pushed out. Intensive breeding of prawns and shrimps creates a polluted 'ecological footprint' estimated at a hundred times the size of the shrimp 'farm'. Oxfam reckons that every kilogram of prawns and shrimps produced kills 20 kilograms of fish, because fish are used as feed, and because factory conditions involve constant use of antimicrobial and other chemical inputs. The 'farmers' abandon the poisoned earth every few years, move on, and destroy more mangroves. Much of the coastline of Aceh province in Indonesia is devastated by shrimp tanks that look like bomb craters.

Here is why the tsunami was not just a natural catastrophe. Coral reefs and mangrove wetlands protect against the force of the ocean. This became big news after the great waves created by the tsunami smashed into the coasts of Indonesia, Thailand, Sri Lanka, India and other countries. Reports from the Andaman and the Nicobar Islands north of Indonesia, and the more distant Maldives, told a pointed story. The reefs and the mangroves that circle these mostly 'undeveloped' islands buffered the impact of the waves, and relatively few communities were destroyed.

Many of those who died were unnaturally close to the ocean. Among them were around 9,000 people from materially rich countries, many more than died in the 11 September attacks on the USA three years earlier. Some of these tourists had their last supper at Indian Ocean seafood restaurants. The devastation caused by the tsunami was geophysical and also geopolitical.

The modern global economy costs more than you may think. International food trade is neither free nor fair. Asian governments need cash crops for dollars to help pay interest on external debts mostly incurred by previous governments. Just before he died, John Maynard Keynes, whose philosophy of economics is currently swept away by a great ideological wave, wrote: 'Prices should be fixed not at the lowest possible level, but at the level sufficient to provide producers with proper nutritional and other standards . . . It is in the interests of all producers alike that the price of a commodity should not be depressed below this level, and consumers are not entitled to expect that it should.' Just over half a century later, the finance and trade policies of the world's most powerful nations have impacted exponentially on the living world and on natural resources, as well as on the welfare, health – and the lives – of producers and consumers.

The right price for food at all stages from production to retail sale is a price that includes the cost of respect, preservation and development of human, living and physical resources. This will protect life as well as livelihoods; and in the case of the tsunami, not only the lives of Asian farmers and fishers, but also of cash-rich people whose experience of catastrophe is usually only what they see on television. This is why the overall price that was paid at the end of 2004 was higher than the price of prawns and shrimps in the shops, and why we need to think about where our food comes from.

Amplifying the possible

The second story is also about global food politics, and it's about breastfeeding. Parents need to know that the best ways to prevent babies and young children becoming fat, which are essential protection against overweight and obesity in childhood and therefore throughout life, are physical activity and extended exclusive breast feeding. This story is told in more detail, because it indicates the relationships between United Nations agencies, national governments, transnational industry, and civil society organizations, in the formulation of food and nutrition policies and practices that in this case affect all families. Also I was there. From time to time I am asked to advise United Nations agencies, or else attend UN meetings as a delegate from international civil society organizations or as a government representative. At the 1992 UN International Conference on Nutrition I was a delegate from the UK. At the January 2001 World Health Organization Executive Board meeting at WHO headquarters in Geneva I was a delegate representing the government of Brazil, and the issue was global policy on breastfeeding – or to be more exact, infant and young-child feeding.

First some background. In the previous chapter I mentioned the new United Nations agreement that babies and young children are crucially protected against overweight and obesity by being exclusively breastfed for six months and more. It's one thing to make this known, and another thing for mothers to achieve it. There are limits to what we can do for ourselves and our own families by ourselves. What is needed to support mothers is an 'enabling environment' in which it is easier – or possible – to make healthy choices.

With breastfeeding this involves governments in the enactment of laws that give mothers – and fathers too – adequate paid time off work. It implies the baby-food industry genuinely accepting that artificial formula feeds are not an adequate substitute for breastmilk except in special circumstances. It requires hospitals, clinics, midwives, physicians and other health workers to encourage mothers in their care to breastfeed exclusively. And in general, an enabling environment for breastfeeding is one in which mothers who breastfeed their children in public are accepted and welcomed.

What is also needed is agreement on the vital value of exclusive breastfeeding, and on the best length of time for mothers to breastfeed their children, at first exclusively and then with complementary food. This gives essential guidance to governments at national, state and municipal level, and to health professionals and parents. Altogether this amounts to visionary yet feasible policies and programmes – what the political philosopher John Rawls calls 'amplifying the possible'.

Needed: energetic civil society organizations

How can this be achieved? Decisions that shape food systems are usually taken by government and industry representatives together with civil servants working for the United Nations system and for other international bodies. Many such decisions are not in the public interest and lead to actions that do not improve public health. Enlightened decisions are more likely if they are informed and influenced by effective and energetic civil society organizations, working on behalf of consumers and citizens – and families and mothers.

By the mid-20th century, in most high-income countries few mothers exclusively breastfed their children for more than a couple of months, and in some such countries many and even most children were never exclusively breastfed. In low-income countries, health professionals and mothers were and still are pushed by the baby-food industry to prefer artificial formula feeds, even when water supplies are unsafe.

Beginning in the 1970s the tide turned, most of all because of the actions of the International Baby Food Action Network (IBFAN), working with Consumers International, Oxfam, War on Want, and other well-resourced civil society organizations. In alliance, these organizations have raised consciousness of the essential value of human milk for human babies, and have inspired a sympathetic response from policy-makers, especially within the World Health Organization (WHO), starting when Halfdan Mahler was director-general.

IBFAN is made up of more than 200 groups in over 100 countries, many of whose members work voluntarily. It guards the 1981 WHO International Code of Marketing of Breast-Milk Substitutes and many other WHO World Health Assembly resolutions on infant and young-child nutrition. Among all international civil society organizations concerned with food and nutrition, IBFAN in my experience is uniquely networked, intelligent and influential. It uses direct action techniques pioneered by Greenpeace, Friends of the Earth and other environmental civil society groups. It has developed phenomenal contacts based on mutual respect within the UN system, with civil servants and politicians within national governments and with the mass and specialist media.

That's the background. The story is about how a group of civil society networks, in combination with national governments throughout the world, and with backing from committed scientists and other experts, succeeded in achieving the current United Nations global strategy for infant and young-child feeding. As approved by all member states in 2002, this includes the agreement: 'Infants should be exclusively breastfed for the first six months of life to achieve optimal growth, development and health.'

Needed: engaged governments

In the year 2000, Brazil had an exceptionally ambitious, knowledgeable and focused Minister of Health, José Serra. Given the good luck of his leadership, officials working in the section of the ministry concerned with food and nutrition policy prepared a draft resolution on infant and young-child nutrition, designed to be supported by WHO member states and thus adopted globally. After a long debate at the WHO World Health Assembly in May 2000 in which delegates from 54 countries participated, the Brazilian position was accepted for further drafting at the next WHO meeting of its Executive Board in January 2001.

The Brazilian draft resolution caused a big stir, because of its assertive and comprehensive presentation and emphasis on ethics. Thanks to information from IBFAN, it took into account all relevant previously agreed WHO resolutions on the topic of infant and young-child feeding. Thanks to solidarity with health ministries throughout Asia, Africa and Latin America it effectively became the position of the South. It insisted that infant and young-child nutrition be put in the context of access to adequate food and nutrition as a basic human right. It urged reinforcement of existing laws, regulations, codes and conventions meant to enable and encourage mothers to breastfeed. It denounced the baby-food industry's use of aggressive advertising and marketing that flouts international codes, including abuse of the internet in ways that mislead health professionals and mothers into believing that artificial formula is as good as or better than breastmilk.

Another clause of the resolution proposed that the recommended period for exclusive breastfeeding be the first six months of life, rather than the then WHO policy of four to six months. This was a contentious clause, one reason being that formula feeding between four and six months, as distinct from the full six months, was reckoned in 2000 to have a value to industry of around $US1.5 billion a year. At that time 61 WHO member-state governments supported a policy of six months; these were all from Africa, Asia, Latin America, the Middle East and former USSR.

In 2000 I became involved, as international food and nutrition policy advisor at the Ministry of Health in Brasília. Late that year the Brazilian resolution was supported at a meeting of member states throughout the Americas held by the Pan American Health Organization in Washington. It was also reinforced by a report of the US Department of Health and Human Services, as a result of indomitable work by women's groups throughout the USA.

With Denise Coitinho and Elisabetta Recine of the Brazilian health ministry food and nutrition policy unit, I worked on the original resolution in order to clarify and update it, and to take into account amendments suggested during the World Health Assembly by many member states. The WHO secretariat undertook a similar exercise, which resulted in different detailed wording, notably on the 'six months versus four to six months' issue. As a result, delegates to the January 2001 WHO Executive Board meeting were presented in Geneva with three variations of the resolution: the version accepted for further drafting at the 2000 World Health Assembly, and the two new 'competing' drafts as amended by Brazil and by WHO, both of which were energetically circulated.

At all stages José Serra was adamant that while the Brazilian resolution should be improved by amendments taking in proposals made by supportive countries, it should not be diluted. Such compromises could for example try to accommodate the position of those countries that, for ideological or commercial reasons, are opposed to laws and other formal processes that impede the baby-food industry's freedom of action and general commercial freedom of expression. Notable among such countries is the USA, which contributes 22 per cent of the income of WHO, and on which many impoverished countries are dependent in one way or another.

Within the UN system the USA usually gets its way on policies considered important by the current US government, or else a compromise is agreed. However, civil society organizations, health professionals and health ministries throughout Asia, Africa, Latin America, and in the Arab and Islamic world, are united in support of extended exclusive breastfeeding, and point out that millions of babies every year who are bottle-fed, especially in areas where water supplies are unsafe, suffer diarrhoeal and other diseases, and often die.

During 2000, in preparation for the World Health Assembly and then the Executive Board meeting, women from the International Baby Food Action Network gave the Brazilian Ministry of Health information, guidance, background documents and other resources. The Brazilian resolution could not have progressed effectively without IBFAN, whose representatives lobbied politicians and senior civil servants in countries all over the world to support the resolution.

What happened in Geneva

In Geneva it was immediately apparent that WHO itself opposed the Brazilian resolution, on the grounds that the scientific evidence on the optimum period for exclusive breastfeeding was unclear. During the opening plenary session of the WHO Executive Board meeting, Gro Harlem Brundtland, then WHO director-general, argued that any discussion on the whole subject of infant and young-child feeding should be delayed until the 'six months versus four to six months' issue was resolved by the findings of a special systematic review of the epidemiological and other scientific literature commissioned by WHO which, she indicated, had not yet been completed.

In a charged atmosphere, Brazil revealed in its response to Dr Brundtland that the Brazilian delegation knew that while the systematic review might not have been finally processed or reviewed, it had already been received by WHO. So why delay? The Brazilian representative urged that Dr Brundtland agree to release the review immediately for examination by Executive Board members. This caused a palpable stir, and after a tense discussion a drafting group was agreed, to discuss the resolution, and to amend and hopefully agree it. I was Brazil's lead representative on the drafting group. Initially planned to take a day, the meeting continued for three days. It was attended by representatives of almost all Executive Board member states and a number of others as well, and also often by Dr Brundtland and an array of WHO senior executives and advisors.

We in the Brazilian delegation knew that the resolution would be opposed by the US delegation, which was being led not by the Department of Health and Human Services, but by officials from the State Department. Friendly European delegates warned us that the European Union nations had collectively agreed that if the US opposition to the Brazilian resolution was supported by even just one country from Asia, Africa or Latin America or elsewhere in the South, the EU block vote would swing to support the USA.

During three days of intense and sometimes heated discussion an increasing number of member states stated their support for the Brazilian position, or else proposed supportive amendments. Finally the resolution based on the Brazilian draft was agreed, suitably strengthened and clarified, with allowance either for 'six months' or 'four to six months' pending the official emergence of the special review.

During this process the US delegation stated that the clause condemning abuse of the internet was unacceptable, insisted on freedom of commercial expression, and repeated that 'we have no flexibility on this point'. Eventually the Brazilian flag was raised and the question asked: 'On behalf of Brazil and also bearing in mind all discussion so far, is there any member state here represented that supports the position of the delegation from the USA?' No flag was raised from the South. No flag was raised from Europe. The chairman of the meeting accepted the clause as drafted, acknowledged that the USA was isolated, and declared that the entire resolution as amended in the drafting committee was agreed.

This was accepted by the whole Executive Board in plenary session. Three months later WHO announced that the special review supported six months of exclusive breastfeeding, which accordingly became part of the new WHO global strategy on infant and young-child feeding, after final debate and agreement at the World Health Assembly later that year and then the next year.

Commenting, the epidemiologist César Victora of the University of Pelotas in Brazil, one of the scientists responsible for assessing the systematic review, said: 'For fifteen years we have been accumulating evidence on the benefits of exclusive breastfeeding, and this has at last led to a change in global policy. The scientist's greatest frustration is when our studies do not result in changes in the real world.'

A VISION FOR THIS CENTURY

Until recently – even into the 1990s – it seemed to make sense to draw a line between what is good for us, and what is good for other people, for the fabric of society, and for the planet. Now these divisions are dissolving in favour of an integrated approach, because of the force of circumstances. As examples, it is now generally accepted that the world's climate is changing, and that non-renewable sources of energy and water are becoming depleted, soil is becoming eroded, degraded and contaminated, forests are disappearing, deserts are growing, and that modern methods of industrial farming cannot be sustained. A 2001 World Bank report states: 'Environmental problems are imposing severe human, economic, and social costs, and threatening the foundation on which growth, and ultimately survival, depend.'

Now the mood of socially responsible scientists is shifting. An increasing number of professionals working in food and nutrition science and policy, and allied fields, are paying special attention to the economic, social and environmental aspects and implications of their work. They are thinking and acting in the spirit of the champions of the great public health movements of the 19th century, who insisted on the social responsibilities of scientists, and who campaigned to ensure that the ruling classes of the time funded great public works, such as closed drains, to protect the health of populations.

In 2002 the Indaba Declaration was agreed on the occasion of the World Summit on Sustainable Development in Johannesburg, South Africa. (In the KwaZulu language *indaba* means 'a gathering to make agreements on important matters'.) This was prepared and signed by representatives of civil society organizations and international agencies from all over the world, together with academics and the

South African Department of Health, and published by the World Health Organization.

It states: 'The nature and quality of food systems, and therefore of diet and nutrition, are fundamental determinants of human health and welfare, and that of the whole living and natural world.' It emphasizes underlying and basic causes of disease, including: 'Inadequate sanitation, polluted water; poverty, inequality, injustice; personal, communal and national debt; unemployment, dangerous environments, precipitate urbanization; unsustainable agriculture, land degradation; poor governance, expropriation, dislocation; the effects of colonialism, unfair terms of trade, subsidy of industry in high-income countries; destruction of indigenous and traditional food systems and culture; commodity speculation, unregulated markets, aggressive promotion of degraded, cheapened and energy-dense food and drink; the use of food aid and trade as an instrument of power; and persecution, terror and war.'

So what is the way forward? 'Successful and accepted public policies for example concerning transport, energy, firearms, tobacco, alcohol and water, include legal, regulatory and fiscal instruments designed to balance the interests of civil society with those of industry and government. The protection and creation of healthy food systems, integral to healthy environments and to human health, also requires the use of law, regulation and pricing policy.'

The urgent need to make decisive moves was then also emphasized in the Giessen Declaration, the product of a 2005 workshop held with the purpose of agreeing new directions for nutrition science. This states: 'For the first time in human experience, the overall size and the economic activity of humankind exceeds the capacity of the planet to supply, replenish and absorb.' (For more on the Declaration and its context, see Annex I.)

Industry is moving

Food systems must and will improve and become fit for this 21st century. This depends on the active and enthusiastic collaboration and indeed leadership of industry, including transnational food manufacturers, supported by international and national government, and always pressed by an intelligent and informed demand from consumers and citizens.

Agreement and action on climate change continues to depend on its acknowledgement by leading oil, fuel, car and associated companies, and action that will be effective only if supported and indeed driven by industry. Likewise, the food systems and supplies that make us fat and diseased will change for the better only when energetic civil society organizations and engaged governments and scientists work together, and are joined by leaders of the transnational food and drink industries determined to change the profile of their products and the shape of their customers. Leaders within the giant food and drink industries know that 'business as usual' is not a feasible strategy.

WHAT YOU CAN DO

In writing this book I have been thinking of you as an individual and also as a member of a family and community. You may yourself want to reduce excess body fat, or there may be people in your life who want to do so. By now I hope I have convinced you that restricting dietary energy from food and drink is not the way. You may also be generally concerned about the phenomenal increase in obesity including among children and young people of your own and most other countries, with the corresponding increase in dieting regimes, and the evidence that the world epidemic of obesity is now out of control.

The actual and potential impact of obesity is less than that of climate change. But the industrialized food systems that drive overweight and obesity are part of the climate change problem. A special 2007 *Lancet* series on energy and health estimated that industrial agriculture contributes over one-fifth of all greenhouse gas emissions, a figure similar to that of all other industry.

Many of the economic, social and environmental causes of obesity, such as the replacement of the family meal by convenience and fast foods, the increase in production and consumption of industrially reared meat, and reliance on cars and other machines to do the physical work humans are designed to do, drain non-renewable energy resources, contribute to environmental degradation, accelerate atmospheric pollution, and for these and other reasons are also a major cause of climate change.

As a global public health crisis I would rate the impact of obesity as well below that of HIV-AIDS, smoking and other uses of tobacco, unsafe water, and multiply drug-resistant 'superbugs'. But it's in that league. And by definition, like all issues of *public* health, obesity is not just about mistaken or unwise personal choices.

It is only the most privileged people, and mostly those who live in the most protected societies, who are able consistently to make choices that will safeguard their health and wellbeing, and that of their family. But nobody is insulated from the impact of external forces. Thus, how can parents protect their children against the ill-effects of sugared drinks on sale in vending machines placed within schools, and how can families who live in cities without parks and other open spaces become physically active as part of their everyday lives?

Obesity is a symptom of the much greater malaise of producing and consuming more than is good for us in ways that abuse other creatures, wreck the environment, and threaten future life on earth. A book on obesity as a sign of our times, its social, economic, commercial, political, environmental and other dimensions, and its being part of a greater whole, is due to be written. Such a book needs also to state what can and must be done by transnational, national and local government and industry, and civil society organizations.

In this and the next chapter I am addressing you as a citizen as well as a consumer, with much more potential power than you have merely as a voter. Speak out! As a shopper, tell supermarket managers why you don't buy cheapened or degraded products. As a parent, press your child's school governors to eliminate machines that sell soft drinks. As an employee, ask your place of work to provide changing facilities. As a traveller, praise the managers of hotels whose stairs are easy to find and agreeable to use. Go further! Write to the big bosses of the companies responsible for products and practices you know are bad, and also those you know are good, stating your views and preferences, and copy the letter to your local legislator. Better still, become an active member of civil society organizations already dedicated to improve public health by means of good food.

Our whole lives

Your wellbeing is good for your sake, and is helpful for your family, friends, colleagues and community. But if we want to believe that we are making any kind of a difference, what else are we doing with our lives? What are the models for wisely led lives that also take into account the circumstances and the aspirations of the peoples of Africa, Asia and Latin America, our place and purpose as humans here on the planet, and what we know now about climate change and the depletion of natural resources? We will do well to think more about where we are going, and why.

Now that I live in Latin America I see North America and Europe differently. Having spent most of my life in London, when I visit its centre now I enjoy what big cities offer – visionary discussions, exciting ideas, parks, books, concerts, theatre, art, architecture, and delicious meals, some based on great cuisines. Now also though I am more aware of the reasons why so many goods in the shops are so cheap. Overall, London's ecological footprint, all the resources the city uses, is 120 times its own size, an area the size of Britain. This cannot continue for much longer. The financial systems that keep the materially rich nations afloat now seem like patched rubber rafts drifting on stormy seas.

If everybody in the world consumed like the average person in the USA, we would need four extra planets. The estimate for the UK is three extra planets. The Global Footprint Network, set up to calculate the impact of human consumption on the earth's resources, calculates that the total ecological footprint of the human species worldwide exceeded the planet's carrying capacity in the 1980s, and by the turn of the 21st century was around 20 per cent above that level. In 2007 the earth was calculated to have gone into 'ecological debt' on 6 October. Near the turn of the century the originators of the ecological footprint concept reckoned that: 'To accommodate sustainably the anticipated increase in population and economic output of the next four decades, we would require six to twelve additional planets.'

Here is hoping that you have your own sense of how life on earth can be, in your lifetime and that of your grandchildren. I have a reason to think about this every day. As I complete this chapter my son Gabriel, who will be four years old when this book is first published, comes up the spiral stairs to my study, gives me the drawing he has just made, and presses a Smilemaker sticky red heart (yes, made in China) on to my hand. I want what I have written to make sense to him. Soon it will be his turn to make sense of being human.

You do not need to move from where you are right now to begin to fulfil yourself. This includes eating and drinking well, as part of acting and living right. Read and reflect, take a walk, and begin with yourself.

Your good health!

6. YOUR SEVEN GOLDEN RULES

There is no sincerer love than the love of food.

George Bernard Shaw

People have a duty to those who are not yet born. That duty is not merely to give them existence but to give them happiness.

Marie Jean Condorcet

Here is how: the system for you to enhance your positive good health and also to reduce excess body weight and fat. These seven golden rules incorporate the most reliable knowledge and wisdom on the best quality food and drink.

Good health is not just physical; it is an aspect of the good life, which includes the enjoyment of food and drink. Here is the way to protect your wellbeing and that of your family and children, of future generations, and of the planet.

For a long time now I have been thinking about how to make what I know and believe about eating and drinking, physical activity, health and wellbeing, work in real everyday life. Here it is. In this chapter, with its seven sections and its notes, I guide you towards getting and staying in good shape, and to being happier, healthier, more energetic, and generally better able to do what you want to do and be who you want to be.

What follows are seven golden rules for how to eat, drink, and act right. They amount to a system for you and for everybody. They will develop your positive health and wellbeing and that of your family. They are also for you if you want to reduce your body fat and weight.

You will not find the word 'should' here, in the sense that you must do this or must not do that. It's up to you. There is no finger-wagging here. What you do – including as a member of a family and community with mutual responsibilities and obligations – is for you to decide.

The rules are a path of self-exploration to put you on the right way to fulfilling your human potential. When you have got into the habit of following the rules, and have worked out how to adapt them to suit yourself, you will be enjoying lots of delicious and healthy food and drink, and will also be enjoying yourself more – maybe more than since you were a child.

Once you have made the rules your own and built them into your way of life, you will be protecting yourself against many diseases the risks of which are affected by food and nutrition. Also, inasmuch as food and drink and physical activity can, your new way of life will help to control any disease you have, before or after it is diagnosed.

The system is also for you as a citizen as well as a consumer. The foods and drinks you will be consuming generally make fewer demands on living and physical resources. The rules are a guide to eating and drinking with respect for the makers of food, for the living and physical world, and for the biosphere of which we humans are a part. What does us good, does good.

THIS IS FOR LIFE

As I have just mentioned, and as indicated in the first words of this chapter, these rules do include a reliable and sustainable way to reduce your body weight. If this is what you want to do, please be patient. As you know from chapters 3 and 4 – and as your experience and thinking may well already have told you – dieting trains the body to become increasingly fat; sedentary people are in artificially low energy balance; and sugary, fatty, energy-dense processed foods and drinks also make you fat. The answer is to train your body to build up lean tissue, to raise your energy balance to a natural level, and to displace energy-dense processed products by consuming lots of naturally satisfying whole fresh and benignly processed foods that do not induce cravings, without restricting dietary energy.

Rules 1 to 6 are all about training yourself to become positively fit and healthy. In this time you may not reduce your body weight, but you will become in better shape and will increase your lean tissue including muscle. It is highly likely that you will reduce your body fat – which is really what you want to do. Your physical activity and the fresh foods and drinks you will be consuming will also change the quality of your skin and flesh, and you will become less flabby.

So yes, you will be rewarded from the start – how much will depend a lot on how prepared you are to follow the rules as specified, in the spirit in which they are set out. These six months are essential training if you want to become and remain lighter, or slim. How much your body weight and shape will change in the first six months will depend on who you are, how old you are, how often you have dieted, your situation and circumstances, and how closely you follow the rules in making them work for you.

This is not a regime to be followed and then set aside while you resume 'ordinary' life, like a dietary equivalent of going to church at Easter, Christmas and when you get married. That's not the idea at all. Think of it as more like learning to switch from using a pen or a typewriter to using a computer. Once you got used to processing words, sending and receiving emails, and using the internet, did you want to go back to relying solely on typewriting, snail-mail and libraries? No, you did not. The same is so here.

There is no such thing as a magic cure. No one system and no one way of life can be completely successful for everybody. Also, many people who start to think about protecting their health in ways other than what's offered by conventional medicine do so after becoming debilitated or disabled. Further, if you are very fat, or crave some forms of processed foods or drinks, or illicit or prescribed drugs, or alcohol or tobacco, or if you are at a bad time in your life or suffer depression, please don't expect a transformed you even in six or seven months. It often takes a long time to lose wellbeing, so give yourself plenty of time to gain it. Also, if you are physically impeded or disabled you will need to adapt the second rule on physical activity. However, none of these are reasons to stop reading at this point and to assume the system is not for you. It is.

We are all mortal

No way of life is proof against disease. Conscious eating and drinking is just one part of an enlightened way of life. No way of life prevents mortality. We will all die. Also, we are all born more or less vulnerable to disease in general and to particular diseases. By the time we choose to live well, all sorts of detected and undetected pathologies may already have developed in our bodies. Healing has limits. There is no elixir against life's blows.

Often people become focused on their own good health and that of others after they realize that they are unusually vulnerable to illness, or because of bad experiences for which conventional medical treatment proved ineffective. You will have your own history to date. We can't trade ourselves in for a new model. We have to make the best of what we have got, which is us as we are now and for the rest of our lives, with all the powers of physical, mental, emotional and spiritual healing we are born with and have developed, and with our unique human ability – when we choose – to live in sympathy with one another and with the whole living and physical world.

THE GENERAL IDEA

The general idea behind these golden rules is as follows. You will develop your good health and wellbeing by consuming more food and drink – in terms of weight and bulk – than is typical where food systems are industrialized. At the same time you will become more physically active, building up to the levels to which humans are evolved and adapted. This is crucial. It is abnormal and unnatural to lead a sedentary life. You will also be more part of your family, social and professional life when your diet – not your dieting! – includes enjoying the feasts that mark special occasions.

You will be adapting and adjusting the system to suit your own way of life, so that you become and remain nutritionally, physiologically and metabolically a normal and natural human being. You will be making good use of the privileges and advantages of living in an environment where food and drink is secure and abundant, as I guess you do. (The notes to this introduction include more information.)

In the first six months please allow yourself to have no intention to reduce your weight, and please do not panic if your weight increases somewhat, especially at first. Simply go with the process and observe what happens. If you have been in the dieting trap you may at first find this system strange and even scary. Remember always that you are becoming fitter and are better nourished, which will protect your health, enhance your pleasure in life, and is essential training in order to be ready to lose body weight reliably. If when you approach the seventh month you still want to reduce your body weight, the seventh golden rule shows you how. Please follow the six-month system before following the seventh rule. By itself in isolation it will not work

Starting, continuing, completing

Introduce the golden rules one at a time. Start with rule 1 and follow it for one month, without making any other conscious deliberate change in your eating, drinking, physical activity, or any other habits. Celebrate every rule, most of which may involve big changes for you. Be aware of what happens as you follow the rules, find out how easy or difficult they are, notice their effects as the months go on, and stay with them as best you can.

If you do not follow any rule for a day, or for longer, for whatever reason, never mind; don't be discouraged. This happens. (Yes, this happens to me.) Don't be self-judgmental. Just observe. Keep a daily record and simply make a note of such days and the reasons why you did not follow the rule, and note these missed days during the month. Also record all the sequences of days when you did follow the rules, and how you felt about this. This system is designed to make you feel good. You will probably find it easier and simpler to follow the rules in the mornings and afternoons, and to reserve most or even all of whatever else you consume to the later part of day and evenings.

Rule 1, as you will see, is about water. The one difference you make in your diet in this first month is the amount of water you drink. That's all. Nothing else. Rule 2 is about physical activity. In this second month continue to follow rule 1, and also incorporate rule 2 into your way of life. And so on. You stay with each of the rules, adding them one by one, throughout the six or seven months. Then you will have incorporated the whole system into your way of life – and, if you take my advice, permanently. Better still, once you have followed the system you will have found out how to adapt it in ways that work best for you.

Once you start to follow a rule, you may want to move to the next rule before the end of the month. Please don't. You will also be tempted to try to practise other habits you think are good, and stop those you think are bad. Please don't. Yes, even smoking. Take one step at a time. You are likely to find that in due course some eating and drinking habits, and other habits, change 'by themselves'. One day you may notice that you don't feel like drinking more than two cups of coffee a day, or are losing your desire for sugared foods and drinks, or can taste chemical taints in packaged foods whose eat-by dates are next month or year. New habits may get you out of old habits. Which these are depends on your nature. In general you will become more sensitive to anything toxic in your internal and external environment. These are not promises, but observations.

Become conscious of any changes in the level or nature of your desires for food, and hunger and appetite. Hunger, appetite and satiety are complex. With time you will become more aware of what your body wants and needs.

Natural needs and desires tend to be obscured, debauched or corrupted when you have habitually consumed foods and drinks formulated to make you want to purchase and consume more and more of them. Remember that the food manufacturing industry employs thousands of technicians whose job it is to formulate products designed to make you want to consume them again and again. There are differences only in degree between foods and drinks that are 'more-ish' and foods and drinks that induce cravings or are in a real sense addictive. Metaphors as in 'I could murder a four-cheese pizza' or 'I'm a chocoholic' or 'I couldn't perform without my morning coffee hit' or 'I'm going out for my sugar rush' are revealing.

Be warned against such foods and drinks. Be careful not to consume more of them than you have in the past as you follow the golden rules. If you lose desire for them and don't feel like eating or drinking them any more, of course feel free to stop, but my advice is not to push yourself to *try* to give them up. Stay with the system and see what happens. Also notice the time you need to get used to the change and its effects on your nature, and also your growing awareness of the social and environmental aspects of the way of life you are now creating for yourself.

Have a little faith

Is it best to follow the rules by yourself, or in company with your partner, a friend or colleague, or your family? People generally become ready to go on journeys at different times and different ways. However, if someone close to you really does want to travel with you, then great, go for it together. Also if you are undertaking this journey alone, you will be helped enormously if those closest to you support you, emotionally and practically.

The first step on a long journey is always the most important. Don't start impulsively. Please read this whole book before deciding to act on this final chapter, and before you do, think about how you can interpret and adapt the rules to make them work for you. If some things don't ring true you can check out the notes to these rules and the previous chapters. An unserious attitude of 'oh well, I'll give it a whirl' won't work. If you have a go and then stop, you will have put up a barrier against starting again.

What you will be doing is learning a skill of living well, while at the same time living as you have done, and consciously emerging from one state to the other. This is different from learning one more skill in addition to those you already have. It is more like a spiritual exercise. Indeed, your heart and spirit are in this, together with your mind and body.

What's easy, what's hard

What about the rules which are easy to follow? Or suppose you are already following some of the rules? But why should all rules be hard to follow? Besides, the whole idea is to follow each rule consciously until it is becoming part of your nature. The change is to what you *do*, and also to your attitude to what you do. This requires attention and should be interesting. Follow each rule as a project, and do some research of your own, on the internet or through your library.

What about the rules which are hard? Suppose some seem impossible, or address habits that you think you can't break? But why should all rules be easy to follow? Some habits are ingrained, especially those of a compulsive nature. The sequence of the rules takes this into account. If you really feel that you can't follow one or more of the rules by yourself, ask your family or colleagues for support. You may enhance their lives too.

Does 'every little bit count'? Will your health and wellbeing improve if you go just some of the way to following any or all of the rules? Yes. Here are two examples. If you are able-bodied but sedentary and unfit, it will take you some time fully to follow rule 2 on physical activity – you may need 'to get into training to get into training'. If this describes you, simply build up to the levels specified week by week within the second month, or take longer if you need to. Similarly, rule 3 on vegetables, pulses (legumes) and fruits almost certainly specifies amounts way above what you eat now. If you are seriously daunted, build up to what's specified, also making allowance for your size, gender and age, a week at a time within the third month.

This said though, I don't agree with the 'softly, softly' approach. You must decide just how important is your positive health and whole wellbeing, for yourself and as an example to others in your life. These days most people in their 60s in high-income countries are suffering from a serious disorder or disease, and for an average of over ten years before they die, their lives are made miserable and often their finances eventually destroyed by the expensive and painful treatments they endure for conditions that are largely preventable. All this is avoidable. So you can see how valuable the information and advice in this chapter is for you. Yes, taken all together, the system does point towards ways of life radically different from the unhealthy and dangerous 'lifestyles' of most people these days. That's the whole idea!

You may now be braced for yet another version of 'how to deprive yourself in order to live longer' regime, but this is not one of those. There is much more to the good life than absence of disease. The first five rules are all about more, not less. You may think as you preview them that the tough ones are the sixth, which is about fasting, and the seventh, which is about how sustainably to reduce body fat and weight, but I predict that once you have made yourself ready for them, you will enjoy them. By that stage you will have had five months of developing and enjoying good habits. Any form of training is hardest at first. In general, when you tackle hard-to-break habits, the first few days will be hard, and even sometimes very hard; and then your body learns and adapts. Combine a little faith with some self-discipline.

The tips and also the text of some of the rules, especially 6 and 7, include the term 'avoid', as for example, 'avoid all branded foods that make health claims'. This is stronger than 'limit', but it does not mean 'eliminate' – unless this is your choice. What it means is 'don't consume these foods and drinks as part of this rule unless you really want to, and if you do, keep them as occasional delicacies or treats'. For adults, delicacies include *delicatessen* (as the word suggests). Thus, I am partial to smoked cheese, and also to tinned sardines, which I enjoy maybe once every two weeks. With children take care with treats though: rewarding them with fatty or sugary junky foods creates a troublesome habit that will be hard to break.

You will learn more from cookery books and from selecting and preparing food yourself, than from nutrition handbooks and dieting regimes, and certainly more than from dieting regimes and recipes. But choose and use cookery books with care: these usually emphasize feast food, and some of them sophisticate original and traditional basic recipes with extra ingredients and added fats and sugars. Pick the simplest recipes for everyday dishes, preferring those using foods you can source locally.

RESOURCES

What do you need to make the system work for you?

Time and money

What about the time and money involved? People who buy books usually have money, time and resources to do what they most want to do. If you really want to buy or do something, you can choose to do so – as well as, or if necessary instead of, other things. Come on, own up!

The comparative costs of the system are not estimated here. To do so might suggest hesitancy about putting a value on developing and protecting your human potential. If that's how you feel you may well not follow the rules, because of infirmity of purpose and lack of self-respect, or simply because you are not yet ready. Following the system may end up costing you more money, or less, depending on the choices you make within the rules. Students and people on low incomes can make them work. Much of what is here I have learned from the traditions and teachings of societies with far fewer material resources than you are likely to have.

And time? Yes, following the system will take up more of your time. This is part of the whole idea, to value food, drink and physical activity and to give them more importance in your life. If now you eat and drink out or eat ready-to-heat meals most days, or if following the system means that you or somebody else buys food and drink just for you while the rest of your household eats and drinks what they are used to, it will take up quite a lot more of your or their time. One of the skills you will learn is how to integrate the rules into your way of life, during which you will discover which of your other time-consuming activities become less interesting. The more skilled you get, the less the system will be an 'add-on extra'. Also, physically active people who eat well often need less sleep and usually sleep well and wake up refreshed.

Measurements

The Zen approach to personal transformation is pure meditation and contemplation, but I am not at that stage, and I doubt you are either. So do keep regular records and notes along the way and summarize them every month. Map these out before you start. Sustained attention creates change for the better.

At this point many self-improvement books print a lot of pages of tables for you to follow and fill in, which bulk out the books and make them look methodical and scientific, but there is no need for this. Here is what I suggest.

If you are healthy in the usual sense there are some physical measurements and checks I recommend you take and make yourself. These are: body weight, waist circumference, heart rate at rest, blood pressure, and frequency and nature of urine and faeces. These are the routine checks old-fashioned physicians make, directly or by enquiry. Of these, blood pressure is the only one for which you need a kit – available at many pharmacies.

Make a note of symptoms like changes in energy levels, imaginative activity and sleep patterns, as well as headaches, faintness and pains – anything that seems remarkable by presence or absence. Measure also how long it takes for your heart rate to return to its resting rate 3, 10 and 20 minutes after physical activity, for colds, sore throats and other transient malaises to resolve, and for wounds to heal.

Keep a daily diary. My method is to use my large-format work diary, and I tick off the items as they are done. (Yes, sometimes there are crosses.) More detailed notes and comments, including monthly summaries, are kept in specially designed folders and files on my computer. You may also find it helpful to record what you discover while researching the topic of each rule as you come to it.

List your sense of your physical, mental, emotional and spiritual wellbeing, rated on a 0–10 scale. As well as this quantified approach, note how you feel and what you want, and summarize these notes once a month. Even if you have to pay special attention to your physical condition because of a diagnosed disease, do pay equal attention to other states. When these are disordered one result is often physical disease, and when they are in harmony the symptoms often fade away. If when you start you don't have a sense of what's spiritual, don't cross this off: list it, leave the category blank, and then see what happens.

What about other measurements? At this point self-improvement books tend to suggest that you consult a professional who will analyse the chemistry of an impressive list of fractions of your body fluids and other bits that are relatively easy to drain or snip. Unless you really do want to become an expert on your personal biochemistry, I advise against taking this route. There is no need, and such professionals are likely to have their own ideas and methods. If you prefer theirs to this system, that's your choice, but don't try both at the same time. Also any quasi-medical approach will tend to turn you into a subject, a patient, with less responsibility for your own life. This system is designed to make you more self-responsible.

If you are already diagnosed with a serious disease, or have any misgivings or doubts, do indeed consult your physician. It is extremely unlikely that this system could do you any harm. What is much more likely, once you and your consultant agree what measurements to take, is that those relevant to general wellbeing, physical good health – and maybe even those specific to your disease – will improve as time goes on. You will be giving your physician something to think about.

If you are undergoing any form of medical therapy, this needs careful monitoring. Your reaction to drugs or other treatments may well change. The most usual change is that your doses will have a more potent therapeutic – and also toxic – effect and will have to be lowered. If you are on medication, do not make any changes to the dose without consulting your physician or other health professional.

What to do when you are unwell, the obvious example being with a viral or bacterial infection that makes you feel rotten, like a cold or a bug in your guts? Here is where this system becomes especially valuable. The best advice is to do what your body is telling your mind; and the further you are into this system, the clearer these messages will be. The best general advice is to rest. Take it easy, look after yourself, and don't force yourself to do anything. Frequent transient infections like colds are a sign that you are too stressed. This does not necessarily mean that you should be less physically active, but it might. If you don't feel like eating, don't, and if you only feel like eating small amounts, do so. When your body is trained and tuned it will give your mind very clear signals about the foods and drinks it needs at times of illness.

THE SEVEN GOLDEN RULES

The seven golden rules that follow are all structured the same way. First there is the principle that guides the rule. Then comes what, followed by why, in which the rule is specified and explained. Then there is how much, meaning what quantities are involved, followed by what effect following each rule is likely to have on your body fat and weight. Next is how you can fit the rule into your life. Then the question is asked, is it safe? This is followed by warnings. Then comes who says, and what is the wisdom of the ages. Then there are some tips, for you and for everybody in your life including children, and finally some big picture stuff.

What's here, what's not here?

If you have looked at books and articles on how to eat and drink well, you may be expecting lots and lots of information about the selenium content of iceberg lettuce, the milligrams per 100 grams of trans-fatty acids in cream crackers, and the number of grams/ounces in a portion size/serving of bouillabaisse. There is none of this here. Self-improvement books also often print pages of tables of energy requirements, so you can learn how many calories or kilojoules are needed by invalids and athletes as well as able-bodied average-type people to stay in energy balance. Such information is needed by dietitians and other nutrition professionals whose job is to plan institutional food supplies or the diets of individual patients or clients. You do not need to know.

The amounts recommended are for most adults and children aged twelve and above. The lower amounts are for people who are relatively small or inactive, or older. The upper amounts are for people who are relatively big or active. For children under the age of twelve, scale down the amounts just like you scale down the portions of food and drink they have now. If you really are unusual, say a big, young, male sporty type, or a small-framed inactive elderly woman, scale up or down to suit yourself.

As you will see, rules 1, 3 and 4 specify weights of foods and drinks. Yes, you will need to measure these and check. Start by weighing the specified foods on scales, because in breaking current habits and making new habits, you do need to check, and you will sometimes be surprised.

Weighing food takes time at first, but it's a lot less tedious than calculating calories, and by the second week of each month you probably will have a good idea of what's involved. It is also a good idea to check weights occasionally, to make sure you are on the right lines.

The section in each rule on 'who says?' gives some information on how the rule relates to expert opinion. Bear in mind though that few people conventionally trained in nutrition and allied sciences have any special knowledge of wellbeing or of mental, emotional and spiritual as well as physical health, or for that matter the relationship between human health and that of the living and physical world. Nobody has academic, professional or other formal qualifications to pronounce on wellbeing. This is more about wisdom than knowledge.

The sections in each rule on the wisdom of the ages may be more enlightening. This mostly refers to ancient and traditional teaching, custom and practice. The world of health does not start in 1980 when scholarship was first collected systematically on electronic databases. Throughout history those philosophers who took a special interest in how to live the good life – among them many of the most learned and scrupulous scholars, observers and teachers of their day – recorded much acute observation and wise advice.

Life as a whole

Until the mid-19th century the discipline of dietetics was all about eating and drinking wisely as a vital part of living well. This is the right attitude. Much of the teachings and practices of natural philosophers was thrown out or went underground with the rise of modern medicine. Some of the ideas of antiquity seem to be of curiosity value only, but many are as accurate and valuable now as then.

The final section of each golden rule is about us as part of the whole living and physical world – the big picture stuff. This book only touches on the answers to the social, economic and environmental and other big issues that relate to food systems and to what we eat and drink. It does ask some of the basic questions, and if you don't know the questions you can't know the answers.

This system is a 21st-century map for transformation through food and nutrition. It distils a lot of knowledge and reflection. I am your guide now, but once you have begun your journey, the first person to trust is you.

Golden Rule 1

WATER
Drink plenty of water

Principle

To get all the water our bodies need, from water.

What

'Water' here includes all safe water: tap water, filtered water, mineral water, and safe spring, well, rain, and river water.

This means water as such. Yes, 98 per cent of the weight of melon, 80 per cent of the weight of cooked rice and potatoes, and well over half the weight of meat is water, and so on and on. No, none of this counts. Nor does the water in soups, yoghurts or in any drink – fruit juices, cola or other soft drinks whether sugared or 'diet', 'energy drinks', milk, coffee, tea, no, none of these count; nor of course do alcoholic drinks. And nor does water with anything added, such as sugar, salt, electrolytes, fruit or herb essences, or chemicals.

Fizzy carbonated water is fine, as of course is cooled and iced water. Water with a twist of lemon is OK. Bottled spring and mineral waters are fine, but water concentrated in minerals, like those you may be offered at health spas, does not count. Nor do tonic waters. If you like the taste of salty bottled waters, limit these to one glass a day as a treat.

Why

We need water for our bodies to function properly, and to refresh and cleanse our body and its vital systems. Water refreshes and cleanses you inside as well as outside.

All systems of the body need and use water, and plenty of water is vital for the digestive system. The average amount of water excreted a day is, for people living in temperate climates, a bit over 2 litres, of which almost half is urine and almost half exhalation from all surfaces of the body. In hot weather and hot climates the amount from sweat increases, sometimes greatly.

When you drink plenty of water, your kidneys, liver and other vital organs are better refreshed. Your urine becomes straw-coloured, as you will see. The flushing of the toxins in tea, coffee and alcohol out of the body increases urine flow; this diuretic effect dehydrates the tissues. More water within the digestive system helps towards a sense of feeling satisfied.

As well as all its other benefits, drinking plenty of water is likely to mean that you will not drink some other things. However, please do not *try* to change any of your other eating and drinking habits. Give your mind a rest and let your body do what it wants to do.

How much

Drink 2 litres (about 4 pints) of water, every day.

This amount is an average. As with all the rules involving amounts, scale this amount down or up according to your size and gender. If you are a small older woman, 1½ litres will do. If you are a big younger man, 2½ litres is better.

This is if you live in a temperate climate. When you feel you need more, for example after exercise in the sun, drink more until you feel satisfied. If you live in a hot tropical climate, drink up to twice this amount. Don't wait until you feel thirsty.

Effect on body fat and weight

People who are weight-conscious are sometimes afraid to drink water because it is heavy – 2 litres weighs 2 kilograms or 4½ pounds. If you are initially dehydrated, drinking more water will certainly increase your weight on the first days – though not of course your body fat. But you will feel and look better.

It is sometimes said that if you drink plenty of water, after a while you will lose weight. The theory is that the bulk of water in your stomach and gut will help to make you feel full, but there is not much evidence that this is so. However, drinking water instead of sugared soft or other sweetened drinks will certainly reduce your weight and body fat.

Fitting it in

Anybody can drink 2 litres of water a day – more or less according to your size, gender and age, as indicated above. Like any new way of being, it takes time to become a habit. Get used to drinking and savouring water when you are not thirsty. Suit yourself how you do this.

Being somewhat into ritual, my own way when I am working at home – like now as I am writing this – is every morning to fill a 2-litre bottle with a handle (that once held cheap wine) from the water filter in the kitchen, and keep refilling a big tumbler also beside me on my desk. You can do the same from the water fountain at work or, if necessary, take bottles of water into work. Jugs of water by the bedside are also a good idea – and see 'tips', below.

Is it safe?

Sure. What do you think might happen? That you burst like a sodden balloon? That your bladder explodes? The chance of you doing yourself some internal injury, even at water intakes much higher than here, falls within the being struck by lightning range of possibility. The more water you drink, the more water is processed by your kidneys, flushed through your system and urinated out – as you will discover. While your body is adjusting you may at first need to get up in the night once or twice to urinate, but once your system becomes accustomed to absorbing and holding more water this will happen less often.

Are there cases of people who retain water pathologically and suffer and even die as a result? Absolutely, the medical term is 'water intoxication', and nutrition textbooks include information like this, which helps nutrition students pass examinations. To take the opposite extreme, the New York marathon winner Alberto Salazar sweated off 2.79 litres of water an hour measured in training for the 1984 event. And this was not a function of speed; running at not much more than half his pace I dropped 10 pounds (4.5 kilos) as a result of running the (generously measured) St Albans half-marathon in my best time of 1.33.39 on a hot June day in 1982, meaning I was sweating at roughly the same rate. Could immediately knocking back six liquor jugs full of water with or without added electrolytes, sugar, alcohol, or whatever, possibly have done me or the great Alberto a serious mischief? This is conceivable, if we had weak or damaged kidneys. But there would be little chance of being unaware of this, besides which everybody who runs long distance now drinks water throughout the race. Give the process time. After a while the best judge of the effect of all these rules will be you.

Warning

As you will see, the golden rules do not include any prohibitions, and rules 3-5 specify consuming more of highly nourishing foods and drinks. You therefore could interpret the rules in unhelpful ways. Take drinks. If you currently drink a lot of sugared soft drinks, or a lot of alcohol, you could interpret this rule by drinking the specified amount of water, and then also drinking even more sugared soft or alcoholic drinks than you did before starting the system. Obviously you can see that this would be a bad idea, but it needs mentioning.

My guess is that you are most unlikely to want to do any such thing and I don't think you need my advice not to do so. But if there are some drinks that you do crave or to which you are addicted, and you delay drinking them until later in the day than usual to ensure you drink all your water, this might cause you to knock back more of them. If this is an issue for you, watch out.

Who says?

Guidelines issued by the World Health Organization and by most national governments and authoritative organizations do not often mention water. Water does not appear as an entry in the food composition tables used by professionals to calculate the nutritional value of foods. Little conventional scientific research is undertaken on water.

In all these cases this is, I suppose, because 'there is nothing in water'. Certainly, it does not contain the energy, carbohydrates, fats and proteins and all their fractions, or vitamins (although it may contain measurable amounts of minerals). However, water is a nutrient by any sensible definition, and it does have weight and bulk.

The official dietary guidelines issued in 2005 by the Brazilian government do, I am pleased and proud to say, include advice on water similar to this rule. In Latin America a few other countries also make a recommendation to drink water. And that is about it.

In the USA the 'healthy food pyramid' issued by the US Department of Agriculture has now become many pyramids for different stages of life. The pyramid for the over-70s, who are reckoned to be at risk of dehydration, recommends consumption of much the same amount of water as here. Some guides also recommend lots of water as therapy for gallstones and kidney stones. My view is that it is better to stop dehydration and furring up of the gallbladder and kidneys before these conditions start.

Wisdom of the ages

Water, one of the four classical elements, has throughout history been recommended as essential to the good life. The 17th-century physician Thomas Sydenham, 'the English Hippocrates', said: 'I had rather undertake the practice of physick with pure air, pure water and good food alone than with all the drugs in the *Pharmacopoeia*,' and: 'I leave you with three great physicians: air, water, exercise.'

As mentioned in chapter 1, in the 18th century spas were built around springs offering external and internal water therapies – the generic name coming from the centre in Spa in Belgium. They became the most fashionable and influential places for treatments of distress, fatigue and disease, and remain popular on mainland Europe. Their reputations have often been based on medicinal claims made for the mineral salts and other elements in their own waters. In most cases it is likely that their good effects, which as with modern 'health farms' were usually ephemeral, came from the whole process of the treatments offered away from everyday habits and temptations. Many bottled waters such as Evian, Vichy and Contréxeville, and in Britain Malvern and Buxton, are named after the centres where they were and sometimes still are offered.

In 1928 Robert McCarrison issued a manual *Food* for the Indian population featuring his 'Food Star', which includes water. He points out that bodies are porous, like earthenware pots. He recommends 'a glass or two' of water on waking and after every meal, and says: 'Water is even more necessary to keep our bodies clean inside than it is to keep them clean outside.' He also says: 'The first rule in dietetics is to drink water in abundance.'

His view is confirmed in editions of *Food and the Principles of*

Dietetics published in 1944 and 1956, which recommend at least a litre of water a day, and also say that 'much more can be taken without the slightest danger'. Amen.

Tips

- Use an adequate filter if you are not sure your water is safe
- Store filtered water, preferably in earthenware containers
- Drink water with all meals and as you work, exercise and relax
- Have a jug of water on tables, desks and by your bedside
- Use the water stand at work or bring in your own water
- Take water in bottles on journeys for you and your family
- Become a local mineral and spring water connoisseur
- Add a sense of occasion by using a special jug and glass
- Make sure that the children in your life drink lots of water
- Drink safe well and river water and do your bit to safeguard it

Big picture stuff

An extra reason for this to be the first of the seven golden rules is that as soon as you start to raise your consciousness about water, you will start to engage as a citizen as well as a consumer. Is your tap water safe? Do you *know* it is safe? You can of course install a filter, if you have not done so already – but do check its ability to eliminate problematic micro-organisms and chemicals.

What about domestic water supplies that are chlorinated and smell like bleach, or are treated with aluminium compounds to make the water sparkle? These chemicals are bad news. There is some reason to be sceptical about reassurances of safety.

You are bound to start to engage as a citizen, and therefore with the social dimension of water, when you start to wonder why domestic water supplies may be significantly unsafe or toxic. What's the underlying issue? Crumbling sewerage systems? Pollution with agrochemicals? Failure to invest in the future? And which system is more trustworthy: ownership by the state using taxpayers' money, or corporate ownership requiring returns for shareholders? For you as a consumer, there are also issues arising from the pricing and metering of water. Then you can start thinking about why it is not advisable to drink well or river water, unless you can be assured by recent thorough analyses.

For many impoverished populations the most basic public-health disasters are lack of basic municipal and communal sanitation and sewerage systems. Lakes, rivers and streams are polluted by chemicals and often become open sewers, leading to waterborne infections that altogether kill millions of young children every year. Over a billion people in the world lack safe water, a figure some say will increase to 5 billion by 2025 – which might well include your family. In China, 90 per cent of surface water in the cities is polluted. The drilling of wells lowers water tables and so kills trees and creates more marginal and desert land. The most valuable resource for rural and urban communities throughout Africa, Asia and Latin America is safe and sustainable water supplies. From this much else can flow.

The quantity of water now being used by humans is, on a global basis, not sustainable. Use of freshwater increased almost tenfold in the 20th century. The vast underground aquifers are now being overdrawn on all continents except Antarctica. Most water withdrawn by humans is used for intensive irrigation on which industrial agriculture depends, and the cost of this is not reflected by prices in the shops.

You may be thinking that all this is a reason to drink less water, not more. Not really. In rich countries every person on average uses anything between 125 and 500 litres of water a day. Consuming an extra 2 litres a day, most of which is recycled through sewerage and filtration systems, is not going to accelerate Doomsday.

Yes, it is best to drink water from the tap. Yes, bottled mineral and spring water is shipped internationally. The top three exporters of bottled water to the USA were, in 2006, Fiji, France and Italy. In the USA alone, 900 million kilograms (2 billion pounds) of plastic bottles are buried in landfill every year. So get your own water filtered and become sensitive to the miles bottled water has travelled before it reaches the shops.

You can begin to make a difference for the better by choosing foods and drinks that need less water to grow, and that make less use of transportation systems – whether by air, sea or roads – using vast amounts of water, and saying that you are doing this and why, and . . . But I am now beginning to write your script, which I do not want to do.

PHYSICAL ACTIVITY

Be active every day

Principle

To maintain our energy balance at the level to which humans are adapted.

What

'Physical activity' here includes all occupational, domestic, transport and recreational activity as energetic as brisk walking, or more so. Moderate physical activity makes you breathe harder and faster after a while, and will then raise a sweat. Vigorous physical activity is more challenging, especially if you are now sedentary and inactive: this keeps you close to being out of breath, and will raise your heart rate to around 70–80 per cent of its maximum.

Occupational physical activity includes most forms of manual labour such as digging, cutting, pounding, hoeing, harvesting, and lifting and carrying loads. Domestic physical activity, which may also be occupational, includes work done by hand rather than just by machines, such as making beds, polishing, ironing, cleaning, gardening, and also walking up and down stairs. Transport physical activity includes walking, running or cycling to and from places of work. Exercise and sport are recreational physical activity. These include brisk walking, jogging and running; cycling, swimming, dancing, football, tennis, basketball, rowing, volleyball, aerobic workouts. Shopping or golf do not count except when you are walking, preferably carrying your bags or clubs.

Most recreational activities can be moderate or vigorous, depending on their nature and how physically fit you are.

Why

It is essential that you are and remain physically active, at natural human levels, to ensure that you are well nourished and also to avoid putting on fat, now and as you become older.

Practically all sedentary people become increasingly fat. This may not be obvious, because as lean tissue gradually decreases and body fat gradually increases, body weight may not change or might even decrease, lean tissue being 20 per cent heavier than fat. Just like fattened animals, the muscle of inactive people becomes 'marbled' with fat. Flabby people may be fairly light, especially if they have wasted their lean tissue through successive dieting regimes.

Sedentary ways of life are a cause of many disorders and diseases. That's more ominous news. More good news is that regular sustained lifelong moderate and vigorous physical activity develops, strengthens and maintains all the body's physical systems. Much current research on physical activity concerns its preventive effects against physical disorders and diseases. These certainly include overweight and obesity, diabetes, high blood pressure, heart disease, colon cancer and osteoporosis.

As well also as being effective against overweight, symptoms of diabetes and heart disease often fade or disappear as a result of sustained increased physical activity. Physical activity also changes the frequency and nature of bowel movements. Runners and joggers can experience the 'when you've got to go, you've got to go' syndrome: remember this before you head outdoors for longer sessions, or note the location of public facilities.

Women commonly report that after becoming physically quite a lot more active, they can eat what and when they like without increasing weight, and that they shed body fat and become more shapely. When people who enjoy life into their 80s and 90s are asked for their secret, two common answers - apart from longevity running in the family - are serenity and walking.

Protection against diseases is just one benefit. Physical activity also enhances wellbeing, relaxes, invigorates and centres thoughts and emotions, and brings us more into the living and physical world. All your senses are enhanced: the experiences of running in a park at first light, or cycling by the side of an ocean, or simply walking in a city and noticing the architecture as if for the first time, are wonderful.

How much

Be physically active for at least an hour five days a week. Begin with moderate physical activity, and gradually increase the proportion of vigorous physical activity so that preferably well before the sixth month you are vigorously active for more than half of this time.

If you prefer to be physically active every day, that's fine too. Specifying five days is partly to be practical, and partly because especially at first you may appreciate rest and relaxation days. Five days also allows for times when exercise really is not possible. If on such days you sometimes join in stretching and balance classes, such as yoga, Pilates or *tai ch'i*, so much the better.

You can divide up the total time you are active any way that suits you. Personally I only count sessions of 10 minutes or more, but feel free to add up shorter periods of time, as long as these really are active. For example, if your house or place of work has stairs, use them, and walk up moving staircases.

You may find this rule hard to follow at first. If you are sedentary, it implies rethinking what you do every day. If now you are unfit, be less concerned at first about the intensity of activity, and focus instead on putting in the hours. As you gain the habit of regular physical activity, become more vigorous. Moderate activity is good in itself, but its main value is training your body and all of you to be able to sustain vigorous activity, which is a lot more beneficial.

If you are physically impeded or disabled please don't be discouraged. Do what you can. Professionally trained therapists or advisors these days usually encourage as much activity as possible, within physical limits.

Effect on body fat and weight

Becoming and staying physically active up to the levels for which humans are adapted is essential to ensure that you will not gain body fat. This judgement is consistent with all the evidence. Its basis is the evolutionary principle. In all physically active populations, overweight is uncommon and obesity is rare. In all sedentary populations, over-weight and obesity are common.

If you want to reduce body weight – though really it is body fat you want to shed – it is essential that you first become more, and probably much more, physically active. Once you are physically active, and are eating lots of nourishing food and drink, it is much more likely that you will not want or need to restrict your energy consumption, simply because you will be in higher energy balance. Once you have been vigorously active for some time you are likely to be both eating more, and carrying less body fat.

Do not, however, expect to reduce weight or change shape as soon as you start to become active. Over time you will gradually reduce fat, and also gain lean tissue. At all times, it's not your weight you should watch, so much as your waist. At the same weight, the waist of an active and physically fit person may be anything between 2–5 inches (5–12½ centimetres) less than a sedentary person.

Becoming more physically active often makes it easier to give up smoking, and in my experience, which has included a *Sunday Times* 'Exercise Against Smoking' project, smokers who become more phys-ically active sometimes quit without much effort or craving. This is in part because exercise releases endorphins, substances that make you feel good, sometimes known as the body's natural opiates. Another reason is that becoming fit and discovering that you are rejuvenating your body will increase your self-confidence and resolve. If you are a smoker you will probably know that after quitting, body weight increases by something like 2–4 kilograms (4½–9 pounds). This is because smoking speeds up metabolic rate by around 200 calories (around 800 kilojoules) a day. The best 'antidote' to this weight increase is increased physical activity.

If being more physically active makes you hungrier – it may, or may not – this is unlikely to cause you to eat so much more that the effect of the physical activity is cancelled out. Reviews of the literature show that most people do not eat or drink more after being physically active. My own experience when I increase my physical activity is that I do not want to eat more. Indeed, after relatively long runs – more than 40 minutes – I generally feel less hungry than I otherwise would. Other people work up healthy appetites.

A bottom line here is that after three or so months of daily including vigorous physical activity as recommended, without making any conscious change in your eating and drinking habits, you may see a reduction in your weight, and certainly your body fat will have decreased. But the main reason to be active is to raise your level of energy turnover.

Fitting it in

Yes, an hour or more a day of physical activity is a lot more than most basically sedentary people undertake. Dedicating at least an hour a day five days a week to physical activity does imply that you rethink how you spend your days, and this is likely to involve discussions and agreements with your family and colleagues.

How you fit physical activity into your everyday life is up to you. Do you think this is impossible? Everybody finds time to do what they really want to do. It may seem easy for me to say this, and hard for you to do. Thus, one of my friends lives in the northeast of Scotland where the winter nights are long. In a previous job she left for work and came home in the dark. She lives miles from the nearest fitness centre or swimming pool, at her work there were no workplace exercise or changing facilities, and limited street lighting makes running or cycling at night hazardous. She wants to exercise for an hour a day, but in that job had no real choice but to compromise.

While seeing all this, my responsibility is to let you know the best level of physical activity. What you then do is up to you. In my friend's case she chose to change her working life in favour of a generally more balanced life, and now has time to stay fit and healthy.

What about the weather? On visits to London when the nights are long I like to get up at first light, run the length of Regent's Park's Broad Walk, round its Inner Circle, and so on back to my lodging at a kind friend's house in Primrose Hill. This makes my days. One of life's unsung pleasures is running in cold rain when you are sure of a hot tub or shower immediately afterwards.

See how you can rearrange your daily life. After three to six months, once your body becomes toned and you are becoming fit, have decreased your body fat and increased your lean tissue, you are likely to be more alert and focused when awake, be sleeping more deeply, and be pleased with yourself.

If your life is basically sedentary and you are not now physically active, you may feel daunted. What is most important is constructing an hour or more a day in which to be active. At first don't push yourself. If the most you feel you can do is walking at a usual pace, congratulate yourself on keeping this up. Women and older people may enjoy company; the 2,139-metre (1.2-mile) circuit road within my local university campus is well populated with walkers and joggers of both genders and all ages most mornings and at weekends.

What suits some people will not suit others. For example, most of the time I work at home in a region of Brazil where the climate is usually pleasant. I am accustomed to jogging, and I like to be methodical. So my daily physical activity is simple: I walk and run 50/50 for 40 minutes first thing in the morning before starting work, and for 40 minutes in the afternoon, which is roughly 10,000 steps. When I am travelling and staying in a hotel I use its fitness centre as soon as I arrive, and a sauna or steam-room which are great for jetlag, and then go there daily.

You may be able to integrate much of your physical activity into your existing routine. If you travel to work, one way is to walk briskly for all or some of this distance. Within a city you may find that this is as quick as using a vehicle or public transport, with the added advantage that you know how long your route will take. When you get keen, carry running gear with you for lunchtimes, find somewhere to change, and keep a change of clothes at work.

Sometimes, including when you are ill, you will not be able to be physically active. Rest instead and simply resume being active as soon as you are able to do so.

Is it safe?

Yes. That said, like all things that need care, including the good things in life and life itself, physical activity is not absolutely safe.

In the 1980s when I was an active citizen runner in London, the best-known advocate of jogging was Jim Fixx, who in his early 50s was found dead by the side of a road. Running and other physical activities in themselves don't kill people. The cause is usually heart disease, almost certainly symptomatic but ignored, which triggers a heart attack during exertion. It is more common, though rarely reported, for constipated sedentary people with heart disease to die on the toilet. Deaths like that of Jim Fixx are remembered because they are so rare. Regular physical activity is safe, like travelling by train is safe – more so.

Warning

It is possible to overdo physical activity. Initially sedentary people who aspire to run long-distance races and who are enthusiastic or competitive may over-train past their limits. They may as a result injure themselves or, more likely, pick up infections. Training to become fit, and then very fit, takes time and patience.

Rearranging your life to give yourself time for physical activity is the big first step. Enjoy this time, be determined but don't push too hard, and remember that the best judge of the effect of physical activity on your health is you.

You should be finishing your activity feeling warm and relaxed, with an overall sense of physical wellbeing. If you are aware of aches and pains at the time or the next day, take care. Keep going, but more gently, or else instead of any vigorous physical activity the next day, do stretching exercises or have a massage. I also advise joining a club that welcomes people at and somewhat above your level, whatever your main activity. Other members will have been where you are and will give good advice.

Who says?

The Swedish exercise physiologist Per-Olof Åstrand, summarizing all that is known about physical activity, says: 'Regular physical activity is necessary for optimal function and health. The health hazards of inactivity are for many reasons much higher than activity: the individual who remains inactive should therefore bother about a health examination much more than the active one.'

All public health reports that I have seen, aimed at high-income, industrialized, or sedentary populations, recommend more physical activity. What's here is similar to recommendations now made by the World Health Organization, the International Association for the Study of Obesity, the UK Department of Health and the US Department of Health and Human Services. Reports that recommend lower amounts of physical activity are compromises. They balance the findings of scientific studies, which generally show that the more physically active people are the better, with a pragmatic view of what can be realistically achieved.

This rule better reflects the evidence. It is based on what is known about the level of physical activity of populations who were or are free of the diseases now known – or suspected to be – caused by habitual physical inactivity. It roughly corresponds to the levels of physical activity of most people most of the time before machines such as cars and television took over the physical work and play for which humans are designed.

It is likely that your life is principally sedentary. If so, this rule is designed initially to build a daily additional 200–300 calories (roughly 840–1,250 kilojoules) of physical activity into your everyday life, which is done by an hour five days a week of brisk walking or its equivalent. That's an excellent start. You then build up to an extra 400–500 calories (roughly 1,700–2,100 kilojoules) a day if you are a woman, and an extra 500–600 calories (roughly 2,100–2,500 kilojoules) a day if you are a man. This requires around an hour and a half every day of moderate physical activity, or half an hour of moderate physical activity plus half an hour of vigorous activity such as jogging and running, or cycling, dancing, swimming, rowing or working out. To be vigorous, physical activity needs to make you sweat, keep you close to being out of breath, and raise your heart rate to 70–80 per cent of maximum.

You may be aware of other systems for measuring degrees of habitual physical activity. In the USA a common system is METs (metabolic equivalents), and internationally the usual system is PALs (physical activity levels).

Wisdom of the ages

Exercise has been incorporated into philosophies of life for thousands of years. In China *ch'i* (also spelled *qi*) means breath, literally and in the sense of energy. Taoism includes the practice of *tai ch'i chuan*, which teaches that learning comes through movement. In India, the Ayurvedic concept of *prana* is similar. Ayurvedic medicine incorporates yoga, and teaches that physical flexibility and proper breathing as well as diet are essential for human mental, emotional and spiritual development.

Physical activity was fundamental within classical Greek and Roman culture. In the 5th century BCE, Hippocrates wrote, no doubt also thinking of women: 'Eating alone will not keep a man well; he must also take exercise. For food and exercise, while possessing opposite qualities, yet work together to produce health.' In the 2nd century CE Claudius Galenus

(Galen) wrote that everybody needs exercise: 'The uses of exercise are twofold; one for the evacuation of the excrements, the other for the production of good condition of the firm parts of the body.'

Tribal societies have included running, dancing, active games, and other exercise, as well as necessary physical activity, as essential parts of their patterns of life and rituals, and as ways to understand the physical and immaterial world. A book on palaeolithic ways of life observes: 'Viewed through the perspective of evolutionary time, sedentary existence, possible for great numbers of people only during the last century, represents a transient, unnatural aberration.'

Tips

- Work your body rather than rely on a machine when you can
- Walk briskly to and from work, all or some of the way
- Take daily breaks for two brisk walks of at least 15 minutes
- Walk up and down stairs at work, and when travelling
- Get energetic with jogging, cycling, dancing, swimming
- Join in team games such as tennis, football, volleyball
- Become more and more vigorously active when you are ready
- Organize your life so that you have plenty of time to be active
- Centre social life and holidays more around physical activity
- Watch television only after you have pre-selected a programme

Big picture stuff

Being physically active in the open air, experiencing the changing seasons and enjoying most weather, is a way of being more in the world. You can also engage as a citizen, on behalf of others.

Now you are following this golden rule, you are a pioneer. Most people will not become physically active until exercise, recreation and sport is accessible, enjoyable and safe. As a citizen and member of a community you can help to make it so.

When you prefer physical activity and exercise rather than relying on a machine you are helping to conserve fuel. An obvious example is walking to work, or part walking and part using public transport, rather than driving your car. In such ways you become a bit more self-sufficient. As you become more physically active, you will become warmer; you will wear fewer layers of clothing, and will prefer room temperatures to be lower.

When you exercise in cities you are likely to become very aware that urban areas are usually designed for motorists rather than for pedestrians and cyclists. Walkers, joggers, cyclists and other active people all over the world are now at the forefront of campaigns to make city streets as well as parks safe and enjoyable for everybody. This can include more pedestrian precincts, more cycle lanes, freedom to cycle on roads and paths within parks, greater provision of outdoor swimming and rowing facilities, subsidized public transport, charges for cars to come into inner cities, and restriction of heavy traffic.

Join the world campaign to restore physical activity in the form of exercise and games to schools. In many countries schools have already sold off their sports and recreation grounds. This is a scandal. Schools need money to educate the bodies as well as the minds of their children. One of my dreams is that to be defined as a school, with the privileges this brings, every place of education must by law include adequate space for sport and recreation, trained teachers, and physical activity built into the daily curriculum. There should be regular sport and games such as running, swimming, football, dancing, tennis and badminton, with priority given to those activities that need the least equipment and organization.

Golden Rule 3

PLANT FOODS

Eat lots of fresh vegetables, pulses (legumes) and fruits

Principle

To obtain most of our nourishment from fresh plant foods.

What

With foods of plant origin, 'fresh' is sometimes taken to mean only wholefoods eaten ripe straight from the tree, bush or ground. You can enjoy such foods when you grow your own, or pick them on farms, or visit farmers' markets. But this definition is too narrow. All plant foods sold in supermarkets are processed in some sense. Fresh vegetables and fruits have almost invariably been selectively bred, which is a form of processing or at least alteration. Many vegetables and fruits, while displayed as fresh, are picked unripe and treated in ways that preserve them after transport, unpacking and display. Pulses (legumes) are usually dried and sometimes cooked before sale.

So here, 'fresh' includes vegetables, pulses (legumes) and fruits, in the whole form in which they are picked, and also dried and then reconstituted before eating, or chilled or frozen, or vacuum packed, or changed from their original state in other benign ways, and eaten raw, or else after being cooked in or by means of water. (There is more on what 'fresh' means in the notes to this rule.)

'Vegetables' here mean all vegetables, all salad vegetables, all roots that are not starchy, and also fungi (mushrooms). Any fruit (botanically) that is eaten as a vegetable or salad counts. All herbs and spices count, as do all sprouts. Here 'vegetables' excludes starchy tubers and roots such as potatoes, cassava or yams. 'Pulses' (legumes) mean all types of beans and peas, and also lentils and peanuts. 'Fruits' mean all types of fruit, including bananas, avocados and olives, and also all types of berry.

Starchy tubers and roots, and other plant foods such as minimally processed cereals (grains), nuts, and seeds, all are or should be nourishing. Of course consume such foods this month, with all the other foods and drinks in your diet, but not as part of this rule – and see rule 4.

'Benign' means methods of changing food from its original state in production, preservation, manufacture and preparation (including cooking) that are beneficial (or at least harmless) for human health. Benign methods of preservation may include bottling and fermentation. Canning is less desirable and foods are often canned with added fat, sugar or salt; unless you can get rid of these additions, prefer food canned in its own juices or water. Any of these methods may preserve the quality of perishable food better than leaving it lying around at room temperatures. Benign methods of cooking in or with water include steaming, boiling and stewing. Many other methods of preparation such as stir-frying, baking, roasting or grilling are all part of great cuisines and of delicious and healthy diets. Enjoy them, but again, not as part of following this rule for this and all following months. See rule 5.

What about vegetable and pulse (legume) soups? The problem with tinned and packaged soups and those served in restaurants is what comes with them; they are often bulked out with degraded ingredients and are often very salty. But if you trust the source, or the soup is made fresh at home with little salt, count the weight of the vegetables used (no, not the added water). Likewise with soups and stews using pulses (legumes).

Why

Fresh foods of plant origin are nourishing, sustaining, and low in energy density. Together with other fresh foods they are the best basis for your diet.

The edible parts of vegetables, pulses (legumes), and fruits, and nuts and seeds, evolved partly as food for predators that, by eating and excreting the seeds, propagate the plant. The human race has co-evolved with these plants. Not all are nourishing, and some have evolved methods of self-protection such as poisons and spines. The value of vegetables, pulses (legumes), and fruits, and also cereals (grains) and nuts, as human food has been magnified over the thousands of years since the beginnings of agriculture through selection and breeding of varieties that are bigger, hardier, and yield more produce, are more readily stored and preserved, and are more delicious.

Eaten in variety and in amounts that make them altogether staples, these plant foods are rich sources of a vast number of bioactive compounds, including vitamins, minerals and trace elements, which protect against deficiency diseases, food-related infections and chronic diseases. Consumed fresh, they are also high in dietary fibre. Together with nuts and seeds, they are practically complete sources of all the nutrients known to be relevant to human health.

If you are overweight, and particularly if you are accustomed to following dieting regimes, this rule may feel counter-intuitive for a while, because fresh plant foods contain a lot of water as well as dietary fibre, and their weight and bulk, together with that of the water you are already drinking, will fill you up, maybe even to the point of feeling uncomfortable for a while. Do not be concerned about this. Your body will adjust. Be patient. If you continue to feel uncomfortably full after a couple of weeks, the best policy is to reduce the amount of other foods and drinks you are consuming, but don't force yourself to do this.

How much

Consume 1 kilogram (roughly 2 pounds) of fresh – including benignly changed – vegetables, pulses (legumes) and fruits, every day. This total is of course for these three types of fresh food taken together. The greater the variety the better.

If you are a small or older woman, somewhat less, say 750 grams (somewhat over 1½ pounds) is OK. If you are a big or young man, somewhat more, say 1,250 grams (around 2½ pounds) is OK.

Following this rule is likely to involve a radical rethink of all your meals, for 1 kilogram is three or more times the amount that most people consume, and more than is recommended in most expert reports.

At first, the really important thing is to get used to thinking – and enjoying – fresh vegetables, pulses (legumes) and fruits. If these amounts daunt you, build up to them a week at a time, in this first month: you could for example start with ½ kilogram (1 pound) a day in the first week, then ¾ kilogram (1½ pounds) a day in the next two weeks, and then the full daily amount in the fourth week and remaining days, and thereafter. Plus you will be adjusting these amounts bearing in mind your size, gender and age.

Effect on body fat and weight

To repeat, the purpose of this rule, and of the three following, is not to reduce your body weight. This rule is meant to accustom you to enjoying lots of fresh plant foods. This month eat and drink what else you like, just as long as you consume the amounts of fresh vegetables, pulses (legumes) and fruits specified above.

If you want to reduce your body fat you may feel impatient, or at this stage have a surge of zeal or enthusiasm and be tempted to start consciously restricting your intake. Please do not. Remember that you now are likely to be a lot more physically active. Trust the process. If you find yourself shifting your eating and drinking habits spontaneously, that's another matter.

Fitting it in

This means two things: fitting into your day, and fitting into yourself.

This rule implies a big change in the quality and nature of what you consume, and in your attitude to and consciousness of food. Suddenly fresh vegetables, pulses (legumes) and fruits have become central in your diet. As with water, a good plan is to get into the habit of consuming almost all of these plant foods earlier in the day, preferably at breakfast and lunch, and as a big salad before your main course in the evening.

Here is what I tend to do. For my breakfast I make a big *vitamina* (smoothie to you, unless you are Brazilian) by liquidizing my favourite fruits in water, in all sorts of combinations. For example, peeled, skinned, and topped and tailed, two bananas, half a mango, a guava, a passion fruit, a chunk of fresh ginger, and a sprinkling of nuts or seeds, altogether weigh over half a kilogram (well over a pound), not counting added water. Later (see rule 4, which includes fresh grains and roots) after relishing this wonderfully yummy mixture, I find out whether I feel like any plain toast, usually from corn bread, or any tea; sometimes I do, sometimes I don't.

At lunch I follow the same principle. What come first are the steamed vegetables. I am very partial to courgettes (zucchini): three big ones also weigh over half a kilogram (well over a pound). I eat them with a drift of olive oil and some balsamic vinegar, and a few crystals of sea salt: also extremely delicious. Favourite alternatives include cauliflower, carrots, onions, spinach and the Brazilian *couve* (a type of cabbage). I may also drink the water used to steam them. My preferred grain at lunch is steamed whole (brown) rice.

Then I eat other food. I may enjoy a snack of a big tomato, with a slice of toast and some cheese, in the afternoon. In the evening I eat and drink as I choose.

When travelling I adapt this method. For example, in London I frequent Nani's of Wigmore Street, which at lunchtimes offers a big container of four salad foods of your choice, including substantial choices such as various beans, chickpeas and lentils. So do many supermarkets. In the evenings I often go to a restaurant in the 'world food' chain Giraffe, whose soups and stew-type dishes, although brought in, are close to fresh. In classier restaurants, if eating fish, poultry or meat, I order double portions of green vegetables. Wherever I am I enjoy juices made fresh in the shop, from whole fruit and vegetables or (in Brazil) from pulp, much of which is trucked down from the hot north. This gives you a rough idea of how I follow this golden rule (and also see rule 4). You will find the ways that suit you.

If you find this rule hard to follow, I guess that you live somewhere where main meals since the time of industrialization have been centred on fresh and processed meat. In the 'meat and two veg' culture, vegetables have become side dishes, salads are usually insubstantial and monotonous, pulses (legumes) almost unknown other than tinned beans, and fruits eaten usually only as occasional snacks. It is very different elsewhere. At a conference at the University of Hangzhou in the Chinese province of Zhejiang we delegates had lunch in one of the refectories for students and staff, which seated maybe 500 people. We had a choice of vegetable soups, and of main courses that included many types of freshly cooked delicious green vegetables, as well as rice, fish and seafood. Students in the UK and the USA are generally not so fortunate.

Is it safe?

Yes. There is no evidence or reason to believe that high levels of consumption of these plant foods, including above 1 kilogram (just over 2 pounds) a day, could do any harm.

If you are worried about pesticide and other chemical residues in plant foods, you have more reason to worry about chemical and micro-biological contaminants in meat and animal foods. If you are worried, prefer food grown and raised to recognized organic standards. Again, see golden rule 4.

Eating a lot more fresh vegetables and fruits than you have been accustomed to will mean that you will open your bowels more often. People who eat mostly processed foods may defecate less often than daily, and their faeces are often hard. Once you start eating lots of fresh plant foods, you may well defecate twice a day, and your faeces will be soft. This is the natural human state. You may also notice that you are passing wind more frequently when you first start following this rule. All of this is perfectly safe – another key change to note in your diary.

Warning

This warning is much the same as that within rule 1. This and the next rule specify more highly nourishing foods and drinks, and prohibit nothing. So you could follow this rule by consuming the specified amounts of foods and, this done, then consuming more energy-dense sugary fatty processed foods than you were before starting this system. Again, you don't need me to tell you that this would be a bad idea. This system is not magic. If you did this you would cancel out some or all of the benefits of the rules.

If there are some sugary fatty foods or convenience, fast or other foods that you crave, it is possible that delaying eating these until later in the day than usual, to ensure you consume your vegetables, pulses (legumes) and fruits, might provoke late-in-the-day binges. If this is an issue for you, watch out, especially in the first three or four months.

Who says?

This rule is for more than is recommended by national governments and by expert reports whose purpose is to prevent obesity, and chronic diseases such as heart disease and cancer. Such recommendations are derived from studies consistently showing that the more vegetables and fruits, and also pulses (legumes) are consumed, the better. But in the countries in which such studies are conducted, average daily consumption of vegetables and fruits is usually roughly 250 grams (a bit more than half a pound), and consumption of pulses (legumes) is almost always very low.

Expert reports have usually recommended at least five portions (servings) a day of vegetables and fruits. A portion (serving) is often reckoned to be around 80 grams (about 3 ounces), so at least five a day adds up to at least 400 grams (14 ounces) a day. Vegetables and fruits are low in energy density, so this might amount to something like 7 per cent of dietary energy, depending on the vegetables and fruits chosen and personal energy balance. By contrast, the specification here, including pulses (legumes) might amount to 20–25 per cent of total dietary energy, depending on what you choose and what is your energy balance.

As with physical activity, the number five chosen in expert reports is a compromise between what is most healthy, and what committees think is feasible to propose for entire populations where current consumption of vegetables – and fruits – is low or pitiful. More recent reports commonly recommend anything up to ten portions a day. This is fairly close to what is specified here. However, such recommendations may or may not include pulses (legumes), may include potatoes, and usually do not specify how these foods may be processed or prepared.

Wisdom of the ages

Until the discovery of vitamins as essential nutrients in the early 20th century, the value of plant foods in general was underrated. Afterwards, vegetables and fruits were classified as one of the main food groups, termed 'protective' (against deficiency diseases), but even after the importance of dietary fibre was acknowledged from the late 1970s, they have still been positioned as ancillary foods.

This mistake has not been made in the oldest established traditional cuisines. The proof of the value of these foods has been in their use. Colin Tudge celebrates the leaves used for Chinese banquets, Southern French haricot bean casseroles, and Egyptian use of broad beans, and rightly (also see rule 4) says: 'In great cooking the world over, the staples prevail: cereals, pulses, tubers. Vegetables and fruits, spices, herbs, fungi and fermented foods are present in huge variety and abundance. Meat the world over (in truly great cooking) is always used sparingly, and always in the greatest possible variety.'

Tips

- Start the day with lots of fresh fruits or a home-made smoothie
- Enjoy big helpings of steamed vegetables with every main meal
- Make meals look good by using different-coloured vegetables
- Use fresh or cooked tomatoes, peppers or onions as toppings
- Enjoy soups of vegetables or pulses (legumes) as a light meal
- Store vegetables and fruits bottled in their juice or in water
- Grow vegetables, herbs and fruits, if you have space for this
- Eat fruits at meals, and as snacks at home and at work
- Give children salads and fresh fruits to eat at school every day
- Lunch on big salads with pulses (legumes) and tasty dressings

Big picture stuff

Plant-based food systems use less fuel and less water, and produce less waste and other pollution, than food systems in which animal foods and feeds are dominant. It is the industrial production of animals that increases greenhouse gases and contributes to climate change. When you switch to a plant-based diet that emphasizes vegetables, pulses (legumes) and fruits, you are taking action that will help to sustain the planet. Favour food grown in your country, preferably your locality, and ideally your garden. When people in your life follow your lead, your influence will multiply.

Another benefit of horticulture is that it is more suited to family-based farms, and needs more human care than intensive animal production. Horticulture can keep more people on the land, and therefore can at least slow down the flight of rural people to the shantytowns and slums of big cities, where so often they live in misery, unable ever to return to the countryside. In Brazil, state and municipal governments now give support – for social, economic and environmental reasons – to co-operatives of farmers and growers whose produce helps to sustain their own and local communities.

These generalizations are not invariably true. For example, when farmers in Africa are forced to grow speciality vegetables or fruits as cash crops for export, and these foods travel many thousands of miles to supermarkets in materially rich countries, the farmers' livelihoods become vulnerable to 'market' prices, and they may no longer be able to sustain their families on the food they grow for themselves. Also, because cash crops typically have to travel so far to supermarkets, their cost in terms of energy used will be high. In cases like this, meat from animals raised, slaughtered and butchered locally might use fewer non-renewable resources. (For more on animal production, see rule 4.)

From the ecological point of view, the choice is not just between animal food and plant food, but also between the ways in which food is produced, grown, processed and distributed. Now there is growing consciousness that intensive agriculture is a dead-end industry. You can play your part in making food systems sustainable by preferring plant foods, and preferably those that are demonstrably the product of low-input organic horticulture, equitably traded. The ideal is that your food and drink can be traced back to the producer. With vegetables, pulses (legumes) and fruits, you can do this by preferring what is organically and preferably locally grown, and by frequenting farmers' markets. You can also grow your own. If all you have is a window box, grow herbs.

You can also shop as a citizen as well as consumer, by making your views known to supermarket managers and by asking them where their foods come from. They are paid to pay attention.

Golden Rule 4

YOUR DAILY DIET
Prefer all whole and fresh foods

Principle

To obtain most of our nourishment from fresh foods.

What

Golden rule 4 adds whole and fresh foods of all types to fresh vegetables, pulses (legumes) and fruits.

This is the month to enjoy every type of fresh food. As well as
continuing to follow rules 1 to 3, now consume all other fresh foods
– cereals (grains), starchy roots and tubers, and other plant foods, and
fresh meat, poultry, fish, eggs, dairy produce, and other animal
foods.

My definition of 'fresh' as applied to vegetables, pulses (legumes)
and fruits, in rule 3, includes foods that are least processed or that have
been changed in benign or relatively benign ways. Applied to other
foods 'fresh' is defined as follows. Some judgement and common sense
is involved, and I have indicated areas where the rule can be interpreted
differently. If your usual diet is vegetarian or vegan, I am not suggesting
that you change. If you choose generally not to eat red meat or all meat,
or animal foods in general, stay with this.

Plant foods

Fresh wholegrain cereals are classified as fresh food. Wholegrain (brown)
rice and wholegrain pasta is best, but parboiled rice and usual-type

pastas and noodles of all varieties – while less good – are included. Usual-type pasta is included because wholegrain pasta is not to everyone's taste. Usual-type white rice is excluded from this rule. Please remember that exclusion does not mean don't consume them at all; rather, don't consume them as part of following this rule.

Wholegrain bread, preferably the relatively solid type, is included, but not if it is spread with any form of fat. Prefer lower-salt varieties. Soft sliced wrapped wholegrain bread is made from wheat, sometimes mixed with other grains, that has been taken apart and put together again, and is inferior to the solid variety. All rolls, and all white and intermediate breads, are excluded. All breakfast cereals, mueslis and granolas are excluded, unless they are wholegrain with no added sugars or fats. All baked goods like biscuits and cakes are excluded.

All starchy roots like yams and cassava and all tubers like potatoes are included, preferably eaten after cleaning and cooking with the use of water or baking. When cooked with added fat – for example, as chips (French fries) or crisps (chips) – they are excluded.

All nuts and seeds are fine, but not if salted; all margarines and other plant-oil-based table fats are excluded.

Animal foods

All meat, poultry and fish, preferably free-range, organically reared, or wild, bought fresh, are included. Can meat from industrially produced animals be 'fresh', given the processing of the animals themselves? If you think not, exclude all such meat. This is a better choice personally, socially and environmentally, but intensively produced meat is not excluded by this rule. (On this point, see the notes to this rule.)

All forms of manufactured processed meat products, including dried, smoked, salted and pickled products, sausages, frankfurters, patés and pastes, are excluded. Dried meat and fish is excluded because typically it is also salted, but if you remove the salt in preparing it for cooking, OK.

Eggs, milk, plain yoghurt and cheese are included; prefer free-range or organic varieties and lower-salt cheese.

Remember that all plant- and animal-based dishes that have been pre-prepared are excluded under this rule, as are any other processed products containing significant quantities of added sugar or fat. To repeat 'excluded' does not mean don't consume them at all, but don't consume them as part of following this rule.

Preparation and cooking

When preparing these foods at home, or choosing them when eating out, include all that are cooked without adding fat, or else with small amounts of butter or oil. Include all that are cooked in or by means of water, by boiling or steaming, and baking. Stewing is fine too, but if fat is added in the cooking the dish does not count as within this rule. Adding stock or wine is fine. Include animal foods cooked by any method that does not add fat: roast, grilled (broiled) and barbecued meat and fish are included, whereas frying is excluded.

Again, some judgement and common sense is involved. Fish fried in batter (remember chapter 1?) is OK provided you eat only the fish. Commercial burgers are prepared and cooked with added fat, and so are excluded. However, if you buy minced fresh meat and make it into burgers at home without adding fat, these are included.

Provided you follow what are now rules 1–4, eat and drink whatever else you want. As before, the simple approach is to follow the rule during the day, and to consume other foods and drinks in the evening.

Why

Fresh foods of animal as well as of plant origin are nourishing, sustaining, and many animal foods, such as lean meat, are not high in energy density.

Humans are adaptable, designed to consume foods of both plant and animal origin, and can thrive on an exclusive diet from either source. We are omnivorous. This is what the design of our teeth and the structure of our digestive tract from throat through stomach to our intestines shows. We are not 'obligate herbivores' like horses, and we are not 'obligate carnivores' like cats. All whole or fresh foods of plant and of animal origin are nourishing.

Fresh foods of animal origin, while not nutritionally superior to whole or fresh foods of plant origin, are usually good sources of a variety of vitamins, minerals and trace elements. For some of these, requirements increase as consumption of animal foods increases, and correspondingly decrease when diets are plant-based. Animal foods contain no dietary fibre. Typically they are good sources of protein, the need for which is usually exaggerated. For comments on plant foods see this section of rule 3.

Meat is not all much the same. There are big differences between a lean grilled (broiled) steak from a grass-fed steer, and a fatty fried rump cut from an animal fed on concentrates. There are also big differences between the meats from farmed and wild animals, and between red meat, poultry, and all types of fish, especially those caught wild. One of this month's tips is to prefer as food the meat and flesh of animals, birds and fish which, when alive, were physically fit. The fat of some game birds and wild fish that protects them against the cold is soft and oily, and high in essential fatty acids. If you eat animal foods, and if in following this specification you decide only to eat fish, or only fish and poultry, or only small amounts of any type of meat, you are probably making a healthier choice. (On these points, see the notes to this rule.)

How much

Consume half a kilogram (a bit more than a pound) a day of fresh – including benignly changed – cereals (grains), roots, tubers, nuts, seeds, meat, poultry, fish, eggs, milk and cheese. Overall, make more than half food of plant origin. The greater the variety the better. The half a kilogram is for the foods prepared and ready to eat, and is of course the total of all these foods.

If you are a small or older woman, somewhat less, say 400 grams (14 ounces), is OK. If you are a big or younger man, somewhat more, say 600 grams (nearly 1½ pounds), is OK.

The main difference between what's specified in this rule and what you may be eating now is not so much quantity as quality. It is quite likely that you are already consuming more than half a kilogram (or a pound) of these foods every day. But unless you now make a point of preferring whole foods, it is unlikely that you will be consuming this amount of fresh foods (in addition to vegetables, pulses and fruits).

Again, you could interpret this rule in unhealthy ways. For example, if you are already accustomed to consuming say 200 grams (just under half a pound) of fresh meat and poultry and no other fresh animal foods a day, which is roughly the average consumed in high-income countries, this rule does not specify any change – indeed, it allows this amount, plus whatever else you are consuming in addition to following this rule. Industrially produced meat is generally fatty. Also, nuts and seeds are energy-dense, as are full-fat milk and most cheeses. So it makes sense to eat these sparingly.

My take on this is as follows. The specification here is for less than 250 grams (10 ounces) a day of all fresh foods of animal origin. It is very unlikely that currently all the animal foods you consume are fresh meat.

Rules that go into great detail are not appropriate and even rather insulting. Once you grasp the general principles, I am sure you will make suitable choices. Plus I don't agree with dietary guidelines that make few if any distinctions between ways in which foods and drinks are processed and prepared. As a general rule to which there are few exceptions, all whole and also fresh foods are healthy.

Effect on body fat and weight

The message here is the same as in rule 3 above. Once again, the purpose of this rule, and of the two that follow, is not to reduce your body weight. This rule's aim is to accustom you to enjoying lots of fresh foods of every type. Continue to eat and drink whatever else you like, just as long as you follow what are now rules 1–4. Trust the process.

Fitting it in

See rule 3.

Is it safe?

Yes. If you are concerned about residues of toxic substances in industrially produced meat and poultry, or in fish, don't eat them. If you don't want to eat animal fat, don't.

Warning

See rule 3.

Who says?

The quantity of cereals (grains) and other starchy foods recommended here may seem a lot less than that recommended by the World Health Organization and many national governments, including those of the USA and UK. Such reports usually specify more than 400 grams (roughly

14 ounces) a day of starchy foods, and may state or imply an upper figure of anything up to around 800 grams.

But the specification here is for fresh foods, as defined. While expert reports generally state a preference for wholegrain or minimally processed starchy foods, I know of none that exclude 'refined' starchy foods made from white flour, as is done here. Besides, you can always choose to consume small amounts of animal foods and more than 250 grams (10 ounces) of starchy plant foods a day, and get closer to the total of 500 grams (a little under 20 ounces) specified for this month, if that's what you want to do. You may also be including starchy foods among those you eat on top of following rules 3 and now 4.

This said, most expert reports do go somewhat over the top. Here is why. Their recommendations for cereals (grains) tend to be 'by difference' – having recommended less fat overall, less sugar, and moderate amounts of protein, starchy foods are almost all of what remains. The main difference with these rules here is that I am specifying much higher amounts of vegetables, pulses (legumes) and fruits in rule 3.

On animal foods, the amount of meat you could eat while following this rule may seem to be a lot more than recommended in some reports. For example, the 2007 World Cancer Research Fund/American Institute for Cancer Research report recommends an upper limit of 500 grams (just under 20 ounces) of red meat *a week*, derived from evidence on colorectal cancer. But the evidence is almost entirely drawn from studies of industrially produced meat cooked in unspecified ways, whereas what's specified here is fresh meat, preferably from free-range or organically reared animals.

This rule may also seem to be at odds with conventional wisdom if you are accustomed to observing current dietary guidelines on fat, or following low-fat dieting regimes, because these are usually severe about meat, milk and dairy products, apart from the lean and low-fat varieties. But depending on how you make it work for you, following this rule, which excludes all processed products containing significant quantities of fat, will not mean that you are consuming a lot of fat. Equally to the point, rules 3 and 4 together are for foods and drinks with no added sugars.

Conventional dietary guidelines are often vague about added sugars, for all sorts of reasons (touched on in chapter 4 and its notes).

Manufacturers of degraded processed foods and drinks, their representative organizations and public relations consultants, and some nutrition and dietetics professionals, have often tried to dismiss those who advocate whole and fresh food as unqualified, eccentric, cranks, or quacks, using phrases like 'the back to nature brigade' or 'the compost school'. Happily, these attacks have faded since the 1990s, with the general realization that greater emphasis on whole and fresh foods is essential nutritionally as well as environmentally. Similarly, discussion on industrialized food systems and the intensive production of animals for food has now become more rational, with the general acceptance that in their present form, such systems are not sustainable.

Wisdom of the ages

Before industrialization writers of course had nothing to say about industrialized food. Since then many influential teachers and writers have advocated whole and fresh foods. In the 20th century in the USA these have included Weston Price and more recently Joan Gussow and Michael Pollan. In Europe these have included Werner Kollath, Max Bircher-Benner, Mikkel Hindhede, Robert McCarrison, T L Cleave, Douglas Latto, and more recently Michael Crawford, Kenneth Heaton, Claus Leitzmann and Colin Tudge. In Brazil they include Clara Brandão.

Tips

- Enjoy meals and dishes that are part of traditional cuisines
- Prefer hot food that is just as delicious when eaten cool or cold
- Prefer animal food from creatures that when alive were fit
- Favour foods from family farms, raised or grown organically
- Prefer foods and drinks that can be traced back to their makers
- Avoid highly processed foods and drinks with long shelf lives
- Avoid products using malign processes or with cryptic ingredients
- Avoid 'fortified' products and others that make health claims
- Ask yourself, before buying any food, 'Would I feed this to a dog?'
- Campaign against processed foods and drinks marketed at children

Big picture stuff

Overall these golden rules specify plant-based diets and emphasize fresh foods and drinks. These are best for your personal health and wellbeing, which is the first purpose of the rules. They will also contribute to your 'treading lightly on the planet', and the more so if you choose free-range, organic and local foods.

Many popular guides to food and health recommend vegetarian or vegan diets, for good health and also often for reasons of animal welfare and to reduce environmental impact. If you prefer not to eat red meat, or any kind of meat, or to be vegan, this fourth rule supports your choice. My own opinion is that mixed 'extensive' agriculture including animals that are reared and husbanded in ways that enable them to lead a natural life is ecologically a better option than farming solely of plants. But this is an ethical issue that allows different opinions. In terms of human nutrition I have a similar opinion, and I eat meat sparingly except at feasts and other special occasions.

Much depends on how you choose to follow this rule. Certainly you will be helping yourself personally, and also helping your family, friends and colleagues, as you become an effective example. How much difference you make ecologically and environmentally largely rests with how you choose your foods of animal origin and the amounts you eat.

Golden Rule 5

FEASTING

Celebrate special occasions with the best food and drink

Principle

To include feasting as a special part of your family and social life.

What

Feasts are special meals consumed in company, to mark special occasions. These include holidays such as Christmas and New Year, Thanksgiving in the USA, and Jewish and Muslim festivals; family and shared special times like births, marriages, anniversaries, birthdays, deaths, a new home or job; or dinner and other parties and special meals for family, friends or colleagues. They are shared celebrations, usually for family, professional, social or cultural reasons. Banquets are feasts. In many cultures family or friends come together on a weekend day and socialize over a feast meal.

Feasts take many forms. Typically they involve consuming more food and drink than usual – measured in terms of energy or mass or weight. They often feature types or quantities of food and drink that are too expensive or uncommon to be consumed from day to day. Feast meals may include more courses than usual. They may have a centre-piece for the main course such as a big whole bird like a turkey, a big whole fish like a salmon, a roast of meat, or a display of plant foods, and may be occasions when unusually large amounts of alcoholic drinks are consumed, depending on the culture.

Feasts are shared occasions. They are different from binges, which are usually solitary, or even secret, and often compulsive. Also there is no need to consume more than usual, let alone gorge, to enjoy a feast.

As you incorporate this rule, get into the habit of reserving feast food for feast days. When people have more than enough to eat and drink, they tend to consume feast food more and more often – aim instead to prefer simple foods and drinks day-to-day.

Why

Humans are social. We are not meant to be alone. Wellbeing includes being with other people. Feasts are times when people who are usually related in some way celebrate their shared lives. The nourishment of feasts is not only from the food and drink, it is also from the conversation and the company, which in turn enhances the quality of what is consumed.

If your weight tends to increase, and especially if you have regularly restricted your dietary energy intake by following dieting regimes, you may be afraid of feasts. This rule lets you be more aware of any such fear, so that you can release it. One deprivation common to most dieting is the exclusion of social feasting on whole, fresh and other healthy food, and one consequence is its replacement by solitary gorging and bingeing on degraded and other processed food, part of the syndrome known as bulimia (see chapter 3). This is no way to live.

How much

Up to once a week in this month, celebrate your family, social or professional life with a feast. These special meals do not need to be enormous. It's enough to share a weekend afternoon with a barbecue and beers, or to relax with family or friends over dinner at your place or theirs or in a restaurant.

There is nothing in the rules you have already been following that suggests you should avoid feasts. The one difference between this month and previous months is that on feast days, up to once a week this month, you continue to follow rules 1 and 2, but you need not follow rules 3 and 4. This of course does not mean that you eat no fresh foods and drinks on feast days, and it's a good idea to note what quantities you do consume.

Effect on body fat and weight

Feasting usually involves consuming more food and drink than usual, and all types of feasting that substantially increase the amount of dietary energy you consume may well have the same type of effect as the overeating that typically follows a dieting regime. Your weight will increase; by how much obviously depends on how much you consume. The increase won't be as dramatic as that after a dieting regime, because your glycogen stores will not have been depleted and you are fully hydrated. When you weigh yourself the day after the feast, you may find you are 1½ to 2 kilograms (3 to 4½ pounds) heavier than you were at the same time the day before.

Do not panic! What happens then depends on your history and your body composition. If you are a lean active person who has never been on a diet regime, your weight is most likely to drop 'by itself' to the pre-feast level in a few days. If on the other hand you have been a flabby sedentary person who has been on a number of dieting regimes, and therefore have trained your body to retain fat, and have not managed to become vigorously active so far, your weight may well remain somewhat increased. If this is you, please do not avoid feasts because their effect scares you. Remember too that you can always feast without increasing your energy intake. Just avoid the sweet or fatty desserts and the fatty foods and drinks. In any case please do not follow a feast by starving yourself in the following days to drive your weight down. That way lies madness. Just accept. Stay with the rules. Trust the process.

When you feast observantly, you may be reminded of the after-effects of restricted-energy dieting regimes. These fears will fade. One of the pleasures in store for you is eating and drinking what you find you most like, every day and on special occasions, with pleasure.

Fitting it in

As mentioned, this rule is not specifying that you have to wait until the fifth month before enjoying feasts. There is nothing in rules 1 to 4 to stop you feasting during the first four months of this system. That's part of the whole idea. In practice, especially if you are still not yet fully following rule 2, you may have found that you have not had much room for feasts, especially in months 3 and 4. The difference is that if you do have a feast in months 3 or 4, please stay with the rules for those months.

It is easier to join in a feast without pigging out if the feast meal is buffet-style or in dishes brought to the table so you can select your own portions. If you are eating out, prefer these styles.

The special feature of this rule is that you continue to follow rules 1–4, except that up to once a week in this month, you follow only rules 1 and 2, and otherwise eat and drink whatever you like, including a special meal. No, I am not suggesting that you organize a blowout a week just for yourself. No, there is no need to party on these days, but do enjoy these feasts, perhaps at weekends. The idea is that you organize or share or join in social feast meals that are arranged for this month, by yourself, your family, friends or colleagues, and eat and drink as much as you like, without any need to follow rules 3 and 4 on fresh foods. If with this extra room inside, you choose to eat and drink a lot, go ahead. Do what you want. But do please continue to follow rules 1 and 2, drinking plenty of water and staying physically active.

You can think of this a bit like a Christmas Day when after the great meal, a member of the family says, 'Right, who's for a walk, then?' – except that you know in advance that you will be going on a walk and may be the person making the invitation. Or you can fit in the walk – and a run – before the feast, if you prefer.

Is it safe?

Yes. The trouble with specifying rules, whether you are by nature obedient or rebellious, is that unless they specify absolutely every possibility however remote, you might misunderstand or see a way to get round them. For example, this rule does not specify 'but when you are feasting, don't drink half a bottle of whisky'. Nor does it specify any limit to the amount of sugar and fat you consume. No, I don't think it is a good idea to get dead drunk, and no, I am not recommending that you eat or drink so much that you become ill. You don't need me to say this.

What about diabetes, heart attacks, some cancers, and so forth? Risk of such diseases is not going to increase significantly as a result of you enjoying occasional feasts.

Warning

If you have chosen to follow rules 3 and 4 in a way that eliminates all the foods and drinks you previously craved, and if in following this new rule you choose on feast days to consume lots of these, you will find it hard to keep off them in the days afterwards. Alcoholic drinks are an obvious example, and so are any processed foods or drinks that give you a rush. So be careful.

If you have already kicked the habit of foods and drinks that you previously craved, it is a bad idea to revert to these during a feast – or for that matter at any other time. Food and drink manufacturers don't like any of their products being compared with cigarettes but here I will make a comparison. If you have kicked a smoking habit, do you think it would be a good idea to revert during a party? No, you don't. It's the same here.

Who says?

As far as I know, nutrition scientists are practically silent on feasting – or any type or pattern of eating and drinking that is out of the ordinary. I can see no good reason for this. On the other hand, food writers are – as you might expect – enthusiastic about feasts, professionally as well as personally. (See the notes to this rule.)

Wisdom of the ages

Just as there is no ode to margarine, no songs are sung about dieting regimes. By contrast, literature is replete with celebrations of special meals. Whole anthologies of quotations on the delights of feasting have been compiled.

The gastronome Jean Anthelme Brillat-Savarin writes of a picnic: 'A shady spot takes his fancy, soft grass welcomes him, and the murmur of the nearby spring invites him to deposit in its cool waters the flask of wine destined to refresh him. Then with calm contentment he takes out of his knapsack the cold chicken and golden-crusted rolls packed for him by loving hands, and places them beside the wedge of Gruyère or Roquefort which is to serve as his dessert.' Of Middle Eastern hospitality, Claudia Roden writes: 'People entertain warmly and joyously. To persuade a friend to stay for lunch is a triumph and a special honour. To entertain many together is to honour them all mutually. It is equally an honour to be a guest.'

Most recently, Michael Pollan wonders why food has become so much confused with its chemical content, and also why thinking and writing about food is so relentlessly focused on prevention of physical diseases. He writes: 'We forget that, historically, people have eaten for a great many reasons other than biological necessity. Food is also about pleasure, about community, about family and spirituality; about our relationship with the natural world, and about expressing our individuality. As long as humans have been taking meals together, eating has been as much about culture as it has been about biology.' He is right. Part of the purpose of this book is to rediscover pleasure in food and drink, including on the special occasions of life.

Tips

- Stay with the rules for water and physical activity on feast days
- Notice how much fresh food you consume on feast days
- Notice how much processed food you consume on these days
- Give guests at feasts choices of salads, fresh fruits and water
- Keep your own jug on the table and drink water during the meal
- If you drink alcohol, also drink a greater quantity of water
- Serve dishes of feasts separately so people can help themselves
- Remember that a feast does not have to involve overeating
- Check your weight before and after feasts, for information
- Note down how you feel for a couple of days after a big feast

Big picture stuff

The big picture here is social. Feasting is convivial. Think of paintings over the centuries showing people at table. When they are solitary are they shown as happy? Usually no. When they are in a group are they shown as vivacious? Usually yes. Feasts bring us closer to partners, family, friends, colleagues. Whether quiet or raucous, whether intimate dinners or vast banquets, whether or not part of parties and music and dancing, they are acts of reaching out and sharing and celebration that mark special times in life. Held at home they are times when the big table and its best ware are used and grand meals are prepared, times of laughter and goodwill and toasts. Held in public places they may be times for awards and speeches. Feasts are also meant to be times marking new paths in life.

Feasts are good times at which to give thanks. Such acknowledgement may be in the form of toasts or speeches to those present. It can also be thanks to the makers of the feast: first to the cooks and all who helped with the meal, and then to the original makers of the food and to the living world whose plants and animals have become our food. As mentioned in the previous chapter, we owe our being to others. Both we and animals depend directly or indirectly on plants for food, and plants owe their being to soil, water, air and light. Feasts are good times to give thanks for the elements, and to remember their value.

Golden Rule 6

FASTING

Build regular abstinence into your life

Principle

To become more conscious of food and drink and its effects.

What

Fasts are abstinence from some or even all food, and some or all drink other than water. All fasting has similarities. Fasts are undertaken for periods of time from a day to months. They may be occasional, as personally chosen and undertaken individually, or regular, as a feature of observance of a religion or philosophy, and undertaken collectively.

Fasts are in some ways the obverse of feasts, and in some faiths precede feasts, as with Lent before Easter, and Ramadan, the holy month before the Muslim festival of Eid. They also take many forms. Pretty much by definition they involve consuming less food and drink than usual overall – measured in terms of energy or mass or weight. They often emphasize simple plain foods and drinks. They may take the form of complete or partial abstinence from specific foods and drinks, or restrict consumption to specified foods and drinks. Radical fasts are those that are most restrictive. The most radical fast is water only, with no food whatever.

No, this rule is not about to specify that you undertake a water-only fast for all of this month. That would be like proposing in rule 2 that you run a marathon without training, besides which most people who are fit are not interested in running long-distance. (For radical fasting, see the notes to this rule.)

Why

As well as its other virtues, fasting of any sort makes you more aware of food and drink and its qualities and effects. Fasting can and does help to break food and drink cravings. Fasting on fresh foods cleanses and refreshes the body, because this allows the body to rest and recuperate, just as the practice of meditation and reflection refreshes the mind and spirit. Like becoming physically active, fasting requires discipline and being prepared to act differently from other people.

Fasting is healthy when it involves whole fresh foods and restriction of energy. The states of mind induced during times of religious observance, of which fasting is traditionally an integral part, may benefit physical health.

During this month you probably – though not necessarily – will be doing much the same, biologically and physiologically, as going on an energy-restricted dieting regime. But the motivation is different. You are not, please, doing this with the expectation of maintaining any reduction of weight or body fat, but solely to pay attention to what happens.

This month you will also be abstaining from some of the foods you most desire. Such foods or drinks may be those most liable to harm you. Anybody who gets the jitters unless they get through a bag of pastries a day or a big chocolate bar or six sugared drinks or half a bottle of liquor, is in trouble. In other ways the relationships between desire, craving, addiction and allergy are more subtle. Are some people hooked on specific branded processed foods? It seems so. We have no way of knowing what are the effects of the more active chemicals within processed foods, singly and in combination, other than by consuming them – or abstaining from them – and observantly experiencing what happens.

How much

For the first week continue as always to follow what is specified in rules 1 to 4, but consume nothing else. That is to say, consume only fresh foods including vegetables and fruits, and water, at the amounts specified, and stay physically active. For the second week, revert to last month's system, and follow rules 1 to 5 together with all the other foods and drinks you choose to consume.

For the third week, stay with rules 1 to 5, except eliminate one type of food and one type of drink that you commonly consume and most desire. Decide what these are and do without them for a week, and then revert, and be super-observant of the process. Notice I am saying 'type'. This means as examples, not steak but all meat, not bread but all starchy processed foods, not one brand but all sugared soft drinks, not wine but all alcoholic drinks. For the fourth week, do as you did in week 2. You get the idea.

In these weeks keep careful records of what you eat and drink, and how you feel, and what happens, and weigh and measure yourself at least three times a week. Use all the ways that work for you of checking yourself out. Make sure your records are organized, so that you can repeat them next time and compare, and be flexible, so you can develop them as your consciousness rises. Note down unexpected things that don't seem to be relevant, because they probably are. Time will tell.

That's 28 days. Follow this by eating nothing for a day. Absolutely nothing, just drink water. You may well feel extremely hungry towards the end of the day. On the thirtieth day, revert to rules 1 to 4 as in the second and fourth weeks, and check yourself out. If this month happens to be February, overlap with the next month.

Effect on body fat and weight

The original purpose of fasting may have been as training to endure and survive times of food shortage and famine, by making the body lay down fat more efficiently at times of plenty. Depending on how restrictive the fast is, you will shed body weight, at first rapidly and then more slowly. Yes, once you end the fast and start to eat and drink as usual, your body weight and body fat will increase rapidly and you will rebound to your pre-fast weight, probably quite quickly. Because you are active you will protect your lean tissue. By now your body will have been trained to get the message that you use and therefore need your lean tissue, and so will conserve it.

When you fast observantly, you will be reminded of the effects of restricted-energy dieting regimes, but without false hope. However, the main purpose of fasting is abstaining from some, most or all foods, to become more alive and gain a deeper sense of being human. Fasting should be a wonderful experience.

Fitting it in

Fasting is not easy within the family or socially, unless you don't mind what other people think, or have support. By this time, though, you probably will be quite a lot more resolute than you were at the beginning of the seven months.

Is it safe?

The fasts specified this month are not radical. The second and fourth weeks are modifications of the rules so far and specify lots of very nourishing food and drink.

In following a one-day water-only fast you may be venturing into the unknown. Most people have likely never done this, except when ill. Radical fasting is associated with hunger strikes unto death, and children being miraculously rescued alive after three days buried under earthquake rubble. If you tell other people you are going on a water-only fast, they are quite likely to express concern – 'are you sure it's safe?', 'do you really think you should?', that sort of thing. Have no fear. Water-only fasting refreshes the body, and for one day is completely safe. You will feel hungry, though, that's true.

Warning

In the first week of this month, and later for one day, you will be restricting the energy from the food and drink you consume, which is biologically the same as going on a diet. However, the fact that this is not your motivation will free you from apprehension and feelings of failure and guilt, and so help you to observe what happens non-judgmentally.

All the same though, coming off an energy-restricted regime is sometimes not easy. You may well feel ravenous after the first week as soon as you start to eat as normal, and also – for different reasons – after the third week. Always – as here – specify how long you will fast and when you will break the fast, and stay with this commitment. Always when you break a fast, follow it by consuming fresh foods – and see rule 7.

Who says?

As with feasting, the conventional nutrition literature draws a veil over fasting. In their combined 1,700 large-format pages, two standard current nutrition science textbooks contain four brief references to fasting. Scientific journals are also almost silent about fasting, or indeed about sustained energy restriction in humans. Little conventional research is undertaken on fasting.

It is commonly assumed inside as well as outside the medical and other health professions that radical fasting is cranky, bizarre and dangerous both in itself and because it could provoke compulsive self-starvation. Perhaps another reason is that in the countries where most research is funded, fasting is not commonly observed, except as a vestigial gesture during Lent.

Unorthodox teachers often recommend fasting. The naturopath Harry Benjamin correctly observes that when animals are unwell they stop eating. 'They will eat nothing perhaps for a week or longer – they may sip a drop of water now and then – until the disease or malaise has run its course.' Writing in the 16th century, Luigi Cornaro said: 'Nature, being desirous to preserve man as long as possible, teaches him what rule to apply in time of illness: for she immediately deprives the sick of their appetite in order that they may eat but little.' In our time, Margaret Visser writes: 'The bodies of both animals and people are biologically gifted not only to do without food for a while should there be none available, but also with a complex mechanism that makes a body deprived of food more alert and in less need of sleep and – some way into the fast – makes the mind much more energetic than usual.' Naturopaths also say that radical fasting encourages the *vis medicatrix naturae*, the body's natural powers of healing. Some say that fasting enables the body to rid itself of accumulated rubbish and also diseased tissue.

Wisdom of the ages

Fasting is still undertaken all over the world by vast numbers of people, usually but not always as an aspect of religious observance. Most if not all ancient philosophies of life, including what we call religions, recommend or enjoin fasting, and it is used as a rite of passage in preliterate cultures. Prolonged fasting enables the visions on which religions are founded and developed. In making fasting part of the preparation for festivals, the ancients understood its benefits for the body as well as for the mind and spirit.

Hindus and Buddhists fast on holidays (holy days). The last day of Yom Kippur is the most important day of fasting in the Jewish calendar.

Jesus, recorded as fasting a feasible 40 days and 40 nights, was within an already ancient tradition. St John Chrysostom declared: 'As bodily food fattens the body, so fasting strengthens the soul . . . to put the heavenly higher than the pleasant and pleasurable things of life.'

The practices of the Greek Orthodox Church remind adherents to value animal foods. These stipulate abstinence from meat, fish, milk, eggs, cheese – and olive oil – for a total of around 150 days of the year. In the periods of fasting, foods of animal origin are prepared and preserved for later consumption, so the practice also has communal, economic and ecological value.

Eastern philosophies, also as interpreted by the human potential movement that took off in California in the 1960s, teach that it is through detachment from desire and intention, and instead simply noticing what is so – especially in changed circumstances – that we best learn.

Tips

- Remember that hunger you will feel at first on a fast will fade
- Stay with the system as here, and please do not be more radical
- Make a note of the foods and drinks you most desire or crave
- Notice also which favourite foods and drinks you don't miss
- Pay close attention to changes in your moods and emotions
- Monitor your weight and other vital signs daily all this month
- Break the fast if you are unable to work or stay physically active
- Plan ahead to avoid temptations at parties or when eating out
- Rejoice in the adventure if this is your first water-only fast
- Break the fast with fresh foods and drinks, not with a feast

Big picture stuff

The big picture is your whole being, personal or in communion with others. The purpose of fasting here is to cleanse and refresh your body and to put you closer in touch with your senses, thoughts and feelings. If you have a sense of a god, you may well feel closer as you fast. If you do not have any such sense, you will gain a sense of communion with your inner and the outer world and with nature.

Golden Rule 7

BODY FAT REDUCTION
Make lower-energy choices that suit you best

Pause for reflection

As said in the introduction to the golden rules, this month is optional. If you have been following the system for the first six months for general health and wellbeing and all the other benefits, and now do not wish to reduce body fat or weight, then yours is a six-month system.

You may have started the system six months ago wanting to reduce a substantial amount of weight, but now that you are in better shape, with less body fat and more lean tissue, you may be wondering whether you now do want to reduce weight. Here is what I think.

First, some people who try and then fail on dieting regimes are really not heavy, but flabby. People can even be light, skinny and nevertheless flabby. So how do you feel about yourself now? How comfortable are you within your skin? If you started six months ago intending to reduce body weight, but now feel that getting in shape is what you really wanted, and that now you do not want to reduce a significant amount of weight but rather continue to get in better shape, then also skip this month.

If you are overweight according to the usual measures, bear in mind chapter 3. Sedentary people who mostly eat highly processed food and who are fat are unhealthy by any definition and more likely to suffer various serious diseases. But this is not because of their extra weight so much as the overall impact of their ways of life. Inactive people of any weight, light or heavy, who consume mostly unhealthy food and drink are also more susceptible to disease. But active people who are a bit overweight, who enjoy lots of good-quality food and drink, and who feel fine, are unlikely to be unhealthy in any sense. Why should they be?

So if you are active and fit, are healthy, feel good, enjoy being the way you are, eat and drink well, and have a body mass index (BMI) a bit over 25, you need not feel any pressure to reduce to a BMI of under 25, let alone 22. If you really want to reduce a substantial amount of weight and more body fat, that's another matter. Go ahead, and use this rule. But if you find that nothing much happens, my advice is that your body is the size it wants to be, and let this be.

However, if six months ago when you started with the golden rules you were fat or frankly obese, and particularly if you have settled mostly just for moderate physical activity such as brisk walking, you will probably want to reduce your body fat now. If that is the case, go for it, and you are now trained to take full advantage of this seventh golden rule, this month and then for always, constantly adjusting to suit your progress, plans and circumstances.

Principle

To reduce body fat, by becoming more physically active, or by preferring from within the types of food and drink you consume, those that are relatively low in energy density.

What

Remember that this rule is optional. Follow it if you still want to lose body fat and weight. If so, start by reviewing your whole diet. Think about what you enjoy, the changes you have made so far, what works best, what has not worked. Then begin. You make this rule work by systematically preferring foods and drinks that are relatively low in energy density

This – emphatically – does not mean that you consume only foods and drinks that are low in energy density. This is not the lettuce and water month. It is not the month to abandon all your favourite foods. It is not the end of alcohol month, unless that's your choice. Rather, it's the month where you adjust your diet, so that it becomes somewhat more heavy and bulky relative to the energy it contains, by making choices that suit you best from within all the types of food and drink you consume.

Energy density

Here again is what 'energy density' means. It refers to the amount of dietary energy (measured in calories or kilojoules) contained in a given weight, or else size, of food or drink. Whole and fresh foods of all types are generally low in energy density, because they contain a lot of water and dietary fibre. The more processed any food is, generally the higher it is in energy density, usually because of added sugar or fat. Other degraded ingredients such as white flour are also energy-dense.

Foods low in energy density, containing a lot of water and dietary fibre, include all fresh vegetables, fruits, pulses (legumes), and also fresh cereals (grains). All fresh fish, and most fresh lean meat and poultry, as part of meals you have prepared yourself, or bought ready to eat, are in themselves low or fairly low in energy density. Water and black coffee and tea (no milk or sugar) contain no dietary energy. Nor do 'no-cal' drinks.

Commonly consumed energy-dense foods – foods high in energy density – are high in fats and sugars added in processing. Most convenience foods and almost all fast foods are energy-dense, as are junk foods. Baked foods such as cakes, biscuits, pies and pastries, fatty and processed meats, and almost all processed snack foods, are energy-dense. Alcoholic and sweetened drinks are energy-dense.

Some fresh foods like lightly processed plant oils are of course concentrated in energy, as are nuts and seeds. Some processed foods are not particularly energy-dense. Burgers, for example, and indeed the complete burger package, are roughly the same energy density as bread. Sorbets have almost the same energy density as boiled potatoes.

Diets in general

Average industrialized diets overall contain anything up to 175 calories (around 735 kilojoules) per 100 grams, whereas diets that follow most current recommendations for good health contain around 125 calories (around 525 kilojoules) per 100 grams. Healthy diets are a lot heavier and bulkier than typical industrialized diets, and all the more so when people are physically active. This is a reason why healthy diets are more satisfying. Another reason, as you know from chapter 3, is that hunger is not just for energy from food but also for nutrients: the more nourishing any diet is, the more readily it will satisfy you.

Books and reports using the energy-density concept draw lines between low and high energy-dense foods (or very low, low, medium, high, or whatever) at different points. A fuzzy line can be drawn at around 225–275 calories per 100 grams. Drinks, being mostly or entirely water, of course contain much lower levels of energy per unit of volume or weight, but the same general approach can also be used, with a fuzzy line drawn at around 30–35 calories per 100 millilitres.

This does not mean that it is best to restrict yourself only to foods and drinks whose energy density is below these lines. This would be boring, for a start. Different types of food by their nature range around different levels of energy density. Fruits are generally more energy-dense than vegetables as defined here, for example, and lean meat is more energy-dense than fruit. This rule is not proposing that you select and consume only foods and drinks low in energy density, but rather that from the various types of food and drink you make specific lower energy-dense choices that suit you best. The one overall helpful general guide is that almost all fresh foods are low or fairly low in energy density, whereas most processed foods are high or fairly high in energy density, and a lot are energy bombs or rocket fuel (see chapter 4).

Specific foods

Now I might give this book some heft with long lists of the energy contents of specific foods and drinks. In the USA the respected nutrition scientist Barbara Rolls includes 'modular food lists' in her calorie-counting dieting books. From these you can learn that 343 grams of 'Asian black bean soup' contains – according to the recipe included – 240 calories, whereas 483 grams of 'Hearty chicken and vegetable soup' contains 290 calories.

To take other examples, according to the standard UK chemical compendium *The Composition of Foods*, boiled brown rice contains 141 calories per 100 grams, whereas egg-fried rice weighs in at 186. Bread generally is around 230 calories per 100 grams, whereas most biscuits and cakes average anything between 400–500 calories per 100 grams. Full-fat milk contains 66 calories per 100 grams, 32 of which are removed by skimming. Rump steak delivers 174 calories per 100 grams, unless it is fried in which case another 52 calories are added. And so on, and on. To convert calories to kilojoules, multiply by four, or if you want to be exact, 4.18.

This system does not require you to get into that kind of detail, and I think such an approach is unhelpful. What is most useful is general information and principles. Once you get the general idea of any of the rules here – or any guidance in life – you are the best judge of what to do next.

You will have noticed that rules 3 to 5 do not rule out any food or drink. What else you are eating and drinking, as well as following these rules, has been down to you, although I have advised you to be careful with anything that you most desire or crave, especially snack, convenience and fast food, and sugary drinks. Before this month you have been enjoying lots of fresh vegetables, pulses (legumes) and fruits, and lots of all sorts of fresh foods, as per rules 3 and 4, and then you have also eaten substantial dinners. Or you may have been making meals with what's specified in rules 3 and 4, together with steamed rice and a jug of water, and preferring not to consume much else at all. I don't know. You know.

Nor do I know how much body weight and body fat you have dropped in the last six months. Other things being equal, rice will lead to weight reduction more readily than strawberry shortcake. But a big man regularly digging into lashings of moussaka or downing a bottle of wine a day, as well as following rules 1–5 and also being vigorously active for an hour or more a day, could shed more body fat in these six months than a small or older woman with little room for any foods and drinks other than those specified, who is only approximating to rule 2, especially if her lean tissue has been reduced by successions of energy-restrictive dieting regimes. At this stage now you are the best judge of what is likely to work for you. Please remember this. Trust what you have discovered for yourself.

The pleasure principle

Colin MacInnes proposed, in one of the columns he wrote for the British social science weekly *New Society*, that everybody can be seen either as a Roundhead or a Cavalier. The legend says that Cavaliers dressed flamboyantly, embraced ceremony, tolerated differences, and enjoyed their food and drink. The legend also says that Roundheads (also known as Puritans) dressed in black, banned theatre and dancing, burned women as witches, and masticated dull and frugal meals. These seven golden rules are on the side of the Cavaliers.

Besides, you are not likely to follow any rule that tells you to give up your favourite foods and drinks, and there is no need. Please don't try to do so. Omelettes made with butter? Stir-fried vegetables with or without strips of chicken? If these are among your favourites (and my mouth is watering as I write this), enjoy them. A dram of single malt whisky savoured in the evening – as by one of my guides, the trim John Neilson of Dumfries, who in 2007 died aged 92 in good health? *Slainte!*

There is a difference between favourite foods and drinks, and those you crave. You will have found out a lot about this in the previous six months. Prefer high-quality favourite foods and drinks that you do not crave, and enjoy them not daily but occasionally.

Why

This is the one golden rule that you can use to reduce body fat. I ask you, very sincerely, please to wait until you have stayed with the first six golden rules before you start with this one – or any variant of it. As I have said above, trust this process.

How much

What you do this month is to make four types of decision. First, decide whether or not you want to become more physically active, and how much more, and if you do, go for it. Second, decide which fatty or sugary foods you won't miss, and stop eating them. Your choice, remember! Third, decide which you would like to modify for less energy-dense versions, like say plain cake, pizza topped not with cheese or meat but with vegetables and some oil, and not ice cream but sorbets. Fourth, decide which energy-dense foods really delight you, and make them an occasional delicacy or treat.

Following the golden rules so far means that the energy density of your diet is almost certainly quite a lot lower than it was when you started. But not necessarily, depending on what else you are now eating and drinking. If the rest of your diet is mostly fresh food, it will be overall a lot lower in energy density than if you are following the rules so far but also consuming cookies, pizzas, ice cream, 'energy bars', chocolate, candies, sugared drinks. I don't need to make a long list. We are talking all processed foods and drinks with added fats or sugars.

This explains the principle of this rule. If you do still want to reduce body weight and fat, the way to do this is to further increase your physical activity or else generally to reduce the energy density of foods and drinks within all the types of food and drink you are consuming, or both. What does this mean in practice? Here is some general guidance on how to modify the golden rules in order to reduce body fat.

RULE 1. WATER
No change.

RULE 2. PHYSICAL ACTIVITY
If you have incorporated at least half-an-hour of vigorous physical activity into your life and are already inclined to be active not five days a week but almost all days, you can step this up. Aerobic exercise like running, cycling and swimming uses body fat as fuel most of all after about half an hour of exercise. So you could go for longer sessions, say of 45 minutes or more if you prefer, say three days a week. Two possible targets are to increase your physical activity overall by 25 or 50 per cent.

RULE 3. VEGETABLES, FRUITS, PULSES (LEGUMES)
There is no need to make any adaptations this month in your consumption of all fresh vegetables, fruits, cereals, or pulses (legumes). Avocados? If you eat avocados but can take or leave them, then leave them. But if for you avocados are part of big, delicious, nourishing and satisfying salads – as they occasionally are for me – stay with them.

RULE 4. ALL OTHER FRESH FOODS

Plant food
Enjoy all fresh cereals (grains) in abundance. Boiled rice, preferably wholegrain (brown) or else parboiled, with vegetables, is a great choice for main meals. Porridge oats is great breakfast food, and even more delicious with added fruits.

Good advice is further to limit your consumption of processed cereals and avoid foods made with processed cereals and those with added fats or sugars. The simplest advice with packaged breakfast cereals is to avoid all of them. Yes, there are some without added sugar or fat, and if you enjoy these, fine. But watch out for products that make health claims (and see below). Granola is an energy bomb, as are cereal or muesli bars.

If as well as following rule 4, you are also consuming some fresh foods made or cooked with fat, cut these down, or cut them out. If you enjoy chips (French fries), following this rule suggests two choices. Either avoid them, or prefer 'fat chips' which are more potato and less fat.

Bread

Now for advice you may not be expecting. The less bread you eat the better. Bread is processed. It is more energy-dense than most fresh lean meat, practically all poultry, and all fresh, including fatty, fish. Sandwiches with added fat spread and fatty fillings are even more energy-dense. The energy density of starch-based dishes like pastas and pizzas similarly depends on what comes with them.

The fact that bread has been made for over 4,000 years does not mean that what's in the shops now has much resemblance to what women in ancient Egypt ground and baked, apart from chemical content. Bread has a terrific press. Nutrition guidelines usually urge us to eat lots of bread both for positive reasons and also on the assumption that the more bread (and other starchy foods) we eat, the less fat and sugar we will consume. Having followed this party line for a long time, I now think this is horrible advice. It suggests that the experts who compile dietary guidelines have never seen sandwiches, let alone checked out their energy density.

If you eat bread – which no doubt you do – always prefer eating bread by itself, meaning only eat bread that is delicious with nothing added. Or make traditional use of plain wholegrain bread, and use it to mop up juices of your main meals including the dressings of salads. This gives you plenty of scope. Sure, I enjoy an occasional wholegrain smoked salmon sandwich with no added fat and three times the usual amount of lemon. But its caloric punch is nothing like a sandwich plus fat containing any kind of processed meat plus mayonnaise.

Animal foods

You can now do better for both yourself and for the environment. Fresh meat continues to have a bad press. Industrially produced meat and poultry involves horrible cruelty and degradation. It is also fatty. As a citizen, and as a consumer, it's a good decision to stop eating it. If you choose to continue to eat red meat, and if as well as following rules 4 and 5 you are sometimes eating chops and steaks with their fat, or fatty processed meats such as sausages or salami or hot dogs, now is a good time to cut all these out and switch to lean meats, game meats like venison or hare and wild fish.

Drinks

If the fuzzy line between low- and high-energy density for drinks is taken to be 30–35 calories (125–145 kilojoules) per 100 grams, then some pure fruit juices and lower-alcohol beer are intermediate, sweetened soft drinks are above the line, and almost all alcoholic drinks are energy-dense. With alcoholic drinks, use the avocado principle. If you drink alcohol, and if what works best for you at this stage – no doubt from previous experience – is to cut out alcohol altogether, feel free. If on the other hand you enjoy alcoholic drinks, then prefer the lower energy-dense versions. The simple tip is to cut out all sweet alcoholic drinks. Prefer lager to stout, dry to sweet white wine, and liquor to liqueur. (See also the note to this rule on alcoholic drinks.)

Processed foods and drinks

If you are prepared to do so, eliminate processed foods and drinks with added fat or sugar – look at the ingredients list – but also apply the avocado (and alcohol) principle. These include all processed food and drinks that make health claims in bigger print on their labels and in advertisements. They also include all such foods that are 'fortified' with vitamins, minerals or other bioactive substances, and so-called 'lower fat', 'low-fat', 'no fat', 'lower-sugar', 'low-sugar' and 'no sugar' processed foods.

If after the first six months you are still consuming some fast or junk foods and drinks, this is not the best month to cut them out completely. Also some types of commercial fast food are, from the personal health point of view, unfairly demonized. For example, a burger with or without salad is a lot less energy-dense than a sandwich with added fat and a fatty filling.

Nothing you most enjoy and that most satisfies you is banned. Nothing is banned. Forget banning. To quote the great Brazilian singer Caetano Veloso, prohibition is prohibited. If after six months of following rules 3 to 5 your daily happiness still depends on a treat or delicacy, this is not the month to make yourself miserable. What you might do is weed these out of your daily diet, and relish them only occasionally – once or at most twice a week, say.

Austere alternatives

There is another way to reduce body weight and fat within these rules, which after reading and following rule 6 on fasting may already have occurred to you. This is simply to repeat the first fasting week for this whole seventh month: follow rules 1 to 4, and eat and drink nothing else. If you did so for all this month you would certainly reduce body fat and weight, simply because all fresh foods are low, or relatively low, in energy density. If they all averaged out at 100 calories (420 kilojoules) per 100 grams, a total of 1½ kilograms (nearly 3½ pounds) would amount to 1,500 calories (6,250 kilojoules) a day.

Given that you are now completely following rule 2, you will probably be in energy balance at well over 2,000 calories (8,400 kilojoules) a day if you are a woman, and well over 2,500 calories (10,500 kilojoules) a day if you are a man. How much above of course depends on your size, your age, and your level of fitness. So you will certainly reduce weight and body fat. Also, because you are now physically active and relatively fit, your body will protect its lean tissue.

You should have an idea of whether this method would work for you, as a result of your first week of fasting – and what happened afterwards. But if you choose this austere alternative for this month, be careful. It amounts to yet one more energy-restricted dieting regime. True, it has the advantage of being made up all from fresh foods, it is also simple to follow, and if you are now fit, your body will conserve more of its lean tissue. But after a while you may feel fatigued, and therefore likely to backslide from rule 2. That is the signal to stop, and revert to the plan outlined above for this month. Also be careful to stay with rules 1 to 6 immediately after this month and thereafter. The golden thread within these golden rules is regular sustained physical activity.

A second somewhat less austere alternative is again to stay with rules 1 to 4, except modify rule 4 and consume more of the fresh food specified – say, instead of 500 grams (just over a pound), you could increase to 750 grams (over 1½ pounds) a day. Provided you make relatively low-energy choices, this might add another 400 calories (1,650 kilojoules) a day and bring you closer to energy balance. This is not an energy-restricted dieting regime – now that you are physically active your energy balance is higher. But it also is somewhat artificial. Throughout these rules, I prefer ways of eating and drinking that are indefinitely sustainable and enjoyable.

Effect on body fat and weight

After a month of following this rule, or its alternatives, you will reduce some body weight, depending on how many changes you make in favour of becoming more physically active, or of lower energy-dense foods and drinks. If you have not, this can only be for one of two reasons. One would be that you are not following the rule.

Two would be because you have been ingenious. Thus I have not recommended that you avoid adding oils to salads, so you might find room for a couple of avocados a day and lashings of dressing as well as everything else you are eating and drinking. If you do something like this and are the same body weight at the end of the month, don't feel bad but don't be surprised.

How much weight and body fat will you reduce? Maybe you will end the month between 1½–3 kilograms (3½–7 pounds) lighter, and one dress or trouser size smaller. Something like that. Nothing dramatic. Maybe less. Maybe more. How much depends on many things, such as your size, how much body fat you have to start with, your body's individuality, and how many changes you chose to make. You will almost certainly be in even better shape.

Fitting it in

You are already choosing and consuming lots of meals and dishes made with fresh foods and drinks. Now that your physical activity and your diet has become a central part of your life, you will be spending more time considering, choosing and preparing food and drink. Great, wonderful! If this month you make a general choice to avoid processed convenience, fast, and junk food and drink, you will be spending some-what more time on your diet. You will find that this is worthwhile. You can make this the month you get seriously into cooking.

Is it safe?

Yes. A related question is: will it work? And here comes the warning.

Warning

A common mistake people make when they try to decrease weight and body fat by changing what they eat and drink is to start out being too enthusiastic. If you have already followed the advice of energy-restrictive diet regimes, you will know for yourself what I mean. If as a result of the way you interpret this rule or its variants, you start to feel fatigued, ravenous or miserable, it is not working. Ease off.

Remember that this rule does not specify that you never consume energy-dense food and drink, only that you prefer the lower energy-dense versions of the types of food and drink you do consume. Continue to enjoy the foods and drinks that you most enjoy, within the rules.

If you find that when you make a change to what you are eating and drinking by following this rule you start to think about food all the time, or want to have naps in the afternoon, or - more telling - start to avoid physical activity, then it's best that you don't make that change. You have likely already found the right balance for you before starting this month. If nevertheless you really do want to reduce more body fat, then I suggest you increase the amount or intensity of your physical activity.

Who says?

The World Cancer Research Fund/American Institute for Cancer Research 2007 report recommends: 'Consume energy-dense foods sparingly' and 'avoid sugary drinks', and 'consume "fast foods" sparingly if at all'. The report judges that low energy-dense food is probably protective against body weight increase, overweight and obesity, and high energy-dense food as a probable cause of increased body fatness, stating that the case is 'compelling on physiological grounds and [is] supported by experimental and observational evidence'.

As mentioned, Barbara Rolls has written books advocating low energy-dense foods as the best way to reduce body fat. Lots of writers are against processed convenience, fast, and junk food and drink, in different degrees and for different reasons. These are usually not so much to reduce weight, as for gastronomic, cultural, economic, social, ethical and environmental reasons, and for general good health. Cookery writers who champion traditional food systems and diets are for this reason all for fresh foods and drinks. The 'slow food' campaign started by lovers of good food in Italy is now a world movement.

Orthodox nutrition scientists focus on nutrients rather than foods and drinks, typically have taken minimal interest in food production, preservation, processing and preparation, and generally see little problem with such foods and drinks unless consumed 'in excess', which is what their manufacturers say. This attitude is usually also reflected in nutrition guidelines issued by United Nations agencies and by national governments, which in this respect are mistaken.

On bread, this rule goes against practically all orthodox guidelines, and may sound a bit like the Atkins Diet. That's because I think that the precursors of Robert Atkins, notably Jean Anthelme Brillat-Savarin (see chapter 2), were basically correct. The idea that carbohydrates are in themselves fattening and that the right way to reduce body weight and fat is to eliminate or severely restrict carbohydrates, is wrong. Forget carbohydrates (and see chapter 4). But 'refined' degraded starches such as white flour, and 'refined' sugar, are fattening, especially when combined with other ingredients, and most of all when combined with added fat.

The issue is not the foods. The issues are identifying types of food with their chemical constituents, and processing that degrades food and turns it into energy bombs. Fresh and preferably lightly processed whole cereals (grains) are healthy staple foods. People in India and China who subsist on great quantities of boiled rice, with vegetables, pulses (legumes) and some flesh foods, do not become fat.

Wisdom of the ages

The ancients have nothing to say about energy density. This was not an issue in the olden days. But both the traditional Chinese and Indian dietary philosophies include the concept of hot and cold. In the traditional Chinese system, foods and drinks are divided into the heating and the cooling, usually reflecting the effect they have on the body.

Meat (flesh and organs), fat, sugar, fried foods, bread, long-baked foods, and alcoholic drinks, are all heating. Water, and most vegetables and fruits, are cooling. Rice and fish are neutral.

Tips

- Continue to enjoy fresh vegetables, fruits and pulses (legumes)
- Prefer fresh cereals (grains) to bread and breakfast cereals
- Enjoy fish and lean meat, preferably from free-ranging animals
- Prefer higher quality meals, snacks, dishes, foods and drinks
- Savour high-quality delicious delicacies within meals and as treats
- Continue to enjoy feasts of whole and fresh foods and drinks
- Avoid processed foods and drinks containing added fats or sugars
- Avoid 'fortified' foods and drinks and others making health claims
- Avoid all energy-dense foods or drinks you no longer really enjoy
- Make this the month that you cook for yourself and your family

Big picture stuff

When you choose a relatively low-energy version of fresh food, you may also be choosing a food produced in ways that are preferable environmentally and in other ways. Meat is a good example. As you know from chapter 4, game animals that lead relatively natural lives are lower in fat and therefore in energy-density than domesticated animals. Free-ranging chickens are lower in fat than factory-produced chickens.

Inasmuch as this golden rule further reduces the amount of processed foods and drinks you consume, it also has a beneficial environmental effect – less packaging and waste, for example. The main benefits are more to do with other choices you make, such as preferring foods and drinks that are produced locally, or that are fairly traded.

The Golden Way

CONSCIOUS WELLBEING
Make the rules your own

When you come to this final passage after you have completed your first six or seven months with the golden rules the experience will be different from before you began the system. You will have learned a lot, your values will have shifted, and you will be more conscious. More than this, you will sense the world differently. People's basic natures stay the same – except perhaps as a result of a great crisis – but you will in a real sense be a renewed person.

So what now? This is a system for life. By now you will have learned many ways to make it work for you, and you will have your own ideas about your degree of success. If you prefer, and certainly if you feel you are still 'in training to get in training' then yes, I suggest you stay with the system as shown here, and continue to learn and refine it. This means staying with rules 1 to 6 as specified indefinitely.

If on the other hand you feel you are fluent with the rules, adapt them more freely. The two obvious examples are rules 2, 5 and 6. Quite a lot of people I know who have changed their lives in favour of their positive health and wellbeing have built recreational physical activity into their lives, as members of citizen running or cycling clubs. Again, a feast day is fine up to once a week any week of the year, and the occasional great occasion that extends over more than one day is OK also – as long as you count this as two days. The same principle applies to fasting. If undertaken by yourself, fast for a week twice a year – or up to say six times a year – any time that suits you. If you follow a philosophy or a faith that includes fasting, fast at those times, reconciling what's specified here with what is enjoined.

Once you make the system your own, do keep on recording your progress and what you discover. In doing this you can help others also.

Reducing body fat

The same consideration applies to body fat. Assuming you have stayed with the system for all seven months, do you now still want to reduce your body fat? As already said, people often undertake dieting regimes believing that they want to weigh less, whereas what they really want is to get into shape, which is not the same thing. Sometimes the underlying motives are more complex, involving general self-dissatisfaction and a feeling that once body weight has been shed, life will improve – another reason why the failure of repeated dieting regimes is depressing. After seven months of the system you may decide that the increased self-confidence and self-respect you have earned is what you were looking for, irrespective of what you weigh. If so, now that you have incorporated the golden rules into your everyday life, stay with the first six; you have no need of the seventh.

But if after seven months you do still want to reduce your body fat, I suggest that you stay with the first six golden rules and experiment with the seventh, say once every three to six months for a couple of weeks, or at any length of time that suits you.

You could, for example, stop consuming energy-dense foods and drinks made from degraded ingredients that now you don't really enjoy. Alternatively – and this is not that much different – you could stay with avoiding fast, convenience, pre-prepared and other highly processed foods and drinks. If such are your choices, don't decrease your physical activity – if anything, become more energetic, so that your overall energy balance remains at a natural level. Other variants are mentioned in the section on rule 7, above.

Rules that work best for you

You may devise a system that works best for you and also that is generally better all round than what's here. You can certainly adapt the rules so that they are ethically and environmentally purer than what's included here, especially in relation to rule 4, which does not exclude meat from industrially produced animals.

You may also decide to vary the amounts specified in ways that suit you. But I suggest you be careful here, and stay with the general principles concerning fresh and processed foods, and also the balance between vegetables, pulses (legumes) and fruits, other fresh foods, and all other foods.

Any such improvements would I think not be radically different from what's here. This system works. Stay with it. It's the basics for your diet in the grand sense – your whole way of life – for always. In saying this I rely not so much on my own knowledge and experience as on that of many teachers and observers whose judgements are consistent, on information about various food systems and supplies and their impact on health and wellbeing, and on common knowledge of human evolution and adaptation and what these imply. Now though you will be finding out for yourself.

ANNEX 1.
THE NEW NUTRITION

The science of food and nutrition is now being born again, in a form fit for the 21st century. This new nutrition is designed to develop and maintain positive health and wellbeing, and to protect the human, living, and physical world.

So many of us get fat, go on diets, get fat again, and become frustrated. One reason for this miserable way of life is that we are mystified about food and nutrition. It's no wonder that we are, because the professionals have also been confused.

Nutrition science was devised in its present form in the 19th century, as a branch of biochemistry applied to humans, animals and plants. Its purpose then and until the middle of the 20th century included building up generations of big tall strong young people; and big has also meant heavy, starting with 'bonny bouncing' overweight babies fed on cow's milk-based formula feeds. Plants, animals and humans were fed artificial growth-promoting feeds devised by scientists, and still are. This was all made possible by the mechanization of agriculture and food manufacture, emphasizing the production of energy-dense processed foods and drinks.

Until the late 20th century the main concern of most nutrition professionals, in materially rich as well as poor countries, has been malnutrition in the 'classic' sense, meaning under-nutrition in general and specific nutrient deficiencies caused by poverty and food insecurity. This understandably remains the main concern of the relevant United Nations agencies, despite the fact that now in almost all countries premature deaths from heart disease and cancer, and in many countries very rapidly rising rates of diabetes, have become important and urgent public-health crises, as has obesity.

WHAT'S NEEDED NOW

In many ways the teaching and practice of nutrition as a biochemical science has become unhelpful in this 21st century. As one example – see chapter 4 – the value of defining foods and drinks in terms of their chemical constituents, such as fats, carbohydrates, proteins and alcohol, has always been limited. A basic cause of the dieting regime wars between advocates of different combinations of macronutrients has been and still is reductionist, mechanistic thinking. Use of the chemical term 'carbohydrate' has made a mess that suits the sugar industry and baffles the public.

Concerns about the nature and direction of food and nutrition policy and practice are now shared by many hundreds if not thousands of scientists and other health professionals throughout the world who are committed to improved personal and public health. These concerns are also shared by agronomists, economists, and social and environmental scientists who are aware of the importance of healthy and sustainable food systems in this era of climate change, continued world population growth, worsening social inequalities, degradation of soil, and draining of non-renewable resources such as water and oil.

This was the context for a workshop meeting at Schloss Rauischholzhausen, a property of the University of Giessen in Germany. The 23 scientists and other participants included the then current and a future president of the International Union of Nutritional Sciences. Ricardo Uauy, IUNS president from 2005 to 2009, states in support of the meeting and its purposes: 'The chemical and biological sciences have provided a strong base for nutrition ... However, these approaches are clearly insufficient to address the main challenges [of] the 21st century. There is a pressing need to include the social, economic and human rights aspects within an ethical framework.'

The location of Giessen has a special significance. It was there that Justus von Liebig developed nutrition science as a specialized biochemical discipline. With Claus Leitzmann of the University of Giessen, I was privileged to convene the 2005 meeting. Its purpose was to re-create nutrition science and its application to food and nutrition policy and practice, ranging from the planning of world food supplies to the positive health and wellbeing of communities, families and individuals.

THE GIESSEN DECLARATION

The first product of the meeting is the Giessen Declaration, drafted, agreed and signed by all present. The Declaration states: 'The purpose of nutrition science is to contribute to a world in which present and future generations fulfil their human potential, live in the best of health, and develop, sustain and enjoy an increasingly diverse human, living and physical environment.'

The Declaration also states: 'The human species has now moved from a time in history when the science of nutrition, and food and nutrition policy, have been principally concerned with personal and population health and with the exploitation, production and consumption of food and associated resources, to a new period. Now all relevant sciences, including that of nutrition, should and will be principally concerned with the cultivation, conservation and sustenance of human, living and physical resources all together, and so with the health of the biosphere.'

Another key statement in the Declaration is: 'Food systems . . . shape and are shaped by biological, social and environmental relationships and interactions . . . How food is grown, processed, distributed, sold, prepared, cooked and consumed, is crucial to its quality and nature, and to its effect on wellbeing and health, society and the environment.'

WE LIVE IN A NEW WORLD

We are now living within a series of global technological, economic, political, social and environmental developments and changes, some auspicious, some ominous, that together amount to a time of revolution.

This new era of human history has profound implications for nutrition science and food and nutrition policy and practice. The electronic and genomic revolutions, deregulation of global flows of trade and money, widening of inequities between and within regions and countries, and depletion of living and physical resources, are examples of inter-related phenomena all of which affect and are affected by nutrition.

Closer to the normal concerns of nutrition science, rates of childhood obesity and early-life diabetes have rapidly increased since the 1980s, as have rates of heart disease and various cancers, while rates of food and nutrition insecurity and inadequacy and even chronic hunger remain outrageously high. For most countries in the world this double burden of chronic disease and deficiency states is politically, economically and socially intolerable, as well as causing misery, suffering, disability and premature death.

Below are some of the questions now being asked by concerned citizens as well as by professionals in the biological, social, economic and environmental sciences. Here they are phrased in the form of 'how?' questions. There are also plenty of 'what?' and 'why?' questions to be asked.

How can exclusive breastfeeding in the first six months of a baby's life become normal, when working mothers are not given adequate paid time off work?

How can traditional ways of life survive the invasion of cheap and highly capitalized and advertised transnational brands of fast foods and drinks?

How can the benefits of local fresh agricultural produce be advocated when political and economic forces are pushing rural populations into big cities?

How can consumers enjoy inexpensive nutritious food while at the same time supporting producers in middle- and low-income countries to sustain equitable livelihoods?

How can policies to prevent childhood food insecurity be harmonized with those designed to prevent chronic diseases throughout the course of life?

How can consumption of red meat and animal fat decrease when subsidies and global food-trade rules and regulations increase their production and supply?

How can consumption of more fish and seafood be recommended when it is known that fish stocks are an increasingly threatened food resource?

How can the human right to adequate nutritious food be achieved in countries devastated by wars and where food trade is used as an instrument of power?

THE FOUR DIMENSIONS

In response the Giessen Declaration begins by stating: 'Now is the time for the science of nutrition, with its application in food and nutrition policy, to be given a broader definition, additional dimensions and relevant principles.'

It continues: 'As originally conceived and as now usually studied and practised, nutrition is principally a biological science. This classic biological dimension of nutrition science is and will remain central.' But: 'Those now concerned with the future of the world at all levels from local to global generally agree that their overriding shared priority is to protect human, living and physical resources all together, in order to enable the long-term sustenance of life on earth and the happiness of humankind. Nutrition science is one vital means to this end. This implies expansion and enlargement of the science, and its identification as a broad, integrative discipline.' The biological dimension should be one of the four dimensions of nutrition science. The other three dimensions are economic, social, and environmental.

PERSONAL, POPULATION AND PLANETARY HEALTH

The Declaration goes on to identify the general context in which food science and technology and the agriculture and nutrition sciences were originally devised in the mid-19th century in Europe. The general social, economic and political context at that time was one of industrial and other material expansion, individual and population growth, and mechanical and technological power, and the exploitation of human, living and physical resources. This was at a time when the global human population was far less numerous and less long-lived than it is now. Further, until relatively recently it has generally been assumed that the world's living and physical resources were inexhaustible.

The Declaration continues: 'Correspondingly, application of the principles that have explicitly or implicitly governed nutrition science has created food systems that have greatly contributed to the sixfold increase of the global human population in the last 150 years ... During this time non-renewable energy use, material consumption and waste generation have increased enormously. This has resulted in the depletion of many living and physical resources and changes to ecosystems, and also has heightened the contrast between and within rich and poor regions and countries in access to material and other resources.'

Food systems have been and are being transformed with accelerating speed, as a result of mechanization, urbanization, and now biotechnology and economic globalization. These have profound effects. The Declaration states: 'Food processing, including refrigeration, has enabled the supply of a wide range of foods across seasons and continents. Food manufacturing, retailing and distribution are now increasingly concentrated in fewer hands. Traditional cuisines are being replaced by new eating patterns framed by new technologies, ways of living and economic structures.' Technological developments 'profoundly affect the relationship between food and the health of people, populations and the planet'.

THE CHALLENGES WE FACE NOW

The Declaration then audits these changes. 'This 21st century in many respects shows prospects of opportunity and prosperity for the minority that enjoys stable entitlements including physical and financial security, adequate, nourishing and safe food, safe water supplies, and good education and health.'

The majority is not so fortunate. They are now 'afflicted and threatened by inter-related deprivations that make social and individual life difficult and sometimes impossible. These include loss of amenities and skills; loss of traditional farming and food cultures; loss of land, property and independence; vulnerability to unemployment, dislocation, and other impoverishments; precipitate urbanization; social, economic and political inequities and turmoil; poor governance, and conflicts and wars of many types.'

At the same time: 'Many planetary environmental indicators are now deteriorating. These include global climate change and the persistent depletion of stratospheric ozone; the depletion and degradation of topsoil;

the accelerated loss of species and of fresh water and sources of energy; and increased use and of persistence of many chemical pollutants. Recent and current modes of food production have made major contributions to such adverse changes.

'If these environmental changes are not arrested, the conditions of the natural world will deteriorate for future generations . . . for the first time in human experience, the overall size and the economic activity of humankind exceed the capacity of the planet to supply, replenish and absorb. The bio-capacity of the natural world is now beginning to diminish.'

NUTRITION: WHAT'S GONE WRONG

Reports published by United Nations agencies and other authoritative organizations since the second half of the 20th century have summarized the state of the world's nutrition and especially under-nutrition, and usually have then gone on to set hopeful targets. But: 'Global food and nutrition insecurity and inadequacy and even chronic hunger have not significantly changed in the last 20 years. These are made worse among the most deprived populations by increased inequity between rich and impoverished nations and populations, most especially in areas of conflict and disaster.

'General and specific nutritional deficiencies increase vulnerability to infectious diseases, especially in women, infants and children. These infections in turn worsen food and nutrition security. Although improved in some parts of the world, nutritional deficiencies and infectious diseases have worsened in many of the more impoverished regions, nations and communities.'

A new challenge is posed by the rapid increases in obesity and of 'diabetes and other chronic diseases, including cardiovascular and cerebrovascular diseases, bone disease and cancers of various sites' now afflicting middle- and low-income countries, populations and communities. 'These diseases, all of which are related to nutrition, impose an enormous burden on healthcare systems.

'Nutrition science can address these challenges, but can do so successfully only by means of integrated biological, social, economic, and environmental approaches. These are also essential if nutrition science is to play its part in addressing the general challenges that now face the human species.'

DEFINITION, PURPOSE, PRINCIPLES

Having set the scene, the Declaration then proposes the principles and the definition of nutrition science. Its principles should be 'guided by the philosophies of co-responsibility and sustainability, by the life-course and human rights approaches, and by understanding of evolution, history and ecology.

'Nutrition science is defined as the study of food systems, foods and drinks, and their nutrients and other constituents; and of their interactions within and between all relevant biological, social and environmental systems.' The economic dimension is also included.

And then: 'The purpose of nutrition science is to contribute to a world in which present and future generations fulfil their human potential, live in the best of health, and develop, sustain and enjoy an increasingly diverse human, living and physical environment.

'Nutrition science should be the basis for food and nutrition policies . . . designed to identify, create, conserve and protect rational, sustainable and equitable communal, national and global food systems, in order to sustain the health, wellbeing and integrity of humankind and also that of the living and physical worlds.'

The principles outlined below have informed the thinking of this book. They are mostly taken from the papers as revised for publication after the Giessen workshop (referenced below) or from workshop discussion. They are not comprehensive and remain work in progress. They are designed to frame nutrition science so that it can be most effective in action. They are meant to engage nutrition scientists as citizens as well as professionals. They are also meant to inspire a whole new way of thinking about food and nutrition suitable for this century and relevant to everybody for whom food and its effects matter – which means everybody. First, ethical principles:

'The overriding responsibility of nutrition science is to work to handing on to future generations an improved human, living and physical environment: healthy people, healthy populations, and a healthy planet.'

'Animals are not merely human resources. They should be able to develop and live a proper life before they serve as our food. The industrial production of animals for human consumption is immoral.'

Next, some suggested evolutionary, historical and ecological principles. Like most of the principles suggested here, they are part of a philosophy, a system of thinking and action which is ethical, evolutionary, historical, ecological, all together.

Evolution

'All nutritional theory, policy and practice should take into account the diet- and nutrition-related evolutionary pressures that shaped the biological evolution of the hominid line and, eventually, *Homo sapiens*.'

'The human species is uniquely evolved to grow slowly and mature late. Policies and practices designed to accelerate human growth and sexual maturity are a mistake from the biological and the social and environmental points of view.'

History

'We can properly understand the food and nutrition issues that face us now and for the foreseeable future only by examination of the historical decisions that have shaped the world's food systems.'

'Food and nutrition practices consistently followed in different cultures in history are probably valid – though not necessarily for the reasons given. They do not require proof to be accepted; they require disproof to be rejected.'

Ecology

'To achieve a world nutritional state that is health-supporting, equitable and ecologically sustainable, it is necessary to understand the interplay between evolutionary, environmental and ecological dimensions and domains.'

'All relevant sciences, including that of nutrition, should be mainly concerned with the cultivation, conservation and sustenance of human, living and physical resources all together, and so with the health of the biosphere.'

Next, some suggested principles for the three dimensions of nutrition science, and for some of the domains of these dimensions.

General

'We are moving out of the era in which human activity has been mainly concerned with exploitation, production, consumption, into a new era in which the main human concerns are of preservation, conservation, sustenance.'

'Nutrition science should follow ethical, evolutionary, and ecological principles, respect history, culture and tradition, affirm human rights, and be committed to preserve and protect the human, living and physical worlds, all together.'

'The responsibility of nutrition science now is to be concerned with the human world (personal, community and population health) and also with the whole living and natural world (planetary health).'

'Nutrition science should contribute to a world in which all people are able to fulfil their human potential, to live in the best of health, and develop, sustain and enjoy increasingly diverse human, living and physical environments.'

Biology

'Nutrition defined as a biological science cannot make much difference to mass epidemics of any type of disease, because the social and environmental determinants of epidemic disease are outside its scope.'

Health (physical)

'The single nutritional factor that most protects human health lifelong is extended exclusive breastfeeding. The practice of breastfeeding is also emotionally vital, socially valuable, and environmentally sound.'

'All nutritional recommendations designed to improve human health should be consistent with and not contradict the need to sustain living and physical resources and to protect the environment.'

'The prevention of malnutrition – most of all of women and children – by dietary means in deprived populations will work only if people have access to foods that are adequate both in quantity and quality.'

Health (mental, emotional, spiritual)

'Nutrition science should once again be concerned with well-being and health in the broadest sense. For humans, mental, emotional, and spiritual health are as important as physical health.'

'The best nutrition is from food eaten as shared meals. Good company and surroundings increase enjoyment and well-being, and enhance the meals' nourishment of physical and all other aspects of human health.'

Society

'Understanding the vast and rapid recent social as well as nutritional and epidemiological changes, and their basic driving forces, is essential for sustained prevention of disease and sustenance of human well-being and health.'

'Choices made by communities, families and individuals play a part in shaping food systems. But social factors, including technological development and economic and political policies and practices, are more powerful driving forces.'

Food systems

'Food and nutrition policies should identify, create, conserve and protect rational, sustainable and equitable food systems, to sustain the health, well-being and integrity of humankind and also that of the living and physical worlds.'

'The most sustainable food systems, and therefore diets, contain a high proportion of foods of plant origin and a low proportion of foods of animal origin and are extremely heterogeneous and biodiverse.'

'Food systems that are biodiverse are superior to those that reduce biodiversity. Biodiverse systems also protect against environmental disasters, as well as providing the most healthy food supplies.'

Technology

'Available technologies determine the nature of food systems. Nutrition scientists should examine all relevant technologies to ascertain that in use they benefit human health and welfare and that of the living and natural world.'

Tradition

'Nutrition policies should take into account that almost all the great cuisines of the world are high in staples (cereals, pulses, roots, tubers), make maximal use of available vegetables and fruits, and are sparing in their use of meat.'

'Indigenous and traditional food systems, when these are known or reliably considered to be beneficial to human health, and which have light environmental impact, should be preserved, reinstated and developed.'

Culture and cuisine

'Nutrition scientists and allied professionals should understand and respect the traditional, cultural, religious and other social factors that drive people's food and health beliefs and practices.'

'There is an absolute one-to-one correspondence between good husbandry, sound nutrition, and great gastronomy. Traditional cooking, rooted in the home, supplies good nutrition, agreeable social life, and autonomy.'

Economics

'New economic models are needed. Progress and development should not be equated with more industrialization and urbanization and more use of money, but personal fulfilment within agreeable and just societies.'

'Food subsidies in rich countries, and tariffs imposed on agricultural products from poor countries, damage human health, social fabric, and the environment, and are a key basic cause of intractable epidemic diseases.'

Politics

'The idea that nutrition can be isolated from economic and political drivers of well-being, health and disease, is a delusion. Like the best of past nutrition, the new nutrition scientists will accept and work within these contexts.'

'The basic causes of epidemics now include the results of decisions increasingly taken without proper democratic process. Action to control and prevent disease requires new structures of governance at international and global levels.'

Environment

Resources (living, physical)

'Industrial food production – amplified by need to earn foreign exchange, and the growing consolidation and power of the food-producing industry – is doing increasing damage to the planet's natural resource base.'

'The only rational food and nutrition policies are those that take account of global renewable and non-renewable resources, designed to sustain renewable resources and not to continue to rely on non-renewable resources.'

'Priority should be given to renewable sources of energy that do not create problems of safety and waste for food systems. These include solar energy, wind power, geothermal energy and tidal energy.'

Agriculture

'Monocultural farming systems can be sustained – though not forever – in rich countries whose people buy imported foods; but in poor countries they cause food insecurity, and increase poverty and instability at all levels.'

'Mixed farming systems suited to climate and terrain that support the natural fertility of the soil by sustainable methods, and make minimal use of chemical inputs, are ecologically and environmentally sound.'

'Industrialized agriculture degrades the nutritional quality of food. As a conspicuous example, the flesh of factory-farmed animals and poultry becomes more fatty, and the quality of the fat deteriorates, becoming more saturated.'

WORK IN PROGRESS

The papers and proceedings of the Giessen workshop meeting were published in a special issue of the journal *Public Health Nutrition;* and the New Nutrition Science project (NNSp) was launched in September 2005 at the International Conference on Nutrition in Durban, South Africa. Ricardo Uauy, president of the International Union of Nutritional Sciences (IUNS) from 2005 to 2009, is a member of the global steering group responsible for progressing the project, as are Mark Wahlqvist and Ibrahim Elmadfa, IUNS presidents from 2001-05 and 2009-13 respectively. The project is a joint initiative of IUNS and the World Health Policy Forum.

After the Giessen workshop meeting and the Durban conference, the principles and scope of the new nutrition science have been developed in more workshops and other meetings in Spain, and in China, Canada, Morocco, Australia and Chile. Guest of honour at the Barcelona conference was José Maria Bengoa, then in his 90s, a founder of the science of public-health nutrition. In his salute to the congress he said: 'One can glimpse a great expansion in the horizons of the science of nutrition. The limited area that we had grown accustomed to is expanding. We are getting closer and closer, like a great magic wheel, to the ideas that the Greeks held about dietetics – the dominion of life itself, both in the biological and social sense. It seems as if we are redefining nutrition as the beginning and end of life itself.'

ANNEX 2. MORE INSIGHTS

Here are detailed notes meant to illuminate and develop the themes of the main chapters. These include references to some of the books and papers used, and also a guide to more sources of information and inspiration.

The notes are not keyed in the main text, which for ease of reading contains no reference marks or footnotes. Instead, the subheadings here are keyed back to the main text.

Assuming you use the internet, there should be enough information here for searching. Many of the people mentioned are subjects of www.wikipedia.com entries, and many of the books are available at Amazon. Full references are given for the most important sources. Specialist journals often give downloadable access to backlisted papers, though for anything published before 1980 you will probably have to visit or access a specialist library.

Epigraphs at beginning of book

The playwright William Shakespeare (1564–1616), or 'William Shakespeare' to those who like my late father believe he is a team, often refers to food and drink and its effects. Thus: 'They are sick that surfeit with too much, as those that starve with nothing.' True enough.

The traveller Edward Hoagland (1932–), born in New York City, celebrates the countryside and, most of all, the world's vanishing wildernesses, as in his *Notes from the Century Before*. His most eloquent statement is simply: 'How shall we live?'

INTRODUCTION. HOW TO USE THIS BOOK

Notes

Diet and dieting

Diet. The word derives from the Greek *diaita*, which means 'way of life' or 'way of being'. This concept, in which food and drink are part of a wisely led life, became progressively narrowed. By the 17th century, as noted by Robert Burton in *The Anatomy of Melancholy*, the other 'outward and adventitious' factors that are part of diet and that modify health and wellbeing are 'retention and evacuation' and 'air, exercise, sleeping, waking, and perturbations of the mind'. This concept remained intact until the early 19th century with the emergence of 'science' in the modern sense, when it became further narrowed to mean food and drink as consumed, of which 'reducing diets', designed to shed excess or unwanted body weight or fat, were one type. In this way, the contribution of food and drink to whole wellbeing became generally forgotten, and professional dietitians emerged mostly as ancillary medical workers whose job was to treat and sometimes prevent diseases agreed by physicians to be affected by food and drink – and also overweight and obesity.

Measures of dietary energy. There are two measures for energy as contained in food and drink. The best understood unit is the calorie (to be exact, the kilocalorie). The 'standard person' accounted for on food nutrition labels in the USA and other countries (such as Brazil) is reckoned to be in energy balance, neither gaining nor losing weight, on 2,000 (kilo) calories a day. In 1960 the *Système International* (SI) was announced. This required the calorie to be phased out in favour of the joule. A calorie is equivalent to 0.004186 joules; the kilocalorie to 4.186 kilojoules. Somebody consuming 2,000kcal a day is therefore consuming 8,374kJ a day (or 8,400 in round numbers). Most scientists obediently use the SI system. Most lay people and some scientists do not. This has created confusion and some chaos, while being good for the pocket calculator business. In this book I use both (kilo)calories and kilojoules.

Weights. Almost all countries now use the metric system. The USA does not, and in the UK both the metric and the old 'imperial' systems are used. With weight, the key unit of conversion to remember is that 1 kilogram is 2.2 pounds; so for example 75 kilograms is 165 pounds. There are 14 pounds in a stone, so for UK readers 165 pounds is 11 stone 11 pounds. In this book I use both kilograms and pounds.

Body weight and body fat. These are different. When people say that they want to 'lose weight', what they usually mean is that they want to reduce their body fat. Fit, physically active people may have little body fat, but muscular and relatively heavy. Lean tissue, including muscle, weighs 20 per cent more than fat. Conversely, sedentary people may be relatively light, but flabby – literally 'out of shape'. It is still sometimes assumed that if you take in less energy from food and drink than your body's requirement, you will get rid of body fat at a rate that arithmetically corresponds to the 'energy gap'. Humans are not machines, and this is not true. See chapter 3.

Measures of body fat. This is now usually estimated in terms of Body Mass Index (BMI), which is weight (in kilograms) divided by height (in metres) squared. BMI under 18.5 is defined as underweight, BMI above 25 as overweight, and anything over BMI 30 as obese, with a BMI of over 40 defined as severely or 'morbidly' obese. Thus for a person of 1.70 metres (5 foot 7 inches) a weight of 60 kilograms (132 pounds) makes a BMI of 21, and a weight of 65 kilograms (143 pounds) a BMI of 23. A weight of 70 kilograms (154 pounds) is beginning to be overweight, at BMI 25; 80 kilograms (176 pounds) is BMI 28; and 85 kilograms (187 pounds) is beginning to be obese, at BMI 30. BMI, being a measure of body weight and not of body fat, is a rough and ready way to measure body fatness. It works for most basically sedentary adults. For children, age has to be factored in. At the same BMI women and older people have more body fat than younger men. The BMIs of muscular people may suggest they are overweight. BMI is also not a great system for people in the USA who don't use kilograms or metres: in this case BMI is calculated as your weight in pounds, divided by the square of your height in inches, multiplied by 704. In the USA the 'cut-off' between 'healthy' and 'overweight' BMI is often taken to be more than 25 – often around BMI 26–27. Conversely, cut-offs recommended in some Asian countries are lower: around 23–24 and above for overweight and around 27–28 for obese. Again, see chapter 3.

Words and meanings. In this book I try not to use misleading or troublesome terms. For example, I avoid 'weight gain' and 'weight loss'. 'Gain' sounds good and 'loss' sounds bad. If you lose something, normally you want to find it or get it back. Could this be a psychological reason why dieting does not work? Technical terms as used by scientists and physicians sometimes have a sense different from or even opposite to their ordinary meaning. If you are in 'positive energy balance' you are increasing your weight, and unless you are in training, body fat. Again, scientists who describe foods as being 'rich in saturated fat' or 'rich in [added] sugar' maybe do not confuse their colleagues, but are liable to confuse the non-technical reader.

Dieting. It will become apparent as you read on that I discuss starvation and fasting, as well as dieting, to explain how and why dieting makes you fat. You know the difference between dieting, which you do on purpose to shed weight; starvation, which is involuntary; and fasting, which is usually to cleanse the body or as a religious requirement or a spiritual exercise. But your body does not know these differences. See chapter 3, and chapter 6, golden rule 6.

What is here?

Reliability of observation and 'folk wisdom'. One of the principles of the new nutrition science (see Annex 1) is that beliefs that have been held consistently and over time within different societies are probably true, though not necessarily in the form they are expressed or for the reasons given. They should not be assumed to be untrue until so proved by modern methods, but should be assumed to be true unless disproved. A good example is nutritional practices developed over many centuries as a result of observation, experimentation and trial and error, particularly when these could make the difference between the life and death of communities during hard times.

What is not here?

Success stories. In the USA, the National Weight Control Registry, founded in 1994 by Rena Wing of Brown Medical School and James Hill of the University of Colorado, has records of around 6,000 people, mostly women, who have kept off 30 pounds (14 kilograms) of shed weight for more than a year. The context of this figure is that in the USA over half of all adults, which is to say around 100 million people, try to shed weight every year. One finding reported by the registry (www.nwcr.ws) is that over 90 per cent of the people they have surveyed now exercise for an hour a day or more. On this, see chapter 3 and chapter 6, golden rule 2.

What can and can't be done?

Spiritual. People trained in conventional science usually reject this concept, because the spirit cannot be measured. Nor can an orange or a rose, in all their aspects. Life is more than the measurable. Nor are things spiritual owned by religion. Animals have bodies, and mental and emotional aspects, albeit evidently simpler than ours. But what marks humans out from other living creatures is not just the opposable thumb, or the use of fire, or language. It is our spiritual dimension which makes us most special. Ethics are not just a matter of thoughts and feelings; and wellbeing has a spiritual aspect. To evade the word and what it means is to reduce us to lesser creatures.

References

For references to the books, reports, articles and papers that have informed this introduction, see the notes to the main chapters.

PART 1. THE DIETING DISASTER

The rock star Lou Reed (1942–) is with John Cale the lead founding member of The Velvet Underground and thus of glam, metal, and punk rock. His cuts delineate the outer and inner lives of people in cities such as New York who are soaked with too much of everything.

The philosopher Ludwig Wittgenstein (1889–1951) is mainly interested in the relationship between language, thought and reality. Paradoxes can be resolved by shifting our point of view or by examining the words we use. This is from his *Philosophical Investigations.*

1. CONFESSIONS OF A RETIRED DIETER

Notes: epigraphs

The *Regimen Sanitatis* (*Regime of Health*) of the first major medical school at Salerno in Italy, first published around 1100 CE, combines the dietetic philosophies of Greek, Roman and Arab masters with current observation, common sense, and good humour.

The philosopher Alan Watts (1915–73), originally British, was one leader of the Californian human potential movement. His main theme is the need for Western thought and institutions to be aware of the wisdom of the East. This is from his *The Wisdom of Insecurity.*

Notes: main text

Dieters as failures

Fatness in infancy and childhood. This is particularly troublesome. Fat children tend to become obese adults. It may be that the number as well as the size of the cells in which body fat is stored increase if infants and young children become overweight. In adult life the number of fat cells probably remains fixed; it seems that energy restriction reduces the amount of fat stored in fat cells, but does not reduce the number of cells. Fat adults who were fat children and who want to reduce their body fatness are therefore fighting their body composition.

Young super-sizer

Fish and chips. Those were the days in Britain before burger 'restaurants', when deep-sea fish were plentiful and cod was cheap. In 1950 there were 30,000 fish and chip shops in Britain. As a basic meal, fried fish and chips (French fries), preferably with a large salad, is nourishing and rather a good choice – all the more so if the fish and the chips are deep-fried fresh and quick in extremely hot oil that is regularly renewed, and the chips are big. Fish and chips make you fat if you eat all the batter as well, and if the chips are thin or made with floury potatoes that soak up oil. White fish and potatoes are in themselves low in energy density. Chips are anything between twice and six times the energy density of potatoes, largely depending on the thickness of the chip. Now there are around 7,500 fish and chip shops in Britain; they have been replaced by burger joints. The problem with the chips served in burger restaurants is that they are very thin. The potato base is just a vehicle to hold fat, like crisps (chips in the USA), and so they are extremely energy-dense. Fish fried in batter is, with the batter, around three times the energy density of the fish itself. There was no way that my mother could get fat on what she ate. See chapter 4, and chapter 6, golden rule 7.

Dietary energy, and weight increase (and decrease). Some academic texts, government-sponsored recommendations, and dieting books and articles even now sometimes persist in saying or suggesting that weight increase is a function of extra dietary energy consumed, and that a weight-reduction plan can be calculated by the amount of dietary energy that falls short of that needed for energy balance. This notion was first proposed in the 19th century, on the assumption that human and animal energy metabolism works like that of a simple machine of fixed capacity, such as a steam train fuelled with coal. It is not true, one reason being that metabolic rate speeds up when extra dietary energy is consumed, and slows down at times of shortfall (such as dieting regimes) so that the body in effect 'defends' its weight. This is why I did not become the Michelin boy. There are other reasons. See chapters 3 and 4.

The textbook is *Human Nutrition and Dietetics* (now *Human Nutrition*), the standard work for British students, including physicians, physiologists and other postgraduate professionals with an interest in nutrition and dietetics. Founded in 1940 by Stanley Davidson, Professor of Medicine in Aberdeen, at a time when British nutrition scientists were still concerned with deficiency diseases in the remaining outposts of Empire, the textbook maintained a mildly Calvinist tone up to the eighth edition of 1986, from whose chapter on obesity the first and second passage is taken (the third passage is taken from the seventh edition of 1979).

The Nibble Diet

The Nibble Diet. It depends on what is nibbled. More and more heavily promoted foods and drinks are energy-dense, including some with a 'healthy' image, like cereal bars and sweetened yoghurts. On a daily diet consisting of just a few snacks many sedentary people will increase weight, and also will feel hungry much of the time. See chapter 4, and chapter 6, golden rule 7.

Christ's Hospital was an especially significant place for human experiments, because its policy was to accept academically promising boys from poor homes who would otherwise be liable to grow up scrawny and feeble. The epidemiologist George Davey Smith found a copy of Dr G E Friend's book describing his experiments, and mounted a study of 'the Christ's Hospital cohort' which at the time of writing is ongoing: see www.epi.bris.ac.uk/chs. As a candidate for inclusion in the study, I can report that acne, foot and crutch rot, impetigo, fevers, and colds, all no doubt incubated in the communal steamy changing, washing and bathing rooms, were rampant.

The Jaffa Diet

The Jaffa Diet. Oranges are not the only fruit that will have this effect. If you eat nothing but fruits, singly or in any combination, plus water, you will drop lots of weight, if only because fruits, like vegetables, are bulky, high in fibre and water, and fill you up long before they supply enough energy to sustain your weight. What happens after you stop any single-food regime is, of course, another story. See chapter 3.

Very low calorie diets (VLCDs). These, sometimes defined as any dieting regime supplying less than 800 calories (3,360 kilojoules) a day, are also known as very low energy diets, or crash diets. They are generally condemned by physicians, nutritionists and their professional organizations as being short of nutrients and therefore dangerous. This is silly. Of course very low calorie diets are inadequate and unbalanced, compared with a normal diet. So what? They are not designed as permanent sustenance. The issue is, do they work, in the sense of leading to permanent decrease of body weight and fat? Answer: no.

Little helpers

Fenfluramine – Ponderax and equivalent brands – was withdrawn in the late 1990s. When combined with phentermine (as 'phen-fen') its efficacy multiplied, and by the mid-1990s it was a roaring success. Then it was found to increase blood pressure and to damage the heart, and faced with class actions, the manufacturers withdrew the drugs. All potent drugs, including those used for weight loss, have adverse effects. See also chapter 2.

Oh! Misery!

Reasons people give for becoming fat. Common reasons given in the 2006 Pew poll were physical inactivity (70 per cent), lack of willpower (59 per cent), and food marketing (50 per cent). Heredity was chosen by 32 per cent. Perceptions have shifted in the last quarter century.

Getting in shape

Energy cost of physical activity. Another well-known example is that running a marathon uses up round about 2,500 calories (10,500 kilojoules), which is more or less the amount of energy that a relatively physically active person needs to keep in energy balance just for one day. But what this discounts is all the energy used in training in order to be able to run a marathon; plus the fact that the everyday energy turnover of an active person is higher than that of a sedentary person weighing the same amount. See chapter 6, golden rule 2.

Running and working out. Running for an average of say 45 minutes a day, and also working out at a health centre three or four days a week, may sound heroic. The total amount of extra energy used might amount to 600-800 calories (roughly 2,500-3,350 kilojoules) a day. While substantial, this is not a great deal more than was used by most men less than a hundred years ago in everyday activity before machines did the work humans are designed to do. On average, energy turnover of women is about 20 per cent lower than that of men. In high-income countries and in most cities, average energy balance has dropped by up to 400-600 calories (roughly 1,700-2,500 kilojoules) a day since the early to mid-20th century. Again, see chapter 3 and chapter 6, golden rule 2.

Hard times

Serpentine Running Club. In 2007 the club had 2,287 members, with John Walker as chairperson. Twice the number one citizens' running club at the *Sunday Times* National Fun Run, the Serpies look after everybody from complete beginner to champion athlete. They welcome guests from other countries. In 2002 I was formally identified as founder – a proud moment. The website is www.serpentine.org.uk.

Plan jams

Surprising big or small weight increase or decrease. This involves emotions and so is distasteful to scientists. The body of somebody engaged in mutual passion seethes with expressed energy. The body of somebody in despair shuts down vital functions. Comfort eating is a disaster not just because of the energy content of the overeaten food. Nobody ever successfully ate their way out of misery. See chapter 4.

The wounded healer

Enlightenment when fasting. The effect may be because after two or three days on a water-only fast the brain's fuel supply is no longer glucose, which has become exhausted, but ketones released from the liver. These seem to have a different effect on the quality and intensity of consciousness, which would account for the practice of fasting to induce mystical states of mind. See chapter 6, golden rule 6.

References

In alphabetical order of authors. Publishing details are usually of first edition.

For other books, reports, papers and features on dieting, see chapters 2 and 3.

Geoffrey Cannon, Hetty Einzig. *Dieting Makes You Fat*. London: Century, 1983. Updated edition, New York: Simon and Schuster, 1985.

Stanley Davidson, Reg Passmore, John Brock, Stewart Truswell (editors). Obesity. [Chapter 28] *Human Nutrition and Dietetics*. Seventh edition. Edinburgh: Churchill Livingstone, 1979.

Department of Health and Social Security/ Medical Research Council. *Research on Obesity*. London: HMSO, 1976.

G E Friend. *The Schoolboy, a Study of His Nutrition, Physical Development and Health*. Cambridge: Heffer, 1935.

Reg Passmore, Martin Eastwood (editors). Obesity. [Chapter 28] *Human Nutrition and Dietetics*. Eighth edition. Edinburgh: Churchill Livingstone, 1988.

School of Salerno. Teachings, translated by John Harington as *The Englishman's Doctor. Or, The School of Salerno. Or, Physical Observations for the Perfect Preserving of the Body of Man in Continual Health*. Translation of the verses of the School of Salerno. London: John Helme, 1608. Obtainable at: www.umanitoba.ca/libraries/units/health/resources/salerno.html.

Alan Watts. *The Wisdom of Insecurity*. New York: Vintage, 1968. First published 1951.

2. THE FABULOUS DIETING BUSINESS

Notes: epigraphs

The epidemiologist George Mann of Nashville, Tennessee, has a long history of opposing conventional wisdom. His own studies of the Maasai nation of East Africa convinced him that people in rich countries do not get fat because their diets are high in fat.

The journalist William Leith (1960–) gets the point of what he calls 'the Cannon conundrum', saying: 'When you diet, something funny happens to your metabolism – it gets better. Better, that is, at making you fat …You think: diet. Your body thinks: famine.' Exactly!

Notes: main text

The obesity boom

Severe obesity. As already mentioned, this refers to body mass indices (BMIs) of 40 and above. At BMI 40 a person 1.65 metres in height (5 foot 5 inches) weighs 109 kilograms (240 pounds, or 17 stone 2 pounds); a person 1.80 metres in height (5 foot 11 inches) weighs 130 kilograms (286 pounds, or 20 stone 6 pounds). Severe obesity is also called 'morbid obesity'. At BMI 40 and above, basically sedentary people are highly likely to suffer from symptomatic diseases of metabolism and the circulatory and musculo-skeletal systems, life expectancy is reduced substantially, and regular physical activity as a method to reduce body fat is unlikely to be feasible at least until after a lengthy period of pre-training. Extremely muscular men such as power athletes who are very heavy while not being fat are well advised to reduce their bulk once their competitive days are over.

Obesity: is it an epidemic? Strictly speaking, because the great increase in overweight and obesity is worldwide, the correct word is pandemic. Again, it depends how the word is defined, and definitions in cases like this are important. People tend to associate epidemics with infectious diseases, although the term now is generally used also to refer to non-infectious diseases when their incidence increases rapidly. On the whole it seems reasonable also to identify rapid increases in physical – and indeed other – disorders as well as diseases, as epidemics, so I do.

The dieting industry boom, boom

Dieting regimes and energy restriction. A systematic review published in 2001 undertaken by staff at the US Department of Agriculture, including Eileen Kennedy (later Dean at Tufts University), concludes that most dieting regimes, whether as specified or as self-selected by dieters, work out at around 1,500 calories (6,250 kilojoules) a day, at which level women (unless they are unusually small and sedentary) as well as men, will reduce weight. This finding seems surprising, because many regimes, such as the Atkins Diet, in effect say 'as long as you follow my rules, eat and drink as much as you like'. The main explanation, discussed in this chapter, is that all diets that restrict whole ranges of foods or macronutrients make you full up or fed up at relatively low levels of energy consumption. So now you know – that's the trade secret of most if not all dieting regimes.

Magic ingredient dieting regimes

The Beverly Hills Diet. Undertaken not in order to reduce weight and fat, but as a type of fast designed to refresh and detoxify the body, a combination of tropical fruits is a good choice. See chapter 6, golden rule 6.

The grape cure. This also can be positioned as a fruit fast. Early versions required the people on the cure to pick their own grapes and so get some genteel exercise. Various fruits, or other raw foods, are still commonly recommended as ways to cleanse the body.

One-food dieting regimes. *Super-size Me* Morgan Spurlock put on 25 pounds (over 11 kilograms) in 30 days of eating McDonald's meals by always choosing the super-size version when it was offered, and in this way consuming around double the energy his body needed to stay in balance. These were meals, not just burgers. As far as I know, nobody has yet been brazen enough to market a dieting regime based only on chocolate or cheesecake (plus water) although either would almost certainly work simply because of inducing nausea. Magic ingredient dieting regimes usually feature foods or dietary components that are bulky or contain a lot of water.

Weight loss on energy-restrictive dieting regimes. The two main reasons why Mrs Eyton's F-Plan in common with many others is mistaken on this point are as follows. First, dieting regimes usually cause initial impressive weight loss, almost all of which is not fat but water. Second, the claim that 'fat contains 3,500 calories per pound, so on an energy deficit of 1,000 calories a day you will lose 2 pounds a week' (and equivalent calculations using kilojoules and kilograms) is just plain wrong, as already indicated. Mrs Eyton is not at fault here. She is simply repeating what nutrition textbooks continued to mis-state. Anybody who persists in dieting needs to know that once the period of water loss is over, further weight loss will be slower – very often much slower – than the '7,000 divided by 3,500 equals 2' calculation suggests. See the next chapter for more detail on these basic points.

Macronutrient manipulation dieting regimes

Dieting doctors. The highest-profile US dieting doctors were colourful and controversial characters. Herman Taller (1906–84) was condemned by the US Food and Drug Administration for his promotion of safflower oil capsules as slimming aids. Irwin Stillman (1896–1975) died of a heart attack. Herman Tarnower (1910–80) was shot dead by his ex-lover. Robert Atkins (1930–2003), who enjoyed boasting about the amount of meat and fat he ate, developed a heart condition, and died after slipping on ice outside his offices in Manhattan.

The Atkins Diet. This remains a subject of furious controversy in the USA. As mentioned in the main text, various medical organizations have condemned the regime as unsupported, unjustified, unhealthy and dangerous. It is hated by supporters of the consensus line on what is a healthy balanced diet, which promotes carbohydrates (or to be more precise, starchy foods). It is hard to say exactly what is the Atkins Diet. Robert Atkins himself shifted his line somewhat over the years, and his 'new diet revolution' is almost a wholefood diet which includes a lot of animal foods but restricts starchy foods and avoids sugar. In its initial 'induction' stage, the diet is absolutely as well as relatively very high in fat and high in protein. But in its maintenance stage the diet includes wholegrains, moderate amounts of starchy roots and tubers and some fruits, while limiting alcohol and warning against sugar. The Atkins Diet in practice usually has the effect of restricting dietary energy to the usual 1,500 calories or so, and so the maintenance stage may well not be absolutely very high in fat, compared with average US and other high-income diets.

Carbohydrates make you fat. 'Refined' carbohydrates, which is to say sugar, sugary foods, white bread, and foods containing a lot of white flour, certainly do raise levels of serum insulin, as do less 'refined' carbohydrates to a lesser extent. Robert Atkins, Arthur Agatston, and others like them, claim that for this reason, starchy and sugary foods derange appetite and cause over-consumption of food and drink, whereas foods mostly containing fat and protein are naturally satisfying. The case for the Atkins Diet (and the South Beach and other diets that restrict carbohydrate) is best made by Gary Taubes.

Cardoons. These are edible thistles, a bit like globe artichokes, whose stalks are eaten raw or cooked like celery. They were a delicacy in classic Greece and Rome, and have been traditionally eaten in some parts of the Mediterranean littoral. Jane Grigson includes some recipes in her *Vegetable Book*.

The Brillat-Savarin and Banting diets. These are much lower in fat than the Atkins Diet, as are the Stillman and Yudkin diets. This is obviously so with any 'drinking man's diet' such as that of William Banting. Also, composition of meat was somewhat different in the 19th century. Some animals were specially fattened, but their fat was a lot less saturated than that of modern intensively produced animals. Research carried out at Maastricht University in the Netherlands suggests that a key factor, as well as high energy balance from physical activity, is that these diets high in protein. By his own account William Banting's regime worked for him; and a much more restrictive regime followed life-long evidently worked for the 16th-century Venetian nobleman Luigi Cornaro. Some very determined people can make what amounts to permanent dieting work for them. On carbohydrates (or sugars and white flour) see the next chapter and chapter 4.

Diet, dieting, and health

The healthy diet. The consensus among scientists and governments developed as from the 1960s is reflected in two World Health Organization reports, both with the title *Diet, Nutrition, and the Prevention of Chronic Diseases*, published in 1990 and then in 2003; and also in the current WHO *Global Strategy on Diet, Physical Activity and Health* (obtainable at www.who.int).

Fat, sugar, and heart disease risk factors. Diets high in saturated fats, found in meat, dairy products, and increasingly in a vast number of processed foods, do indeed increase levels of 'bad fats' in the blood, such as low-density lipoprotein. Between the 1950s and 1980s, John Yudkin was almost alone in insisting that diets high in sugars are also troublesome because they raise blood levels of triglycerides, another type of fat. There is no doubt that high-sugar diets do have this effect, but the medical-nutritional establishment decided that saturated fat is where it's at. It is now pretty much generally accepted that raised blood triglycerides do increase the risk of heart disease – or perhaps this is better put by saying they are a sign of heart disease. In this respect Robert Atkins is now supported by many researchers, whose views, however, do not yet amount to a serious challenge to the general consensus.

Nathan Pritikin. Like Robert Atkins, his ideas have a long pedigree. They have a lot in common with the 19th and early 20th century teaching and practice of Sylvester Graham, John Harvey Kellogg, Horace Fletcher, Russell Chittenden, and the naturopathic movements in Europe as well as North America and elsewhere.

Dieting as a sign of the times

Dangers of dieting. The immediate danger of dieting is grossly exaggerated. The long-term dangers are underestimated: see the next chapter.

References: books, reports

In alphabetical order of authors. Publishing details are usually of first edition.

Arthur Agatston. *The South Beach Diet. The Delicious, Doctor-Designed Foolproof Plan for Fast and Healthy Weight Loss.* New York: St Martin's Press, 2003.

Robert Atkins. *Dr Atkins' Diet Revolution.* New York: Bantam, 1972.

Robert Atkins. *Dr Atkins' New Diet Revolution.* New York: Avon, 1992, paperback 1999.

William Banting. *A Letter on Corpulence Addressed to the General Reader.* 1862. The third edition is obtainable by Googling the name and title.

Jean Anthelme Brillat-Savarin. On Obesity. [Meditation 21]. *The Physiology of Taste. Or Meditations on Transcendental Gastronomy.* MFK Fisher (trs). Washington DC: Counterpoint, 1999. First published in French, 1825.

Jane Brody. Why 'diets' don't work. [Chapter 16]. *Jane Brody's Nutrition Book.* New York: Bantam, 1981.

Consumers' Association. *'Which' Way to Slim.* London: CA, 1978.

Luigi Cornaro. *The Art of Living Long.* Milwaukee, WI: William F Butler, 1905. First published in Italian as *La Vita Sobria,* 1558.

Allan Cott. *Fasting: the Ultimate Diet.* New York: Bantam, 1975.

Audrey Eyton. *The Complete F-Plan Diet.* London: Penguin, 1982.

Audrey Eyton. *The F2 Diet.* London: Bantam, 2006.

House of Commons Health Committee. *Obesity.* London: The Stationery Office, 2004.

International Food Policy Research Institute. *The World Food Situation: New Driving Forces and Required Actions.* Washington DC: IFPRI, 2008.

Gina Kolata. Epiphanies and hucksters. [Chapter 2]. *Rethinking Thin. The New Science of Weight Loss – and the Myths and Realities of Dieting.* New York: Farrar, Straus, Giroux, 2007.

Kamala Krishnaswamy. *Obesity in the Indian Middle Class in Delhi.* Scientific Report 15. New Delhi: Nutrition Foundation of India, 1999.

William Leith. *The Hungry Years. Confessions of a Food Addict.* London: Bloomsbury, 2005.

Robert Linn, Sandra Lee Stuart. *The Last Chance Diet.* New York: Lyle Stuart 1976, Bantam, 1976.

Richard Mackarness. *Eat Fat and Grow Slim.* London: Fontana, 1961.

Judy Mazel. *The Beverly Hills Diet.* New York: Buccaneer Books, 1994. First published 1982.

Dean Ornish. *Eat More, Weigh Less.* New York: Harper Collins, 2001.

Pew. Prevalence of overweight and obesity in the US, 1999-2004. Obtainable at: www.pewresearch.org.

Nathan Pritikin. *The Pritikin Program for Diet and Exercise.* New York: Bantam, 1979, paperback 1984.

Shirley Ross. *Fasting: the Super Diet.* New York: Ballantine, 1976.

Royal College of Physicians of London. *Obesity.* London: RCP, 1983.

Royal Prince Alfred Hospital Weight Management Program. *Never Say Diet Again. Lose Weight the RPA Way.* Sydney: Park Street Press, 2006.

Amanda Sainsbury-Salis. *The Don't Go Hungry Diet. The Scientifically Based Way to Lose Weight and Keep it Off Forever.* Sydney: Bantam, 2007.

Barry Sears. *Enter The Zone.* New York: Harper Collins, 1995.

Irwin Stillman, with Samm Sinclair Baker. *The Doctor's Quick Weight-Loss Diet.* New York: Putnam, 1967.

Herman Taller. *Calories Don't Count.* New York: Simon and Schuster, 1961.

Herman Tarnower, with Samm Sinclair Baker. *The Complete Scarsdale Medical Diet. Plus Dr Tarnower's Lifetime Keep-Slim Programme.* New York: Bantam, 1979.

Gary Taubes. *Good Calories, Bad Calories. Challenging the Conventional Wisdom on Diet, Weight Control, and Disease.* New York: Knopf, 2007. (Published in the UK as *The Diet Delusion*: London: Vermilion, 2008.)

E S Turner. Shadow of a regal paunch. [Chapter 18] *Taking the Cure.* London: Michael Joseph, 1967.

UK Government Office of Science. Foresight. *Tackling Obesities: Future Choice. Trends and Directions of Obesity.* London: Stationery Office, 2007. Obtainable at: www.foresight.gov.uk.

US Department of Health and Human Services. *The Surgeon General's Report on Nutrition and Health.* Washington DC: US DHHS, 1988.

US Institute of Medicine. *Preventing Childhood Obesity: Health in the Balance.* Washington DC: National Academies Press, 2005.

US Institute of Medicine. *Progress in Preventing Childhood Obesity. How Do We Measure Up?* Washington DC: National Academies Press, 2007. Obtainable at: www.nap.edu.

US National Research Council. *Diet and Health. Implications for Reducing Chronic Disease Risk.* Washington DC: National Academy Press, 1989. Obtainable at: www.nap.edu.

Edward O Wilson. *The Diversity of Life.* Cambridge MA: Harvard University Press, 1992.

World Health Organization. *Prevention of Coronary Heart Disease.* Report of a WHO expert committee. WHO technical report 678. Geneva: WHO, 1982.

World Health Organization. *Diet, Nutrition, and the Prevention of Chronic Diseases.* Report of a WHO study group. WHO technical report 797. Geneva: WHO, 1990.

World Health Organization. Prevention and management of overweight and obesity in at-risk individuals. [Chapter 10]. *Obesity: Preventing and Managing the Global Epidemic.* Report of a WHO consultation. WHO technical report 894. Geneva: WHO, 2000.

World Health Organization. *Diet, Nutrition, and the Prevention of Chronic Diseases.* Report of a joint WHO/FAO expert consultation. WHO technical report 916. Geneva: WHO, 2003. Obtainable at: www.who.int.

John Yudkin. *This Slimming Business.* London: MacGibbon and Kee 1958, London: Penguin, 1970.

References: papers, features

In alphabetical order of authors:

American Medical Association. A critique of low-carbohydrate ketogenic weight reduction regimens: a review of 'Dr Atkins' Diet Revolution'. *Journal of the American Medical Association* 1973; 224(10): 1415-19.

Anon. Pupils' trousers with 42-inch waists. *Daily Telegraph*, 10 April 2007.

Bray G. Preface. In: *Recent Advances in Obesity Research. Proceedings of the Second International Conference on Obesity Research.* London: Newman, 1978.

Campbell D. Obesity crisis to cost £45 billion a year. *Guardian*, 14 October 2007.

Datamonitor. www.nutraingredients.com/news/ng.asp?id=37340-keep-dieters-dieting.

Freedman M, King J, Kennedy E. Popular diets: a scientific review. *Obesity Research* 2001: 9 (supp 1): 1-40.

Jorge M. *Não existe solução mágica. Veja*, 24 October 2007.

Kennedy I, Bowman S, Spence J, Freedman M, King I. Popular diets: correlation to health, nutrition and obesity. *Journal of the American Dietetic Association* 2001; 101(4): 211-20.

Lejeune M, Kovacs E, Westerterp – Plantenga M. Additional protein intake limits weight regain after weigt loss in humans. *British Journal of Nutrition* 2005; 93: 281-9

Mann G. Diet and obesity. *New England Journal of Medicine* 1977; 296: 812.

Misra A, Pandey R, Devi J, Sharma R, Vikram N, Khanna M. High prevalence of diabetes, obesity and dyslipidaemia in urban slum population in northern India. *International Journal of Obesity and Related Metabolic Disorders* 2001; 25(11): 1722-29.

Monteiro C, Conde W, Popkin B. Is obesity replacing or adding to undernutrition? Evidence from different social classes in Brazil. *Public Health Nutrition* 2002; 5(1A): 105-12.

Monteiro C, Conde W, Popkin B. The burden of disease from undernutrition and overnutrition in countries undergoing rapid nutrition transition: a view from Brazil. *American Journal of Public Health* 2004; 94(3): 433-4.

Monteiro C, Conde W, Popkin B. Income-specific trends in obesity in Brazil 1975-2003. *American Journal of Public Health* 2007; 97: 1808-12.

Mudur G. Scientists identify obesity gene. *Telegraph,* Calcutta, 14 April 2007.

WHO European Ministerial Conference. European Charter on Counteracting Obesity. Istanbul, Turkey, 15-17 November 2006. Obtainable at: www.euro.who.int.

Younge G. Airlines lose life-vests to fat flyers. *Guardian,* 13 August 2005.

3 WHY DIETING MAKES YOU FAT

Notes: epigraphs

The poet George Gordon, Lord Byron (1788–1824) is a well-documented early case of yo-yo dieting. His biographer Fiona MacCarthy notes that 'he kept up a more or less obsessive dependence on dieting and purgatives all through the years of his celebrity'.

The geneticist Theodosius Dobzhansky (1900–75), who emigrated to the USA in the 1920s, has done as much as anybody to reintroduce the principle that evolutionary principles govern biological phenomena. He never repudiated his (Orthodox) Christian culture.

Notes: main text

Frequently asked questions answered

Authorship of 'dieting makes you fat'. The phrase and the idea in the form of a reasoned thesis is mine, to the best of my knowledge. The idea that dieting characteristically does not work is of course not new. This is now often stated in expert and popular writing, and is the experience of almost everybody who goes on dieting regimes.

'Diet' and 'dieting'. It is unfortunate and muddling that these two terms are so similar. The old-fashioned term 'reducing diet' is clearer, but is not used here because it implies that dieting regimes are effective.

Dieting makes you fat as a paradox. It has also been put to me that this is like saying 'stopping smoking makes you smoke'. Arguments by analogy may or may not indicate a valid point. Where this analogy breaks down is that the equivalent of eating and drinking healthily is never smoking, the equivalent of dieting is starting to smoke, and the

equivalent of quitting smoking is quitting dieting. See the rest of this chapter.

Methods used to reduce weight. Many people who reduce weight by taking drugs or undergoing surgery prefer not to say so. While people are entitled to their privacy, this can have the unfortunate effect of making other people think the reduced weight is because of a dieting regime.

Dieters who succeed. There is no way that people who reduce weight on a dieting regime can stay at the lower weight unless they continue to restrict the energy from food and drink, or else become more physically active, or both. If they revert to their previous eating and drinking habits and are not more active, they will increase their body weight and fat for the same reasons these increased in the first place before they went on the dieting regime. The other reasons why dieting itself will accelerate and exacerbate this process are explained in the main text.

Who can you believe? In the USA, a substantial proportion of the most influential academics in the field are funded by, and often consultants to, the pharmaceutical or dieting industries, and may also run obesity clinics committed to specific weight-loss techniques. It is safe to say that in general, findings in the scientific literature on treatments of obesity, whether by surgery, drugs or dieting, are biased in the direction of emphasizing their safety and efficacy and downplaying their risks and failures.

Physicians. A number of health professionals who are physicians are experts in energy balance and obesity or nutrition and health. This is not because of their medical training, which teaches them how to diagnose and treat physical diseases, but because they have taken a personal interest in these topics, or have decided to specialize.

Our bodies are more than machines

Humans are not machines. The triumph of modern chemical and biological science is built on a war that was won in the 19th century by materialists over 'vitalists' – thinkers including scientists who insisted on the fundamental importance and implications of what being alive means. Vitalism was always more influential in Germany than in English-speaking countries, and further declined with the eclipse of German science in the 20th century. Materialists do not necessarily believe that the body is a machine, but they do believe it is most fruitful to work and think as if it is.

Calories are fuzzy counters

David Ludwig is referring to the contrast between high- and low-glycaemic index foods, less technically expressed as the contrast between highly processed foods and fresh and benignly processed foods. This example of a calorie not being a calorie is a rationale of 'GI' (glycaemic index) dieting and healthy eating books, and others that focus on resistant starch. It is also a rationale of regimes such as the Atkins Diets that severely limit sugars and starches. There are other examples. George Bray of Louisiana State University finds that high-fructose corn syrup as contained in soft drinks in the USA is preferentially converted to body fat.

Emergency feeding. Even in acute situations it is not true that semi-starving people need only energy from food. If as often happens they are fed processed energy-dense rations, such as mixtures of starches, sugars, fats or oils, they will remain malnourished.

Bulky foods. This is the rationale of dieting regimes and also general dietary recommendations that emphasize foods like vegetables, fruits and wholegrains, all of which when ready to eat are high in dietary fibre and water. See chapter 6, golden rules 3 and 4.

Hunger is not just for energy

Hunger for nutrients. This point was made by Arvid Wretlind, then of the National Institute of Public Health in Stockholm, Sweden, in the 1960s. He gives the examples of calcium (lack of which may cause brittle bone disease) and iron (lack of which causes lassitude and impedes learning ability), and also vitamin A.

Craving, compulsion, addiction. These are types of deranged hunger or appetite. The terms are often used loosely or metaphorically. We might say 'I am addicted to movies starring Mel Gibson', or 'she is compelled to buy shoes', or 'I crave solitude', but that is not what is meant here. An addictive substance is one whose consumption creates changes in the body as a result of which the substance is craved, so that its consumption becomes compulsive and its withdrawal is likely to cause suffering. Some addictive substances are illegal. Many are not. As well as tobacco and alcohol, many people will say that coffee is liable to be addictive, and also sugars especially when consumed in the form of sugary and sugared foods and drinks. Also see later in this chapter.

Do obese people overeat?

Do fat people eat more than thin people? As stated in the text, the phrasing of this question is unhelpful. In the first version of this book I cited studies evidently showing that fat people consume less dietary energy than thin people. In 1979, Professor Harry Keen of Guy's Hospital, London, reported 'highly significant inverse correlations between food energy intake and adiposity, a relation found in both sexes'. In 1984, George Sopko, then of the St Louis Medical Center, reported a 'strong inverse relationship between caloric intake and body fatness'. Interviewed by me, Peter Wood of Stanford University said that 'generally speaking, fatter people eat less than thinner people'. I also quoted John Garrow as saying that there was then no evidence 'that obese people ate more than thin ones. The cause of obesity is astonishingly difficult to pin down.'

How much people eat and drink now. It's commonly supposed that we are consuming more overall energy from foods and drinks now than a generation ago. The amount of available food and drink has steadily increased all over the world and consumption has actually increased in many middle- and low-income countries. But estimates of available food and drink are misleading, especially in materially rich countries, one reason being that they do not allow for waste. In high-income countries the increases generally are in food and drink that is discarded.

Primal hunger

Building up a case in science. Scientific theses are generally prompted by observations, known in the trade as 'anecdotal evidence', that lead to relevant types of controlled studies, which in nutritional science include epidemiological and also laboratory investigations. Some scientists say the process starts by accumulating data and ends with a theory (the inductive approach). Others say the process starts with an idea which is then tested by investigation (the deductive approach). Justus Liebig (1803-1873) says: 'An experiment not preceded by a theory –

that is, by an idea – stands in the same relation to physical investigation as a child's rattle to music.'

Hugh Sinclair (1910-90) is best known for his theory that a key dietary cause of cardiovascular disease is not too much saturated fats but not enough essential fats. These are mostly found in wholefoods, and are systematically lost in the processing of food in order to give it longer shelf life. As founder and director of the Oxford Nutrition Survey from 1941-46 he was one of the architects of Britain's wartime food policy, and after the war he studied the effects of the Dutch 'hunger winter' (see note on semi-starvation below). Yes, he concluded that starvation followed by unrestricted feeding is a cause of overweight and obesity in humans as well as pigs.

Catch-up growth and body weight – and body fat – overshoot. Small infants and young children have been fed formula feeds and energy-dense foods to 'catch up' their growth and weight, in order to conform to growth charts that were issued by the United Nations and national governments, until they were replaced in 2006. These charts are based on the growth and weight of formula-fed children. The result is an increase in overweight and obesity. The lesson is that breastfeeding is indispensable and that these growth charts are wrong. David Barker of the University of Southampton is associated with the theory that small babies are more likely to become obese later in life and to suffer from the metabolic syndrome which includes diabetes, stroke and heart disease. Expressed in this way the theory is wrong. The risk is increased not by low birth-weight alone, but low birth-weight followed by excessive feeding with artificial formula and energy-dense diets. See also chapters 4 and 5.

Energy restriction: the classic experiments

Francis Benedict, with his mentor Wilbur Atwater, constructed the 'calorimeters' – exactly controlled metabolic chambers – still used to measure energy input and output reliably. Less exacting methods are far less reliable. Much current work involving lots of subjects relies on what people say they eat and drink, which is often, even usually, remarkably different from what they actually eat and drink.

Ancel Keys. A book by Todd Tucker on the Minnesota Experiment was published in the USA in 2006. Both Gina Kolata and Gary Taubes feature the experiment in their 2007 books on food, diet, dieting and health. The body mass indices (BMIs) of the participants in the Minnesota Experiment dropped from an initial average 21.7 to 16.6.

Semi-starvation is one form of energy restriction. Others are famine, and conditions in concentration camps. These have both been studied. Probably the most studied famine is that of the Dutch hunger winter of 1944, when the German army blockaded the northern part of the Netherlands, leaving its entire population short of food. People were restricted to 1,000 calories (4,200 kilojoules) a day or fewer. At the time they shed weight, of course. Researchers have investigated the effect of this semi-starvation on the later incidence of disease. Children of mothers who were undernourished in the first three months of their pregnancy were more likely to become overweight and obese as young men and as middle-aged women. They were also more likely to have high blood pressure, suffer heart disease, and be mentally and emotionally disturbed. The macabre observation 'people never got fat in a concentration camp' has a twist. Survivors were liable to binge on food and to be flabby or fat in later life.

Dieting: the modern evidence

The *British Journal of Nutrition* review. In my response I said: 'The body is evolved to adapt to periods of energy restriction as if these are periods of scarcity or famine, by means of mechanisms that after the restriction is over, trigger hunger, inhibit satiety, and preferentially conserve body fat ... It is hard to see how *Homo sapiens* could have evolved and survived without some such adaptive mechanisms.' See later in this chapter.

Systematic reviews. These summarize all relevant accessed scientific and other expert literature and therefore are a basis for reliable conclusions and recommendations. Necessarily they can only be as good as the research studies on which they are based. In the field of obesity, reviews of the epidemiological and biological literature are impressive, but studies from evolutionary, ecological, cultural and historical points of view have not been and probably could never be reviewed methodically.

Roy Walford. Born in 1924, he died in 2004. I knew him: he and I ran side by side in the 1980 Paris Marathon – well, we did for a while, for he finished ahead of me and over dinner said that he completed the run on general fitness without special training. He was 56 then. As a young man he paid his way through medical school with winnings from beating the system at a Reno gambling house. He was best known for experiments in which he extended the lives of laboratory animals by restricting their dietary energy. He was a character – in the 1980s he shaved his head and grew a Fu Manchu moustache.

The biospherians. The body mass of five ranged from BMI 19.1 to 21.2, one was BMI 23.7, the other two were BMI 25.6 (a woman) and 28.8 (a man).

What happens when you go on a diet

The fundamental fallacies. The textbook (referenced below) was edited by Reg Passmore and Martin Eastwood. Obesity was Reg Passmore's field. It's safe to say that he wrote this passage. It more or less repeats what was said in the previous 1979 edition, also co-edited by him with others.

Body fat – more precisely termed adipose tissue – is not pure fat. It contains a small proportion of water, and also other tissue. Its energy value is around 3,000 calories a pound or 6,600 calories a kilogram. Because of the energy needed to metabolize food, it takes about 4,500 calories to lay down a pound of body fat (or 10,000 calories per kilogram).

Glycogen. The energy value of human (and animal) lean tissue, at roughly 100 calories (400 kilojoules) per 100 grams, is the same as glycogen bound up with water. This is one-eighth the energy value of body fat, and for the same reason – most of its weight is water.

Proportions of muscle and fat reduced by dieting. Most studies do not detect that the bodies of fit and active people protect muscle tissue. This is probably because fit people do not go on dieting regimes, and would not be interested in being the subjects of experiments. Why should they? They may be 'normal' weight, or they may be overweight and carry quite a lot of body fat, but physically fit people usually like the shape they're in. The same point applies to the time after dieting regimes are ended. Studies have been made of wrestlers who reduce and increase weight, but not, as far as I know, of boxers, jockeys, dancers or actors. If carried out on such fit people over a long period of time the results might well be illuminating, but

professionals like these are not likely to give energy-metabolism studies priority over their work. Almost all research in this whole field is done on sedentary unfit obese people who long to reduce their body weight and body fat.

What happens when you come off a diet

Metabolic rate. The first version of this book stated that metabolic rate remains depressed after a dieting regime, and that successive regimes accentuate this effect. Since then a substantial number of studies on humans, including one carried out by Andrew Prentice of the London School of Hygiene and Tropical Medicine and colleagues published in 1991 (referenced below) have not found this. Bearing in mind that animal experiments do show this effect, there are a number of explanations. One is that rats are not people. Another is that the effect occurs in humans only as a result of severe dieting regimes, which rats endure, having no choice. In my opinion the most likely explanation is that the effect does occur in humans, but would be found only in long-term studies. Neither investigators nor human subjects can replicate the situation either of animal studies or of what happens in real life to humans over substantial periods of time as their body composition changes to become relatively more fat. The mechanism that accounts for the preferential accumulation of body fat that follows dieting may well be microbial.

Increased weight. John Garrow has documented another case – himself. For 1,000 days between 1973 and 1976 he overate, later went on a reducing diet, and checked to see what happened. In April 1973 he weighed around 75 kilograms (165 pounds, or 11 stone 11 pounds). 'I had remained at that weight without conscious effort for many years.' In July he started to overeat, and in August had driven his weight up to 81 kilograms (178 pounds), in part by consuming many plain chocolate digestive biscuits, 'to which I am very partial'. He had assumed that as soon as he stopped overeating, his weight would drop to 75 kilograms. It did not. Between September 1973 and March 1974 it was usually between 79 and 80 kilograms. He then went on a dieting regime, and by May had driven his weight down to 75 kilograms; this was 'not as easy as I had expected'. Between July and December he was weighed 'blind' (himself not knowing the result) and his weight drifted up to 76 kilograms (167 pounds), at which level it remained until April 1975. He then went on a low-energy diet and dropped 7 kilograms (15½ pounds, or over a stone) in 31 days. Thereafter his weight continued to rise, and before the end of the year his clothes were tight. His weight increased not by 6 kilograms, back to the weight he had maintained without effort for many years, but by 10 kilograms (22 pounds), to 79 kilograms (174 pounds). After his overeating and dieting his weight had increased by 4 kilograms (9 pounds), and he became somebody who had to watch his weight.

Gut microbial ecology. There is more at stake here than Nobel prizes. If our symbiotic bacteria are the drivers of body-fat sparing and body-fat deposition, and if their ecology can be effectively manipulated by a safe intervention, here could be the treatment of choice for overweight and obese people who have access to and money for bug replacement therapy.

Adapting to fatness

Set-point theory. Richard Keesey of the University of Wisconsin first proposed this idea. Based on rat work, he explains: 'Laboratory animals, like human beings, appear to regulate body weight around a stable level or set-point. If their weight is reduced by restricting their calorie intake, rats rapidly restore body weight to the level of unrestricted controls when allowed to feed freely . . . Thus, as in man, the stability and the vigorous defense of its body weight by the rat suggests the presence of a set-point regulator.' In its usual form the theory depends on assuming that people's weight normally does not change much over time, like rats in controlled settings. This is not true. The idea was dusted off when the role of the hormone leptin in regulating appetite and therefore body weight was identified. Researchers supposed that, synthesized and injected, leptin would be the Big Daddy appetite suppressant. It works on rats but not on humans. The next discovery was of ghrelin and various other substances secreted in the stomach that drive the sense of satiety. Manipulating these also controls the feeding habits of rats, but no drug has been devised that works on humans. Rats, one might say.

Set-point as moveable. This is a basis for a number of dieting books, including *The Shangri-La Diet* by the inveterate self-experimenter Seth Roberts, best known in the USA, and *The Don't Go Hungry Diet* reviewed in the previous chapter, best known in Australia.

Over-feeding experiments. These show that when people overeat their weight does not increase to the level that would be expected if this was just a function of extra energy input. This is why I did not become the Michelin boy (or man). The classic experiments on over-feeding were done by R O Neumann at the beginning of the 20th century on himself in Germany, and by Ethan Sims in the 1960s on prisoners in the USA.

Others, including Derek Miller and Michael Stock in the UK and Claude Bouchard in the USA, have investigated over-feeding. The results are always consistent.

Why physical activity is crucial

Human energy requirements at rest. The categories in the table of 'lean', 'average', 'fat' and 'very fat' do not correspond to the body mass index (BMI) system which is based only on weight and ignores body composition and degree of physical fitness. They are more sophisticated. Crucially, they allow for people having different weights with the same body composition, and different body compositions at the same weight. Acknowledgements and thanks to John Durnin. The responsibility for the table as adapted here and for its interpretation is mine.

Overall human energy requirements. Basically sedentary women now are often in energy balance at around 1,750–1,850 calories a day – more or less largely depending on weight and age. The average figure of 1,800 calories a day is included in the 2005 official US dietary guidelines. The mid-century energy requirement calculated in 1950 for the Food and Agriculture Organization of the United Nations for an average woman of 60 kilograms was 2,451 calories a day. The contrast between energy requirements at BMIs of 1.45–1.75 given in the most recent FAO report published in 2004 is not as wide as that suggested here, and for women and men is around 400–450 calories a day. This may be because of not allowing for the 'fitness factor' – the additional energy turned over by the body of a physically fit person all the time.

The range of 400–600 calories a day. This is found by comparing current energy requirements with those meticulously compiled in the mid-20th century for United Nations agencies, and also notably by John Durnin and Reg Passmore. I am also grateful to James Hill for pointing out that the difference in energy turnover now of US Amish communities, whose way of life avoids mechanization, and typical US communities, is the same range – 400–600 calories a day.

Why dieting makes you fat

Evolution is the study of the origin, development and adaptation of all life forms and in particular the environmental and other influences that enable the appearance and differentiation of living things. It is concerned with primordial and later forces that account for the relative success or failure of species.

Ancestral diets. Loren Cordain, S Boyd Eaton and colleagues propose that the diets to which we are adapted go back further than 200,000 years ago when *Homo sapiens* emerged, and first developed among the various lines of hominid (now termed hominin) lines that emerged perhaps 5–7 million years ago.

Human adaptability. In the opinion of the biological scientist Lynn Margulis, living organisms are likely to be 'far more responsive to immediate environmental forces' than is usually supposed. In which case, maybe humans will in time – at least to some extent – adapt to food supplies that are bountiful and always accessible, without becoming fat. In parts of the world where food is abundant they now have the selective advantage. Epidemics arise and then decline as vulnerable people have fewer offspring and die and their bloodlines dwindle, so that less vulnerable people become dominant. It is hard to believe that humans will adapt to becoming sedentary and to consuming sugary fatty processed foods and drinks, without increasing in weight. But just maybe, some time in the future, obesity will become uncommon again. This assumes that staple foods will remain cheap, but in 2007 and 2008 the trends and projections were that food will become a lot more expensive. But maybe food-secure populations will even be able to restrict their energy from food, by fasting or dieting, without provoking their bodies to store more fat. Maybe one day dieting will not make you fat. Maybe one day humans will colonize Mars. This won't happen in my lifetime, or yours, or that of your children and grandchildren.

Is Dieting Dangerous?

National Institutes of Health task force on the prevention and treatment of obesity. Competing interest disclosures showed that of this panel of nine people, seven were directors of weight-loss clinics, six were advisors to commercial weight-loss organizations, and eight were advisors to manufacturers of drugs designed to reduce weight. Such links are usual in this field and may simply indicate special commitment to the improvement of public health. They also indicate that collectively the task force supported weight-loss regimes. Then and now, it would be hard to create a committee from eminent experts in this field who had no competing interests.

Weight-cycling studies. The 1989 paper was by Peggy Hamm, Richard Shekelle and Jeremiah Stamler, of the University of Texas at Houston and of Northwestern University in Chicago, Illinois (using the Western Electric cohort). The 1991 paper was by Lauren Lissner of Goteberg University, Sweden, and colleagues (using the Framingham cohort). The 2005 study was by Vanessa Diaz of the Medical University of South Carolina at Charleston, and colleagues (using National Health and Nutrition Examination Survey – NHANES – data).

Adjusting for pre-existing disease. Another paper published in 1999 is sometimes cited as refuting the evidence that weight cycling is risky. This was by Simone French of the University of Minnesota at Minneapolis and colleagues including from CDC, from the Iowa Women's Health Study. This separated unintentional and intentional weight loss. It concluded that unintentional weight loss was associated with increased death from heart disease and all causes, whereas 'intentional weight loss was not associated with increased total or cardiovascular disease mortality risks'. But in fact the study showed that intentional weight loss was associated with a 22 per cent higher rate of total deaths. The reason for the authors' conclusion was that the result was not 'statistically significant', meaning there was a 5 per cent possibility that it was due to chance, expressed as a 'confidence interval' of 0.98 to 1.51. Had the lower number been two percentage points higher at 1.00, the tone of the study's conclusions would be different. Besides, this study is not about weight cycling! The comparisons made were between 'at least one' substantial change in weight. That's not weight cycling.

Weight cycling and heart attacks. Remembering that body fat is metabolically active just like all the body's tissues, the best policy is gradually to change its composition, by switching to a diet mostly made up from fresh and benignly processed foods, which is therefore very low in saturated fats and trans-fatty acids, and to reduce body fat gradually by increased physical activity. This is one of the rationales for golden rules 1–4 in chapter 6.

Compulsive self-starvation. So-called 'anorexia nervosa' is basically a metabolic disorder. The anorexia-bulimia syndrome, cycles of starvation followed by gorging, is an extreme and violent version of yo-yo dieting. Without bulimia, the starved body feeds on its own fat and then on its own lean tissue, and unless there is a change or intervention death follows. Obviously anorexia has psychological aspects, as does dieting, but the driver of the disorder is metabolic.

What's wrong with being fat

Methods of calculating degrees of body fatness. The first systematic method was devised by the statistician Louis Dublin in the USA for the Metropolitan Life Insurance Company. Tables of 'desirable' or 'ideal' weight ranges for 25-59-year-old people were first published in 1943, have been revised up to 1985, and can still sometimes be found screwed on to weighing machines in pharmacies. Since the late 1970s the body mass index (BMI) method has been preferred.

BMI in the USA. In this case BMI is calculated as your weight in pounds, divided by the square of your height in inches, multiplied by 704. In the USA the 'cut-off' between 'healthy' and 'overweight' BMI is often still taken to be more than 25 – often around BMI 26-27. Cut-offs recommended in some Asian countries are lower: around 23-24 and above for over-weight and around 27-28 for obese.

Estimating fatness. A simpler way to measure body fat is by waist circumference. Currently waist measurements of 94 centimetres (37 inches) for men, and 80 centimetres (31.5 inches) for women are suggested as advisable upper limits. This of course can't be right. One circumference cannot fit all. What's needed is a scale related to height. Graded waist measurement would be a better gauge of fitness and health, and indeed of body fat. Another method is waist-hip ratio.

Currently waist-hip ratios of 1.0 for men and of 0.85 for women are suggested as advisable upper limits. An even simpler method, recommended in the UK by Margaret Ashwell, is to keep your waist circumference below a half of your height.

Obesity, overweight, and the risk of chronic diseases. University-based professionals in the USA who challenge the generally accepted view now include Paul Campos, J Eric Oliver and Glenn Gaesser, who have written books for the general reader. Paul Ernsberger, Paul Haskew, Richard Koletsky and a substantial number of co-authors have been publishing in academic journals on this topic, and also on weight cycling, since the late 1980s. Relevant books and papers are referenced below.

Body size and cancer. Overall there is good evidence that being big, including being fat, itself increases the risk of some cancers. All the lines of evidence point to relationships judged to be convincingly or probably causal, and justifying public health recommend-ations. Also, relatively heavy birth-weight, accelerated growth, and early sexual maturity are certainly associated with higher risk of breast cancer. Further, bigger fatter girls and women have higher levels of circulating hormones that affect the risk of post-menopausal breast cancer. The taller you are the more cells you have, and there-fore the more chance of an error in cell division that may lead to cancer. All this shows that fatness itself increases the risk of some cancers, and maybe cancer in general. The source here is the 2007 World Cancer Research Fund/American Institute for Cancer Research report, referenced below.

Ideal body weight. It is sometimes suggested that the lighter you are the healthier you are, as long as you don't become underweight. This idea has little merit. True, Asians with little family experience of food security who now are consuming more processed food and are much less active, tend to become diabetic at BMI levels in the low 20s, both in their native countries and when immigrants to other countries. But this does not apply to adults who live in parts of the world where food supplies have been secure for some generations.

References: books, reports

In alphabetical order of authors. Publishing details are usually of first edition.

General, including for the general public

William Bennett, Joel Gurin. *The Dieter's Dilemma. Why Diets are Obsolete: the New Set-Point Theory of Weight Control.* New York: Basic Books, 1982.

Paul Campos. *The Obesity Myth. Why America's Obsession with Weight is Hazardous to Your Health.* New York: Gotham, 2004.

Department of Health and Human Services. *The Surgeon-General's Call to Action to Prevent and Decrease Overweight and Obesity.* Washington DC: DHHS, 2001.

Glenn Gaesser. *Big Fat Lies. The Truth About Your Weight and Your Health.* New York: Gurze, 2002.

House of Commons Health Committee. *Obesity.* Third report of Session 2003-04. London: The Stationery Office, 2004.

Gina Kolata. The girl who had no leptin. [Chapter 7]. *Rethinking Thin. The New Myths of Weight Loss – and the Myths and Realities of Dieting.* New York: Farrar, Straus, Giroux, 2007.

Ray Moynihan, Alan Cassels. *Selling Sickness: How the World's Biggest Pharmaceutical Companies are Turning Us All Into Patients.* New York: Nation Books, 2005.

Marion Nestle. A digression into calories and diet. [Chapter 24]. *What to Eat.* New York: Farrar, Straus, Giroux, 2006.

J Eric Oliver. *Fat Politics. The Real Story Behind America's Obesity Epidemic.* Oxford: University Press, 2006.

Todd Tucker. *The Great Starvation Experiment. The Heroic Man Who Starved So That Millions Could Live.* New York: Free Press, 2006.

Specialist. Usually these include evidence that is both biological, including evolution mechanisms, and also social, including epidemiology

Aristotle. *The History of Animals.* Book 8. D'Arcy Wentworth Thompson (trs).

Per-Olof Åstrand, Kaare Rodahl. Nutrition and physical performance, [Chapter 14] *Textbook of Work Psychology.* Second edition. New York: McGraw-Hill, 1977.

David Barker. *Mothers, Babies and Disease in Later Life.* Edinburgh: Churchill Livingstone, 1998.

Francis Benedict, R Miles, P Roth, M Smith. *Human Vitality and Efficiency Under Prolonged Restricted Diet.* Publication 280. Washington DC: Carnegie Institute, 1919.

William Brock. Philosopher of science: the Bacon affair. [Chapter 11]. *Justus von Liebig. The Chemical Gatekeeper.* Cambridge: University Press, 1997.

John Durnin, Reg Passmore. *Energy, Work and Leisure.* London: Heinemann, 1967.

Paul Ernsberger, Paul Haskew. *Rethinking Obesity. An Alternative View of its Health Implications.* New York: Human Sciences Press, 1988.

Mary Gale, Brian Lloyd (editors). *Sinclair. The Founders of Modern Nutrition* (3). London: McCarrison Society, 1990. Obtainable from www.mccarrisonsociety.org.uk.

John Garrow. *Energy Balance and Obesity in Man.* First edition. Amsterdam: Elsevier, 1974. John Garrow. Factors affecting energy intake. [Chapter 4]. *Energy Balance and Obesity in Man.* Second edition. Amsterdam: Elsevier, 1978. John Garrow. The physics and the physiology of obesity. [Chapter 3]. *Take Obesity Seriously. A Clinical Manual.* Edinburgh: Churchill Livingstone, 1981.

Ancel Keys, Josef Brozek, Austin Henschel, Olaf Mickelsen, Henry Taylor. *The Biology of Human Starvation.* 2 volumes. Minneapolis: University of Minnesota Press, 1950.

Lynn Margulis, Dorian Sagan. Darwin revisited: species in the evolutionary dialogue. [Chapter 13]. *Acquiring Genomes: A Theory of the Origin of Species.* New York: Basic Books, 2002.

Reg Passmore, Martin Eastwood (eds). Energy. [Chapter 3]. *Human Nutrition and Dietetics.* Eighth Edition. Edinburgh: Churchill Livingstone, 1986.

Royal College of Physicians of London. *Obesity.* London: RCP, 1983.

US Department of Health and Human Services/US Department of Agriculture. *Dietary Guidelines for Americans 2005.* Washington DC: USDHHS/USDA, 2005.

World Cancer Research Fund/American Institute for Cancer Research. *Food, Nutrition, Physical Activity and the Prevention of Cancer: a Global Perspective.* Washington DC: AICR, 2007. Obtainable at: www.wcrf.org, or www.aicr.org.

World Health Organization. *Obesity:*

Preventing and Managing the Global Epidemic. Report of a WHO consultation. Technical report series 894. Geneva: WHO, 2000.

World Health Organization. *Diet, Nutrition and the Prevention of Chronic Diseases.* Report of a joint WHO/FAO Expert Consultation. Technical report series 916. Geneva: WHO, 2003.

References: papers, articles

In alphabetical order of authors:

The main categories here are biological (including evolution and biological mechanisms) and social (mostly epidemiological studies, and some behavioural). Some papers cover both biological and social aspects.

General

Anon. Fazer regime engorda. *Veja*, 18 April 2007.

Cable News Network. Fat chance. Transmitted 4 May 2002. Transcript obtainable at: www.CNN.com_Transcripts.mht.

Henig R. Fat factors. *New York Times*, 13 August 2006.

Kiely K. Governor's healthy state. *USA Today*, 11 July 2004.

Leith W. Health warning: all diets make you fat. The *Daily Telegraph*, 11 April 2007.

'Plutarch'. What if Huckabee's 'signature issue' is a scam? Obtainable at: www.freerepublic.com/focus/f'-chat/1937730/posts.

Rouse B. Most dieters 'end up heavier'. The *Independent*, 10 April 2007.

Biological including evolution mechanisms. May also include epidemiology

Apfelbaum M, Bostsarron J, Lacatis D. Effect of caloric restriction and excessive caloric intake on energy expenditure. *American Journal of Clinical Nutrition* 1971; 24: 1405-9.

Astrup A. The satiating power of protein - a key to obesity prevention? *American Journal of Clinical Nutrition* 2005; 82(1): 1-2.

Blackburn G, Wilson G, Kandera B, Stein L, Lavin P, Adler J, Brownell K. Weight cycling. The experience of human dieters. *American Journal of Clinical Nutrition* 1989; 49: S1105-09.

Bray G, Nielson S, Popkin B. Consumption of high-fructose corn syrup in beverages may play a role in the epidemic of obesity. *American Journal of Clinical Nutrition* 2004; 79(4) 537-43.

Brownell K, Rodin J. Medical, metabolic and psychological effects of weight cycling. *Archives of Internal Medicine* 1994; 154: 1325-30.

Cannon G. Dieting. Makes you fat? *British Journal of Nutrition* 2005; 93: 1-2.

Cogan J, Ernsberger P. Dieting, weight, and health. Reconceptualising research and policy. *Journal of Social Issues* 1999; 55(2): 187-205.

Cordain L, Boyd Eaton S, Sebastian A, Mann N, Lindeberg S, Watkins B, O'Keefe J, Brand-Miller J. Origins and evolution of the Western diet: health implications for the 21st century. *American Journal of Clinical Nutrition* 2005; 81(2): 341-54.

Dobzhansky T. Nothing in biology makes sense except in the light of evolution. *American Biology Teacher* 1973; 35: 125-9.

Dore C, Hesp R, Wilkins D, Garrow J. Prediction of energy requirements of obese patients after massive weight loss. *Human Nutrition: Clinical Nutrition* 1982; 36C:41-8.

Dulloo A, Jacquet J, Girardier L. Autoregulation of body composition during weight recovery in humans: the Minnesota Experiment revisited. *International Journal of Obesity* 1996; 20: 393-407.

Dulloo A, Jacquet J, Girardier L. Poststarvation hyperphagia and body fat overshooting in humans: a role for feedback signals from lean and fat tissues. *American Journal of Clinical Nutrition* 1997; 65: 7-23.

Dulloo A, Jacquet J, Montani J-P. Pathways from weight fluctuations to metabolic diseases: focus on maladaptive thermogenesis during catch-up fat. *International Journal of Obesity* 2002; 26: S546-57.

Dulloo A, Jacquet J, Seydoux J, Montani J-P. The thrifty 'catch-up fat phenotype: its impact on insulin sensitivity during growth trajectories to obesity and metabolic syndrome. *International Journal of Obesity* 2006; 30: S23-35.

Dulloo A. Suppressed thermogenesis as cause for resistance to slimming and obesity rebound: adaptation or illusion? [Editorial]. *International Journal of Obesity* 2006; 30: S1-3.

Ernsberger P, Haskew P. Health implications for obesity: an alternative view. *Journal of Obesity and Weight Regulation* 1987; 6: 58-137.

Ernsberger P, Koletsky R. Biochemical rationale for a wellness approach to obesity: an alternative to a focus on weight loss. *Journal of Social Issues* 1999; 55(2) 221-60.

Garrow J, Webster J. Effects on weight and metabolic rate of obese women of a 3.4MJ (800kcal) diet. *Lancet* 1989; i:1429-31.

Garrow J. The safety of dieting. *Proceedings of the Nutrition Society* 1991; 50: 493-9.

Hill J. Understanding and addressing the obesity epidemic: an energy balance perspective. *Endocrine Reviews* 2006; 27(7): 750-61.

Hirsch J. Obesity: a perspective. [Chapter 1]. In: Bray G (ed). *Recent Advances in Obesity Research: II*. Proceedings of the 2nd International Congress on Obesity. London: Newman, 1978.

Hirsch J. An interview with Jules Hirsch. 1991. Available at: www.archive.sciencewatch.com/interviews/jules.hirsch3.htm.

Hoffman D, Sawaya A, Verreschi I, Tucker K, Roberts S. Why are nutritionally stunted children at increased risk of obesity? Studies of metabolic rate and fat oxidation in shantytown children from São Paulo, Brazil. *American Journal of Clinical Nutrition* 2000; 72: 1025-31.

Jenkins D, Wolever T, Collier G, Ocana A, Rao A, Buckley G, Lam Y, Mayer A, Thompson L. Metabolic effects of a low-glycemic index diet. *American Journal of Clinical Nutrition* 1987; 46: 968-75.

Keen H. Nutrient intake, adiposity and diabetes. *British Medical Journal* 1979; 1: 655-8.

Keesey R. A set-point analysis of the regulation of body weight. In: Stunkard A (ed). *Obesity*. Philadelphia PA: WB Saunders, 1980.

Langley-Evans S. Developmental programming in health and disease. *Proceedings of the Nutrition Society* 2006; 65(1): 97-105.

Leibel R, Rosenbaum M, Hirsch J. Changes in energy expenditure resulting from altered body weight. *New England Journal of Medicine* 1995; 332: 621-8.

Leitch I. *Growth and health. British Journal of Nutrition* 1951; 5: 142-51.

Ley R, Turnbaugh P, Klein S, Gordon J. Microbial ecology: human gut microbes associated with obesity. *Nature* 2006; 444: 1022-3.

Ludwig D. Dietary glycemic index and obesity. *Journal of Nutrition* 2000; 130: S280-3.

Macias A. Experimental demonstration of human weight homeostatis: implications for understanding obesity. *British Journal of Nutrition* 2004; 91: 479-84.

National Institutes of Health. Weight cycling. Publication NIH #01-3901. Updated 2006. Available at: http://win.niddk.nih.gov/pubs/cycling/htm#conclusions.

National Institutes of Health. National Task Force on the Prevention and Treatment of Obesity. Weight cycling. *Journal of the American Medical Association* 1994; 272: 1196-1202.

Neel, J. Diabetes mellitus: a thrifty genotype rendered detrimental by progress. *American Journal of Human Genetics* 1960; 14: 353-62.

Neumann R. Experimentelle Beiträge zur Lehre von dem Taglichen Nahrungsbedarf des Menschen unter besonderer Berücksichtigung der Notwendigen Eiweissmenge. Archiv für Hygiene 1902; 45: 1-87.

Ong K, Ahmed M, Emmett P, Preece M, Dunger D. Association between postnatal catch-up growth and obesity in childhood: prospective cohort study. *British Medical Journal* 2000; 320: 967-71.

Prentice A, Goldberg G, Jebb S, Black A, Murgatroyd P. Physiological responses to slimming. *Proceedings of the Nutrition Society* 1991; 50: 441-58.

Prentice A. Fires of life: Struggles of an ancient metabolism in a modern world. *British Nutrition Foundation Bulletin* 2001; 26: 13-27.

Sims A. Experimental obesity, diet-induced thermogenesis, and their clinical implications. *Clinics in Endocrinology and Metabolism* 1976; 5(2): 377-95.

Sims E, Danforth E, Horton E, Bray G, Glannon J, Salans L. Endocrine and metabolic effects of experimental obesity in man. *Recent Progress in Hormone Research* 1973; 29: 457-96.

Singhal A, Lucas A. Early origins of cardiovascular disease: is there a unifying hypothesis? *Lancet* 2004; 363: 1624-45.

Tappy L, Binnert C, Schneiter P. Energy expenditure, physical activity, body-weight control. *Proceedings of the Nutrition Society* 2003; 62: 663-66.

Turnbaugh P, Ley R, Mahowald M, Magrini V, Mardis E, Gordon J. An obesity-associated gut microbiome with increased capacity for energy harvest. *Nature* 2006; 444: 1027-31.

van Baak M. Adaptive thermogenesis during over- and underfeeding in man. *British Journal of Nutrition* 2004; 92, 329-30.

Weigle D, Breen P, Mattys C, Callahan H, Meuuws K, Burden V, Purnell J. A high-protein diet induces sustained reduction in appetite, *ad libitum* caloric intake, and body weight, despite compensatory changes in diurnal plasma leptin and ghrelin concentrations. *American Journal of Clinical Nutrition* 2005; 82: 41-8.

Westman E, Feinman R, Mavropoulos J, Vernon M, Volek J, Wortman J, Yancy W, Phinney S. Low-carbohydrate nutrition and metabolism. *American Journal of Clinical Nutrition* 2007; 86(2): 276-84.

Weyer C, Walford R, Harper I, Milner M, MacCallum T, Tataranni P, Ravussin E. Energy metabolism after 2 y of energy restriction: the Biosphere 2 experiment. *American Journal of Clinical Nutrition* 2000; 72(4): 946-53.

Wilson P, Osbourn D. Compensatory growth after undernutrition in mammals and birds. *Biological Reviews* 1960; 37: 324-63.

Wooley C, Garner D. Dietary treatments of obesity are ineffective. *British Medical Journal* 1994; 309: 655-6.

Wretlind A. Nutrition problems in healthy adults with low activity and low caloric consumption. In Blix G (ed). *Nutrition and Physical Activity.* Symposia of the Swedish Nutrition Foundation V. Uppsala: Almqvist and Wiksell, 1967.

Yajnik C S. Obesity epidemic in India: interuterine origins? *Proceedings of the Nutrition Society* 2004; 63: 387-96.

Social including epidemiology, behaviour

Allison D, Fontaine K, Manson J, Stevens J, Van Itallie T. Annual deaths attributable to obesity in the United States. *Journal of the American Medical Association* 1999; 282 (16): 1530-8.

Drapeau V, Provencher V, Lemieux S, Depres J-P, Bouchard C, Tremblay A. Do 6-y changes in eating behaviour predict changes in body weight? *International Journal of Obesity* 2003; 27: 808-14.

Favero A, Rodella F, Santonastasco P. Binge eating and eating attitudes among Nazi concentration camp survivors. *Psychological Medicine* 2000; 30: 463-6.

Freedman M, King J, Kennedy E. Popular diets: a scientific review. *Obesity Research* 2001: 9 (supp 1): 1–40.

French S, Jeffery R, Forster J, McGovern P, Kelder S, Baxter J. Predictors of weight change over 2 years among a population of working adults. *International Journal of Obesity* 1994; 18: 145–54.

French S, Folsom A, Jeffery R, Williamson D. Prospective study of weight loss and mortality in older women: the Iowa Women's Health Study. *American Journal of Epidemiology* 1999; 149(6): 504–14.

Garner D, Wooley S. Confronting the failure of behavioural and dietary treatments for obesity. *Clinical Psychology Review* 1991; 11: 729–80.

Gordon T, Kannel W. The effects of overweight on cardiovascular diseases. *Geriatrics* 1973; 28: 80–8.

Hamm P, Shekelle R, Stamler J. Large fluctuations in body weight during young adulthood and twenty-five year risk of coronary heart disease in men. *American Journal of Epidemiology* 1989; 129: 312–18.

Hill A. Does dieting make you fat? *British Journal of Nutrition* 2004; 92: S1: 15–18.

Jeffrey R, Drewnowski A, Epstein L, Stunkard A, Wilson G, Wing R. Long-term maintenance of weight loss: current status. *Health Psychology* 2000; 19: S5–16.

Juhaeri, Stevens J, Chambless L, Tyroler H, Harp J, Jones D, Arnett D. Weight change among self-reported dieters and non-dieters in white and African-American men and women. *European Journal of Epidemiology* 2001; 17(10): 917–23.

Kassirer J, Angell M. Losing weight – an ill-fated New Year's resolution. *New England Journal of Medicine* 1998; 338: 52–4.

Kennedy I, Bowman S, Spence J, Freedman M, King I. Popular diets: correlation to health, nutrition and obesity. *Journal of the American Dietetic Association* 2001; 101(4): 211–20.

Klesges R, Isbell T, Klesges L. Relationship between dietary restraint, energy intake, physical activity and body weight: a prospective analysis. *Journal of Abnormal Psychology* 1992. 101: 668–74.

Klesges R, Klem M, Epkins C, Klesges L. A longitudinal review of dietary restraint and its relationship to changes in body weight. *Addictive Behavior* 1991; 16: 363–8.

Kolata G. Asking if obesity is a disease or just a symptom. *New York Times*, 16 April 2002.

Korkeila M, Rissanen A, Kaprio J, Sorensen T, Koskenvuo M. Weight-loss attempts and risk of major weight gain: a prospective study in Finnish adults. *American Journal of Clinical Nutrition* 1999; 70: 965–75.

Lissner L, Odell P, D'Agostino R, Stokes J, Kreger B, Belenger A, Brownell K. Variability of body weight and health outcomes in the Framingham population. *New England Journal of Medicine* 1991; 324: 1839–44.

McGuire M, Wing R, Hill J, Klem M, Lang W. What predicts weight gain in a group of successful weight losers? *Journal of Consulting Clinical Psychology* 1999; 67: 177–85.

Mann T, Tomiyama J, Westling E, Lew A-M, Samuels B, Chatman J. Medicare's search for effective obesity treatments. Diets are not the answer. *American Psychologist* 2007; 62(3): 220–33.

Martins P A, Hoffman D J, Fernandes M T B, Nascimento C R, Roberts S B, Sesso R, Sawaya A L. Stunted children gain less lean body mass and more fat mass than their non-stunted counterparts: a prospective study. *British Journal of Nutrition* 2004; 92, 819-25.

Metropolitan Life Insurance tables. Obtainable at: www.obesitycare.com/1983 MetropolitanLifeInsuranceTable.htm.

Perri M, Fuller P. Success and failure in the treatment of obesity: where do we go from here? *Medicine, Exercise, Nutrition and Health* 1995; 4: 255-71.

Ravelli A, van der Meulen J, Osmond C, Barker D, Bleker O. Obesity at the age of 50 in men and women exposed to famine prenatally. *American Journal of Clinical Nutrition* 1999; 70(5): 811-16.

Ravelli G, Stein Z, Susser M. Obesity in young men after famine exposure *in utero* and early pregnancy. *New England Journal of Medicine* 1976; 295(7): 349-53.

Roseboom T, de Rooij S, Painter R. The Dutch famine and its long-term consequences for adult health. *Early Human Development* 2006; 82(8): 485-91.

Stice E, Cameron R, Killen J, Hayward C, Taylor C. Naturalistic weight-reduction efforts prospectively predict growth in relative weight and onset of obesity among female adolescents. *Journal of Consulting Clinical Psychology* 1999; 67: 967-74.

PART 2: CONSCIOUS WELLBEING

Epigraphs for Part 2

The physicist David Bohm (1917-92), having worked with Albert Einstein and Robert Oppenheimer in the USA, settled in London where his main interest became the nature of reality, life and consciousness. This is from his *Wholeness and the Implicate Order*.

The anthropologist Margaret Mead (1901-78) was dedicated to understanding the human condition within our natural environment. She also says: 'Never doubt that a small group of thoughtful people could change the world. Indeed, it's the only thing that ever has.'

4. EVERYTHING ELSE THAT MAKES YOU FAT

Notes: epigraphs

The journalist Eric Schlosser (1959-) also says: 'The obesity epidemic that began in the United States in the late 1970s is now spreading to the rest of the world, with fast food as one of its vectors . . . wherever America's fast-food chains go, waistlines start expanding.'

The pathologist Rudolf Virchow (1821-1902) was at the age of 27 asked by the rulers of Prussia to identify the causes of an outbreak of typhus in Upper Silesia. He reported that its basic cause was the outrageous living conditions of impoverished communities.

Notes: main text

The medical model

The medical model. This sees public health in quasi-medical terms. Physicians are trained in human physiology and pathology, and in diagnosis and treatment of diseases at an individual level. Since the late 19th century, the medical profession has become increasingly powerful, and the health professions concerned with public health have become relegated and positioned as one branch of medicine. Many if not most influential nutrition scientists are physicians, physiologists or biochemists who have gained an interest in nutrition, or who work within hospitals or academic medical departments. Identification of overweight and obesity as mainly a medical matter, is professional empire-building. Epidemiologists are trained to think of diseases in their economic, social and environmental contexts, but most nutrition scientists are not epidemiologists.

Causes and significant causes. What's said here about obesity applies to all sorts of disorders and diseases. Professionals tend to give most value to what they best understand. 'To a man with a hammer, every problem is a nail.' Modern orthodox medicine treats symptoms and diseases, so medical professionals think in terms of physiology, biochemistry and pathology, and emphasize what can be called the immediate (or proximal) causes of diseases. But disorders and diseases also have underlying and basic (or distal) biological, economic, social and environmental causes. These are the main types of cause of disease, health and wellbeing. Immediate causes are not the issue when disorders or diseases become epidemics – as Rudolf Virchow insisted.

Medical and surgical approaches. Modern orthodox medicine is allopathic, meaning that it is based on the treatment of diseases and their symptoms. This is useful and can be vital. In general though, I agree that 'to administer medicines to diseases which have already developed is like the behaviour of people who dig a well after they have become thirsty, or of those who make their weapons after they have already engaged in battle'. This saying is attributed to the legendary Chinese Yellow Emperor Huang Ti (or Huangdi), said to have founded the Han dynasty in the third millennium BCE. The Chinese tradition, like the Indian tradition, teaches the fundamental value of the balance of diet in health and healing, and the supremacy of prevention.

It's not all in the genes

Drugs for obesity. New drugs are known to work in cases of rare genetic malfunctions that cause gross obesity starting in infancy. All new drugs are very expensive, because of the cost of developing them, and the profits to their manufacturers that are at first protected by patents. Because we are evolved with a hunger drive that is crucial for survival, effective appetite suppressants are likely to be powerful and so to have serious adverse effects.

In defence of industry

Food and drink and allied industries. Allied industries include the agrochemical industry, whose products make industrial agriculture possible; the pharmaceutical industry, which supplies antimicrobial drugs to the agriculture industry, and natural and synthetic vitamins and other bioactive substances to food manufacturers; the manufacturers of cosmetic additives – colours and flavours – and other chemicals used in food manufacture; and the manufacturers of 'purified', 'refined' homogenous starches, sugars, fats, and other ingredients in processed products; and suppliers of machinery. There are others.

Giant food and drink manufacturers, retailers and caterers. Both as consumers and citizens, we have to decide how to act in this world of big food business. People who for ethical or other reasons never shop in supermarkets, or never consume commercial processed or animal food, deserve respect. This is not my case. Also as I indicate here, to be hostile to 'the food industry' makes no sense. It is also counterproductive. What is now the general awareness shared by governments on the big issues of climate change has come about partly because of civil society engagement with the energy industries, and also because the leaders of some of these industries have seen that strategically, 'business as usual' is not an option. There is more on this in the main text of the next chapter, and its notes.

Basic reasons why we get fat

Food systems. These include the planting and breeding, production, harvesting and slaughter, storage, preservation and transport of food, and also its manufacture, processing, packaging, trade, distribution, sale and preparation, as well as its composition, consumption and metabolism, and also inter-related processes flowing within the contexts of evolution, history, resources, environment, tradition, culture, cuisine, health, technology, economics and politics. Traditional food systems necessarily make use of available resources adapted to local climate and terrain. Long-evolved food systems include that of the Mediterranean littoral, from southern Spain, France and Italy, to Greece and Turkey, Lebanon, Palestine, and Egypt and the other Maghreb countries of North Africa. Derived from Persian, Egyptian, Greek, Roman, Arab and other cultures, Mediterranean food systems have a history of over 3,000 years, and in their ancient and modern forms are celebrated by nutritional and culinary authorities. It is now known that a reason for the fall of empires is the depletion of natural resources: for example, Rome fell after the soil of North Africa, which had been the Empire's granary, became exhausted.

Evolution as the guiding principle for biology. The credo of Edmund Brisco Ford (1901–88) pre-dates the famous statement of Theodosius Dobzhansky quoted at the beginning of the previous chapter. E B Ford rightly goes further, with his emphasis also on history. On a personal note, he influenced my attitude to modern science: the quotation is from his preface to the first book I ever bought, as my present to me on my 14th birthday: *Butterflies*, in the Collins *New Naturalist* series.

Hunger for sugar and fat

Desires. What about alcohol? Most human societies eventually discover that almost any plant food when suitably fermented becomes alcoholic, and throughout history and all over the world, a feature of feasting, fighting and social rituals is drinking alcohol. Most societies enjoy parties. But the desire to get stoned is not specific to alcohol. Other cultures use other psychotropic substances. Islam forbids alcohol but permits hashish, and Mesoamerican shamans rely on hallucinogens. I think consciousness-altering substances are a different case, as are stimulants

like coffee, tea, *maté*, other herbal infusions, *guaraná* and ginseng.

Sugars consumption. The 100 pounds a year figure comes from estimates of the amount of sugars entering food supplies, minus around 10 per cent for waste and non-food uses. As a general rule, the more processed any food supply, the higher its proportion of sugars. Thus, consumption is higher in the USA, the UK and northern Europe, than in France, Italy, Greece and the Mediterranean region. It would be easier to estimate the amount of added sugars people consume if manufacturers were required to give this information on all food labels.

Fat (and oil) consumption. The Maasai of East Africa and the Inuit of the Arctic are adapted to diets very high in animal fat, and the traditional Cretan diet is said to be high in fat mostly from olive oil. When active these peoples rarely become overweight. Fats from free-ranging and wild animal sources, and relatively unrefined oils from various plant sources, are nourishing.

Hard-wiring of desires. To say that we cannot alter our built-in desire for sweetness and succulence is not to say we are doomed. First, awareness of the reason for these desires itself brings about change. Second, as in so many other ways, we can train our bodies to prefer these tastes from natural sources. My experience is that after about three months of avoiding foods containing added sugars, fats, and also salt – in any and all combinations – the body adjusts. This is one rationale for the golden rules of chapter 6.

The chemicalization of food

Carbohydrates. The only respect in which all carbohydrates are biochemically similar in effect explains the initial illusory effectiveness of dieting regimes like the Atkins Diet, which as explained in chapter 3 severely restrict carbohydrates and cause substantial reduction of weight in the first week or so. As stated in the previous chapter, this is because they most efficiently deplete the body of its own immediately available store of carbohydrate in the form of glycogen bound to water. The resulting impressive drop in weight, which might amount to 4½– 7 kilograms (roughly 10–15 pounds), is almost all due to dehydration.

Sugar and blood chemistry. Sugar as contained in wholefoods such as fruits is released into the bloodstream at a natural rate. But sugar as added to sweet processed products, especially soft drinks, floods into the bloodstream, and blood-sugar levels soar above natural maximum levels. In response, the pancreas releases insulin into the bloodstream, which pushes blood-sugar levels down, sometimes to unnaturally low levels. The impact on mood is a sense of euphoria followed by a sense of emptiness and craving for more – or to put it more plainly, an upper followed by a downer. Hence people referring to their 'sugar rush'. Fat in foods does not have this effect. As an adult I have not consumed sugary soft drinks. I have also learned to beware of chocolate, which I am liable to eat compulsively – my solution is only to eat high-quality varieties with 70 per cent plus cocoa content. A sugary food and drink habit overuses and abuses the homoeostatic insulin reaction and, some researchers say, eventually causes the pancreas to pack up – result, insulin-dependent diabetes. Other researchers state that sugars as contained in industrialized diets are not a cause of diabetes and that fluctuations in blood-sugar levels as caused by sugary foods and drinks are normally nothing to worry about. This is a controversial issue, confused by the fact that the sugar industry defends its product energetically and funds a lot of scientific research.

Infant and young-child feeding. If I had to rank the reasons why the human race is becoming fat I would put feeding with artificial formula at number one. In the backlands of Amazonia in Brazil I have seen children conscientiously weighed and measured by health professionals and volunteers, to ensure that their weights and heights conform to the United Nations charts based on the growth patterns of formula-fed US children.

The degradation of food

Glycaemic indices. At this point diet and dieting books now often include lots of information about the glycaemic index, and indeed some dieting books have 'GI' in their titles. Wholefoods including those high in starch are assimilated by the body at a natural speed, whereas products containing lots of processed starch as well as sugar, particularly when these are in relatively 'free' forms, shock the body and cause big-dipper effects in blood sugar, as summarized above. Glycaemic indices rate foods according to how slow or fast they are in having such effects. Basically all you need to know is that the human body is adapted to fresh foods and is not adapted to products high in processed starch, sugar, or both.

Mistreatment of animals. Feeding concentrates to animals has usually been seen as separate from issues of animal welfare, and of the environmental impacts of the factory farming of animals. Now, no longer, as a result of 'mad cow disease', especially in the UK, and the overwhelming evidence that the systematic use of antimicrobial drugs, essential in the factory farming of animals, is a cause of multiply drug-resistant human infections. Some defenders of animal rights say this is in effect a revenge of the mistreated animals.

The illusion of comfort

Energy balance then and now. These are average figures. Men and big and young people turn over more energy than women and small and old people, other things being equal, but in general, as stated in the main text, people now in energy balance turn over roughly 20 per cent less energy than people did up to the mid-20th century. It follows that if you consume the same amount of energy from food and drink as somebody like you in energy balance did up to the first half of the 20th century, you will become increasingly overweight, unless you become as physically active as it was natural to be in those times. See chapter 6, golden rule 2.

The cheapening of food

Spending on food and drink, and rates of obesity. As the available income of people increases, the proportion of available income spent on food and drink decreases. This is known as Engels's Law, after Friedrich Engels, the political philosopher, social reformer, and close colleague of Karl Marx. The most significant figures are those showing differences between people with roughly similar available incomes in different countries. These don't prove that a root cause of obesity is cheapened, degraded food, but they point in that direction. Relative rates of obesity in European countries are uncertain: OECD figures showing rates of obesity in France and Italy of under 10 per cent in the early 2000s are likely to be underestimates because based on self-reporting, whereas the UK figure of 22.6 per cent (and the US figure of 30.6 per cent) are based on actual measurements. There's no doubt that obesity rates in the UK are higher than in France and Italy, but the difference is likely not to be as dramatic as the OECD figures suggest.

Income, money, time, and obesity. In middle-income countries such as Brazil, South Africa and Thailand and low-income countries like India and China, the same general rule applies to middle-class people. Impoverished communities necessarily spend high proportions of their available income on food and drink. Depending on the relative resilience or fragility of their own food cultures, some still rely on traditional basic staple foods (such as rice, beans and cassava in Brazil), others increasingly turn to heavily promoted packaged convenience products whose main ingredients are processed starches, sugars or fats. These cost more than traditional staples, but are advertised as part of the good, active and healthy life and take little or no time to prepare.

'Fast food' – and also 'convenience food'. This means processed foods and drinks that are ready-to-eat or ready-to-heat, that characteristically are energy-dense, high in sugars, fats or salt. It does not refer to fruits or to dishes or foods low in energy and high in nutrients that can be consumed immediately or quickly. It can also be taken to refer to alcoholic as well as soft drinks. It may also refer to street food, when this is both served fast and is also energy-dense, fatty, sugary or salty, and relatively low in nutrients. Ready-to-eat food can be nourishing, varied and delicious. In London an example is the eat-in or eat-out chain Fresco Juices™, whose outlet in Westbourne Grove serves the best falafel I have ever tasted, and whose fresh carrot and beetroot juice plus ginger makes my heart zing. In Rio de Janeiro state the Queijão ('big cheese') chain of shops which include snack bars specialize in locally sourced produce, and their *empadas*, flaky pastry filled with chicken or shrimp, melt in the mouth. Patronize such places.

Junk food. This means foods and also drinks that are energy-dense and also low in or empty of nourishment other than calories. More specifically, junk food is foods and drinks that are high in added sugars or 'refined' starch or saturated fat, or salt, and also low in nutrients. Processed sugars, which contain nothing but energy, and most products mainly made with added sugar, are by this definition junk foods. 'Refined' starch, like white flour, is also pretty junky; most of the nutrients in the whole grain have been removed or greatly reduced. Likewise added processed fats. As a general rule the more processed any foods and drinks, the more junky they are. Nobody needs junk food, except in special circumstances when in urgent need of easily digested energy-dense food.

Economic and cultural globalization

Globalization in its modern form, accelerated by the electronic revolution, also creates new freedoms. The electronic revolution is at least as potent a force for communication of information and ideas to and from the common people as was print and the radio. Non-government organizations in the South, including those representing the interests of impoverished people, are now potentially much more potent because of the internet. The issue here is not globalization in general but economic and cultural globalization.

Structural readjustment. This is the system whereby countries already in debt to the World Bank, the International Monetary Fund and other lenders, receive further money and other aid only on condition that they reduce public spending and convert their internal economy in ways considered appropriate by the Washington-based international banks. Among other effects this tends to privatize public-health systems and so reduce independent advice on food and health. The best-informed critical account is by Nobel prize winner Joseph Stiglitz, also former World Bank chief economist.

Food industry concentration. This refers to the tendency for food and drink manufacture, distribution and sale to become concentrated in the hands of fewer and fewer increasingly giant and usually transnational companies with massive marketing and advertising budgets. In the 2000s, the total individual promotion spend of the largest companies, such as Nestlé, McDonald's and Coca-Cola, is up to or over $US1 billion (yes, billion) a year. This distorts the market and influences choice.

The dogma of individual supremacy

Information and education. One of the principles of public health is that citizens have a right to expect to be protected by governments, which in the case of food, drink and physical activity should include legal, fiscal and other formal policies and programmes that make healthy choices the easier choices. Authoritative guidelines are needed, but information and education by itself is ineffective.

References: books, reports

In alphabetical order of authors. Publishing details are usually of first edition.

Advisory Council for Applied Research and Development, *Report on the Food Industry and Technology.* London: HMSO, 1982.

Robin Blackburn. *The Making of New World Slavery. From the Baroque to the Modern, 1492–1800.* London: Verso, 1997.

Manuel Castells. *The Information Age. Economy, Society, and Culture.* 3 volumes. Second edition. Cambridge: University Press, 2000.

Michael Crawford, David Marsh. *The Driving Force.* London: Heinemann, 1989.

Food and Agriculture Organization of the United Nations. *Calorie Requirements.* Nutrition Studies 5 and 15. Washington DC: FAO, 1950; Rome: FAO, 1957.

Food and Agriculture Organization of the United Nations. *Globalization of Food Systems in Developing Countries: Impact on Food Security and Nutrition.* FAO Food and Nutrition Paper 83. Rome: FAO, 2004. Available at: www.fao.org.

Food and Agriculture Organization of the United Nations. *Human Energy Requirements.* Report of a joint FAO/WHO/UNU consultation. FAO: Food and nutrition technical report series 1. Rome: FAO, 2004. Available at: www.fao.org.

Michael Jacobson. *Liquid Candy. How Soft Drinks are Harming Americans' Health.* Washington DC: Center for Science in the Public Interest, 2006.

John Maynard Keynes. The international control of raw material prices, 1946. In: *Collected Writings,* vol XXVII. London: Macmillan, 1980.

Tim Lang, Michael Heasman. The food wars business. [Chapter 4] *Food Wars. The Global Battle for Minds, Mouths and Markets.* London: Earthscan, 2004.

Claus Leitzmann, Geoffrey Cannon (eds). The New Nutrition Science. *Public Health Nutrition* 2005; 8(6A): 667–804.

Donella Meadows, Jorgen Randers, Dennis Meadows. *Limits to Growth. The 30-Year Update.* White River Junction, VT: Chelsea Green Publishing, 2004.

Sidney Mintz. *Sugar and Power. The Place of Sugar in Modern History.* London: Viking Penguin, 1985.

Marion Nestle. *Food Politics. How the Food Industry Influences Nutrition and Health.* Berkeley CA: University of California Press, 2002.

Oxfam. *Rigged Rules and Double Standards. Trade, Globalization, and the Fight Against Poverty.* Oxford: Oxfam, 2002. Available at: www.maketradefair.com.

Michael Pollan. Corn, and The consumer: a republic of fat. [Chapters 1 and 6]. *The Omnivore's Dilemma. The Search for a Perfect Meal in a Fast-Food World.* London: Bloomsbury, 2006.

Mark Prendergrast. *For God, Country & Coca-Cola. The Definitive History of the Great American Soft Drink and the Company That Makes It.* New York: Basic Books, 1993.

Eric Schlosser. *Fast Food Nation. What the All-American Meal is Doing to the World.* Boston MA: Houghton Mifflin, 1991.

Amartya Sen. *Development as Freedom.* New York: Basic Books, 1999.

Adam Smith. *An Inquiry into the Nature and Causes of the Wealth of Nations.* London: Strahan, 1776.

Joseph Stiglitz. *Globalization and its Discontents.* London: Allen Lane, 2002.

UK Government Office for Science. Foresight. *Tackling Obesities.* Released 18 October 2007. See also www.foresight.gov.uk.

UK House of Commons Health Committee. *Obesity.* Third report of Session 2003–04. London: The Stationery Office, 2004.

US Department of Health and Human Services. Office on women's health. *Breastfeeding.*

HHS blueprint for action on breastfeeding. Washington DC: USDHHS, 2000.

US Institute of Medicine. Health, diet, and eating patterns of children and youth [Chapter 2]. *Food Marketing to Children and Youth: Threat or Opportunity?* Washington DC: National Academies Press, 2006. Available at: www.iom.edu.

John Vidal. *McLibel. Burger Culture on Trial.* London: Macmillan, 1997. See also www. mcspotlight.org.

Mathis Wackernagel and William Rees. *Our Ecological Footprint: Measuring Human Impact On the Earth.* Gabriela Island BC: New Society Publishing, 1996. See also www. footprintnetwork.org.

Walter Willett. Surprising news about fat. [Chapter 4]. *Eat, Drink, and be Healthy.* New York: Free Press, 2001.

World Cancer Research Fund/American Institute for Cancer Research. *Food, Nutrition, Physical Activity and the Prevention of Cancer: a Global Perspective.* Washington DC: AICR, 2007.

World Health Organization. *Obesity: Preventing and Managing the Global Epidemic.* Report of a WHO consultation. Technical report series 894. Geneva: WHO, 2000.

World Health Organization. *Globalization, Diets, and Non-Communicable Diseases.* Geneva: WHO, 2003.

World Health Organization. *Diet, Nutrition and the Prevention of Chronic Diseases.* Report of a joint WHO/FAO expert consultation. Technical report series 916. Geneva: WHO, 2003.

World Health Organization/United Nations Children's Fund. *Global strategy for infant and young child feeding.* Geneva: WHO, 2004.

References: papers, articles

In alphabetical order of authors:

Anon. Argentina, Brazil join WTO complaints against US corn subsidies. *New York Herald Tribune Business,* 22 January 2007.

Aykroyd W. Sugars in history. In: Sipple H, McNutt K. *Sugars in Nutrition.* Published for the Nutrition Foundation by New York: Academic Press, 1974.

Blair T. Healthy living. Second lecture in series 'Our nation's future'. Accessible at www.number-10.gov.uk.

De Onis M, Garza C, Victora C, Bhan M, Norum K. The WHO Multicentre Growth Reference Study: rationale, planning and implementation. *Food and Nutrition Bulletin* 2004; 25: S1–S89.

Englyst K, Englyst H. Carbohydrate bioavailability. British Journal of Nutrition 2005; 94: 1–11.

Fang C, Beghin J. Urban household oil and fats demand in China: evidence from household survey data. *Journal of Comparative Economics* 2002; 30(4): 732–53.

Fischler C. The 'McDonaldization' of Culture. [Chapter 40]. In: Flandrin J-L, Montanari M (eds). *Food: A Culinary History.* New York: Penguin, 2000. Originally published in Italian. 1996.

Food and Agriculture Organization of the United Nations. *Food Outlook 2007: Global Market Analysis,* Rome: FAO, November 2007. www. fao.org/docrep/010/ah876e/ah876e07.htm.

Goody J. Industrial food. Towards the development of a world cuisine. In: Counihan C, Van Esterik P (eds). *Food and Culture.* London: Routledge, 1997.

Highfield R. Scientists find the gene that makes you fat. *Daily Telegraph*, 13 April 2007.

Kleinman M. We'll have a Big Mac, fries and a green pea pie. *Daily Telegraph*, 24 November 2006.

McMichael A J, Powles J, Butler C, Uauy R. Food, livestock production, energy, climate change. *Lancet* 2007; 370: 1253-63.

Meade B, Rosen S. Income and diet differences greatly affect food spending around the globe. *International Market Trends* September–October 1996: 39-44.

Monteiro C, Conde W, Popkin B. The burden of disease from undernutrition and overnutrition in countries undergoing rapid nutrition transition: a view from Brazil. *American Journal of Public Health* 2004; 94 (3): 433-4.

Popkin B, Horton S, Kim S. The nutrition transition and prevention of diet-related diseases in Asia and the Pacific. *Food and Nutrition Bulletin* 2001; 22(4) (suppl): 1-58.

Sample I. Gene map will lift lid on diseases. *Guardian*, 23 January 2008.

Schwartz P, Ogilvy J. *The emergent paradigm: changing patterns of thought and belief.* Values and Lifestyles Program. VALS report 7. Menlo Park, CA: SRI International, April 1979.

Singhal A, Lucas A. Early origins of cardiovascular disease; is there a unifying hypothesis. *Lancet* 2004; 363: 1642 -5.

Sobal J, Khan L, Bisogni C. A conceptual model of the food and nutrition system. *Social Science Medicine* 1998; 47(7): 853-63.

Sweney M. Plan for junk food ad ban dropped. *Guardian*, 22 January 2008.

US Department of Agriculture. The influence of income on globalized food spending. Washington DC: USDA Economic Research Service. *Agricultural Outlook*, July 1997: 14-17.

US Department of Agriculture. Percent of income spent on food in the US. Washington DC: USDA Economic Research Service, 2007. Obtainable at: www.ers.usda.gov.

Ward L. Life through a lens. How Britain's children eat, sleep and breathe TV. *Guardian*, 15 January 2008.

Watts J. China's rise in wealth brings fall in health. *Guardian*, 21 September 2004.

Wretlind A. Nutrition problems in healthy adults with low activity and low caloric consumption. In: Blix G (ed). *Nutrition and Physical Activity*. Symposia of the Swedish Nutrition Foundation V. Uppsala: Almqvist and Wiksells, 1967.

5. THE PLACE OF FOOD IN OUR WORLD

Notes: epigraphs

The gastronome Mary Francis Kennedy Fisher (1908–92) writes about food and drink as central to the good life, with flair and passion. This passage is taken from *The Gastronomical Me*. She is also the classic translator of Jean Anthelme Brillat-Savarin.

The writer Michael Pollan (1955–) also says: 'Eating is an agricultural act . . . it is also an ecological act, and a political act too.' In *The Omnivore's Dilemma* he examines three food systems, industrial, organic, and hunter, the last requiring him to shoot a wild pig.

Notes: main text

The real value of food

Cooking and cookbooks. Book publishers do a roaring trade in cookbooks as well as dieting books. This may suggest a general revival in cooking and the origins of food. For some readers, who use cookbooks, it does. For most buyers and for people who have cookbooks bought for them as presents, these often beautiful productions are more for show. Where are they kept and what state are they in? Do you find them in the kitchen, well thumbed and interleaved with markers and notes of home variations? Books like those used by my beloved stepmother Elise, who when I was adolescent nourished me with delicious dishes of hearts, livers, kidneys and other parts of animals now ground into chow for dogs and cats? Or do you find them in the living room, stacked with books on art? I rest my case.

The best things in life

Free-range and battery eggs. The German philosopher Klaus Meyer-Abich writes of the 'visible meal', which is what we see, and the 'invisible meal', which includes where the food comes from. 'The visible meal may be vegetables and fish or meat; the invisible meal may be cruelty to animals in factory farming or fairness in organic farming; selfish interests or corporate social responsibility in food business, and so on.' He continues: 'Does this excellently prepared fish still taste good when we remind ourselves that it was taken from a poor country which was not adequately compensated for it? Moreover, the fish may have been caught by over-fishing.' People are becoming increasingly conscious of such issues. It is not only battery eggs that are distasteful.

The theologian Leonardo Boff (1938–) is one of the courageous Catholic priests who created 'liberation theology' which, in the name of Jesus and the New Testament gospels, champions the rights of dispossessed landless communities in Brazil. Forced out of the priesthood on instructions from Rome, he continues to teach and write.

Our privileges and choices

Comparison of gatherer-hunter, peasant-agricultural, and industrial-urban ways of life. This also does not mean that gatherer-hunter, pastoral, and peasant-agricultural communities will be better off if they live like us. For a start, they do not: now they usually lose what they have, and often live in misery. As customers and consumers we can make choices that protect the livelihoods of people who do not live in cities.

Food security. In settled gatherer-hunter, pastoral, and peasant-agricultural societies, food supplies originally were usually secure, if only because this was the first purpose of these societies, whose populations fluctuated with circumstances. The first European arrivals in the Americas consistently remarked on the rich variety of food cultivated and enjoyed by the native peoples. The fruit and nut trees still abundant in the Amazon rainforest are probably wild versions of orchards cultivated by riverine communities who were massacred by the Europeans or else retreated into the forest fastnesses. In the USA the Thanksgiving feast is an adaptation of the foods shown and given to early English settlers by the natives. Black Hawk, chief of the Souk and Fox, said: 'We always had plenty, our children never cried from hunger, neither were our people in want. The rapids of Rock River furnished us with an abundance of excellent fish, and the land being very fertile never failed to produce good crops of corn, beans, pumpkins and squashes.' Speaking then of the time after the Europeans came, he said: 'If a prophet had come to our village in those days and told us that the things were to take place which have since come to pass, none of our people would have believed him.' Food insecurity is usually a consequence of oppression. But now there are few populations untouched by industrialization.

Supermarkets. Some friends and colleagues with whom I have discussed this book and its themes think I should not consume food from supermarkets, or at least that I should feel bad for doing so. People who avoid supermarkets for ethical reasons including solidarity with small producers, and concern about 'food miles' and the waste of resources caused by long-distance travel of food, deserve respect. My view is as follows. My first responsibility in writing this book is to readers who want to improve their health and enhance their wellbeing. Yes, as I say in

this and the next chapter, in the full sense health has social and environmental and above all ethical dimensions, and yes, conscious consumers shop in sympathy with the makers of food, and in awareness of environmental impacts. Yes, buying cash crops whose producers are paid outrageously small amounts of money and who are not able to grow food for their own families is ethically problematic. Yes, powerful supermarket chains are notorious for driving small traders out of business and for pauperizing farmers. But I think it is a better choice to engage. As a consumer you can do this by preferring produce that is local and fairly traded and by telling your supermarket manager that this is what you do. As a citizen you can help to make supermarket chains more socially and environmentally responsible. The environmental movement teaches us that simply demonizing or rejecting big business does not work and if anything creates more problems. But these are not clear-cut issues. You will make your own decisions and choices. One bottom line is that supermarkets stock plenty of fresh and benignly processed foods, including some that are locally sourced. Seek these out.

The bigger picture

Ecological footprint. This is based on calculations of the energy cost of your housing, transport, food and drink, fed into a computer program that calculates the number of acres of the world's resources you consume in a year. That's the size of your ecological footprint. The program then multiplies this up by the number of the world's population.

Amplifying the possible. José Serra was the unsuccessful centre-right candidate for the presidency of Brazil in the election of 2002 won by the workers' party candidate (known everywhere in Brazil as 'Lula'). Like many senior Brazilian politicians, José Serra has a background as a socialist and a courageous opponent of the mid-1960s to mid-1980s Brazilian military dictatorship.

The power of the USA within the UN system. Diplomacy is a sophisticated version of horse-trading. For example, Brazil wants to be a member of the UN Security Council. If the USA had felt strongly that the baby formula and food industry must not be impeded, word could have gone from the US State Department to the Brazilian foreign ministry that if Brazil abandoned its resolution on infant and young-child feeding, its larger ambition would be supported by the USA. For all I know such a hint was dropped. Most of what goes on in international and national politics is 'behind the curtain'.

A vision for this century

The Giessen Declaration. In April 2005 a group of 23 scientists and other experts met at Giessen in Germany, with the aim of integrating the four dimensions of nutrition and food policy – biological, economic, social, environmental – in effect to make new maps. As a result the New Nutrition Science project has been established, initially to re-create nutrition science according to new principles. See Annex 1.

Our whole lives

Sources of urban wealth, and the monuments of empires. Once I asked a Brazilian friend if, when admiring splendid London buildings of the 17th to 19th centuries, she was aware that they were built with treasure looted from Asia, Africa and Latin America, including profits of the Brazilian sugar trade that depended on slave labour and that perverted Britain's food systems. She politely said that yes, she knew. Conscious people from Asia, Africa and Latin America are well aware that the sources of the wealth of Europe and North America are their own countries.

References: books, reports

In alphabetical order of authors. Publishing details are usually of first edition.

Geoffrey Cannon, Claus Leitzmann (eds). *The New Nutrition Science.* Cambridge: Blackwell, 2009 (in preparation when this book was first published).

Geoffrey Cannon. *The Fate of Nations. Food and Nutrition Policy in the New World.* London: Caroline Walker Trust, 2003. Obtainable from www.cwt.co.uk.

Michael Crawford, David Marsh. *The Driving Force.* London: Heinemann, 1989.

Elizabeth David. *An Omelette and a Glass of Wine.* London: Robert Hale, 1984.

M F K Fisher. *The Gastronomical Me.* New York: Farrar, Straus, Giroux (South Point Press), 1989. First published 1943.

Susan George. *Ill Fares the Land.* London: Penguin, 1990. First published 1984.

International Food Policy Research Institute. *The World Food Situation: New Driving Forces and Required Actions.* Washington DC: IFPRI, 2008.

John Maynard Keynes. The international control of raw material prices, 1946. In: Keynes J M. *Collected Writings,* vol XXVII. London: Macmillan, 1980.

Claus Leitzmann, Geoffrey Cannon. The New Nutrition Science. *Public Health Nutrition* 2005; 6(A): 667–804.

John Boyd Orr. *Food Health and Income. A Survey of Adequacy of Diet in Relation to Income.* London: Macmillan, 1936, 1937.

Michael Pollan. *The Omnivore's Dilemma. The Search for a Perfect Meal in a Fast-Food World*. London: Bloomsbury, 2006.

Colin Tudge. *So Shall We Reap*. London: Allen Lane, 2003.

Colin Tudge. *Feeding People is Easy*. Pari Publishing. Pari, Italy, 2007.

UK Government Office of Science. Foresight. *Tackling Obesities: Future Choice. Trends and Directions of Obesity*. London: Stationery Office, 2007. Obtainable at: www.foresight.gov.uk.

US Department of Health and Human Services. *Blueprint for action on breastfeeding*. Washington DC: DHHS, 2000. Also see www.4women.gov, and www.cdc.gov. breastfeeding.

Mathis Wackernagel, William Rees. *Our Ecological Footprint. Reducing Human Impact on the Earth*. Gabriola Island BC, Canada: New Society Press, 1996. See also www. globalfootprint.org.

World Bank. *Making Sustainable Commitments: An Environmental Strategy for the World Bank*. Washington DC: World Bank, 2001.

World Health Organization/ United Nations Children's Fund. *Global Strategy on Infant and Young Child Feeding*. Geneva: WHO, 2004.

World Wide Fund for Nature. *Ecological Footprints. A Guide for Local Authorities*. WWF UK, 2002.

References: papers, features

In alphabetical order of authors:

The Giessen Declaration. *Public Health Nutrition* 2005; 6(A): 783-6.

Kemp K. Food – and how it's going to change the world. *Sunday Herald* (Scotland), 10 January 2008.

Li D, Premier R. Cuisine: Hangzhou foods and their role in community health and nutrition. *Asia Pacific Journal of Clinical Nutrition* 2004; 13(2): 141-6.

MacLennan R, Zheng A. Cuisine: the concept and its health and nutrition implications – global. *Asia Pacific Journal of Clinical Nutrition* 2004; 13(2): 131-9.

McMichael A J, Powles J, Butler C, Uauy R. Food, livestock production, energy, climate change. *Lancet* 2007; 370: 1253-63.

Meyer-Abich A. Human health in nature – towards a holistic philosophy of nutrition. *Public Health Nutrition 2005*; 8(6A): 738-42.

World Health Organization. Infant and young child nutrition. Draft resolution prepared by the delegation of Brazil. A53/A/ Conf.Paper no 3, 17 May 2000.

World Health Organization. Global strategy for infant and young child feeding. Report by the Secretariat. Executive Board 107 session, provisional agenda item 3.1.eB107/3. 15 December 2000.

World Health Organization. The optimum duration of exclusive breastfeeding. Results of a WHO systematic review. Note for the press. Geneva: WHO, 2001.

World Rainforest Movement. Thailand: uncertain future for the world no 1 exporter. Available at: www.wrm.org.uy/bulletin/51/ Thailand.html.

Yamey G. Baby food industry lobbies WHO on breast feeding advice. *British Medical Journal* 2000; 321: 591.

6. YOUR SEVEN GOLDEN RULES

Notes: epigraphs

The playwright George Bernard Shaw (1856–1950) was also a leading socialist. Vigorous into his 90s, he was a champion of public sanitation, personal hygiene, plain speaking, and diets without meat. The quotation is from *Man and Superman*, Act I.

The philosopher Marie Jean, Marquis de Condorcet (1743–94) believed that the solution to rising population was birth control. He said: 'The time will come when the sun will shine only upon a world of free men.' He was arrested for his opinions and died in prison.

Notes: introductory text

Principles. What's behind the principles is as follows. First, the issue is not food and drink, so much as what is done to foods and drinks before we consume them. The issue is methods of production and processing. But this does not mean that processing is intrinsically bad. Such an idea makes no sense. There are benign, harmless, and malign forms of processing. Second, while quantification has value, what's most valuable is the quality of food and drink. As a general rule, the fresher foods and drinks are, the higher their quality. Third, for people living where food systems are industrialized, the way to good health and wellbeing is to increase the weight and bulk of foods and drinks consumed; to become physically active; and to reduce the energy-density of diets. This means avoiding foods and drinks processed with added 'refined' starches, sugars, fats and chemicals, including most 'convenience' and 'fast' foods and drinks as defined in chapter 4.

Hunger, appetite, satiety, desire, craving, addiction. If you consume a substantial amount of highly processed foods and drinks, it is likely that your normal sense of hunger (for food in general) and appetite (for specific foods) has become confused. This is almost inevitable. Your desire for various processed foods and drinks will be provoked by their fat or sugar content, or else by chemical cocktails formulated by food scientists whose job is to make processed foods more desirable, and you will find it increasingly difficult to sense when you are satisfied. Any food or drink that is not just desired but craved is likely to be over-consumed. This also explains some of the thinking behind these golden rules. The best way to dissolve cravings for and addictions to processed foods and drinks is to consume lots of fresh foods and drinks which, being whole or benignly processed, may be delicious but are never craved, strengthen your body's systems, and restore natural appetite. See also chapters 3 and 4.

Quantities of foods and drinks. Golden rules 1, 3 and 4 specify weights of foods and drinks. Here is the explanation. Sedentary people are in artificially low energy balance – which is why they are liable to become overweight and obese. Industrial food systems, because of their use of added sugars and fats, are more energy-dense – which is why people who consume industrialized diets are liable to become overweight and obese. Most sedentary people now consume industrial-type diets, hence the world epidemic of overweight and obesity. Again, the way out of this trap is to become physically active and to enjoy diets high in nourishment and relatively low in energy. Industrialized diets deliver around 160 calories (675 kilojoules) per 100 grams. It follows that a sedentary woman in energy balance at say 1,750 calories (7,350 kilojoules) a day, will gain weight if she consumes significantly more than 1 kilogram of industrialized-type food a day.

Healthy diets as indicated by the World Health Organization average around 125 calories (525 kilocalories) per 100 grams a day. Following the golden rules in this chapter will probably bring the overall energy density of the diet down to closer to 100 calories (420 kilojoules) per 100 grams, because of the large amounts of vegetables and fruits specified, but also it depends on what other foods and drinks you consume. An active woman on energy balance at 2,250 calories (9,500 kilojoules) a day, enjoying a healthy diet averaging say 125 calories (525 kilojoules) per 100 grams, can consume close to 2 kilograms of food a day without gaining weight. This is the rough average weight of food human females are evolved to consume, varying of course according to size and age. Amounts for men average about 20 per cent higher.

Golden rule 1

Robert McCarrison (1878-1960) became the first director of nutrition research in India until his retirement in 1935. His work is now continued in India at the National Institute of Nutrition in Hyderabad. Like his British contemporaries John Boyd Orr and Jack Drummond, he had a broad view of nutrition and dietetics. With them he played a part in the UK 1939-45 wartime food policy, at which time the nation remained well fed and there was a decrease in the rates of disease of which bad diets are an important cause.

Golden rule 2

Moderate and vigorous physical activity. There is no clear dividing line between any intensity of physical activity. Strolling uses more energy than standing, which uses more energy than sitting, which uses more energy than lying down. The more you are on your feet the better. Strolling is not moderate physical activity: the test is that you are breathing faster and can feel the effect. The test of vigorous physical activity is often taken to be around 80 per cent of your maximum heart rate, which is reckoned as 220 beats a minute minus your age. Thus if you are 40 your maximum heart rate is around 180, of which 80 per cent is 144 beats a minute. If you are 60 your maximum rate is around 160, of which 80 per cent is 128 beats a minute. This is also known as '80% VO$_2$Max', meaning 80 per cent of maximum oxygen uptake. As you become more fit, your heart rate at rest and during physical activity will drop, and the time it takes for your heart rate to return to its resting rate after exercise will also drop. Blood pressure is also very likely to drop.

The 10,000 steps a day. This helpful guideline is also recommended by Barbara Rolls. Amanda Sainsbury-Salis (see chapter 2) recommends 8,000-12,000 steps a day. At first it's a good idea to count your steps and also to time them. Thereafter the simplest check is time. If you want to use a pedometer go ahead, but I think this is too fussy, unless maybe you are accumulating your physical activity in a lot of short sessions, or just like to know this kind of detail. The more of these steps are in the form of vigorous activity the better.

The 500 calorie a day guideline. An hour of moderate physical activity will use around an extra 250-350 calories (about 1,050-1,450 kilojoules) a day, depending on whether you are a woman or a man, on how big you are, and on how energetic you are. An hour and a half of moderate physical activity, or an hour more than half of which is vigorous physical activity, will use around an extra 400-600 calories (roughly 1,650-2,500 kilojoules) a day. If you are physically active at such levels not every day but five days a week, this evidently does not add up to an average 500 calories a day. The additional energetic expenditure comes from the 'training effect' once you are fit and are regularly vigorously active. This keeps your lean tissue metabolically active when you are exercising, and afterwards as well. In the USA Amish communities, whose ways of life exclude cars and much 20th-century technology, and who walk a lot, are in energy balance 400-600 calories a day higher than typical sedentary people in the USA. I am grateful to James Hill of the Colorado School of Medicine for pointing this out. Also see the next note.

Recommended physical activity. This corresponds with calculations made by Peter Wood and colleagues at Stanford University. They have compared the energy intake of men and women aged 35-59 jogging or running 35-40 miles a week (a higher level of physical activity than specified here) with the energy intake of an equal number of sedentary people. The active groups were leaner and lighter than the sedentary groups. But the active groups were consuming a lot more. The active men were turning over 2,959 calories (12,368 kilojoules) a day, compared with 2,361 (9,869) for the sedentary men. The active women were turning over 2,386 calories (9,973 kilojoules) a day, compared with 1,817 (7,595) for the sedentary women. But although the active women were consuming more energy than the sedentary men, they were a lot slimmer and lighter. There is nothing odd about this. Muscle, being designed to work, is more metabolically active than body fat – much more so when people are active on a daily basis. People who remain fit by continuing to be physically active get into higher energy balance, and so can consume more food and drink without gaining weight. The amounts recommended here are also similar to those found to be most protective against chronic diseases and most likely to prolong active life in the classic work done by Ralph Paffen-

barger in the USA and Jerry Morris in the UK, and by Steven Blair, Roy Shephard and others. Lower levels of only moderate physical activity also improve health, but to a lesser extent.

Physical activity levels. These, abbreviated as PALs, are a measure of how active you are. Basal metabolic rate (BMR), which measures energy used simply being alive, can be taken to be 1.0. A bedridden person has a PAL of about 1.2. Most sedentary people are on around PAL 1.40-1.50 or maybe a bit more. Following this rule will increase the PAL of basically sedentary people to above PAL 1.70, the level recommended in a number of expert reports.

Golden rule 3

Changed, or modified, in benign ways. This is not a ringing phrase but I can't think of a better one. The alternatives, of 'lightly processed' or 'minimally processed', often used in books and reports, are not satisfactory. Both these phrases suggest that totally unprocessed whole food is best, and this is a meaningless notion. Both focus on processing in the sense of methods used by food manufacturers, whereas methods of production (including breeding), preservation, and preparation (including cooking) are just as important. Both imply that no method of changing or modifying food from its original state – whatever this may be taken to mean – can improve its nutritional quality, and this is not so. There are many examples. Fermentation, used to modify many foods including vegetables, pulses (legumes) and fruits, and drinks, and to create others like yoghurt, can positively improve their nutritional quality. Bacteria introduced in the fermentation of cabbage to make sauerkraut enhances its content of beneficial bioactive substances. Also some nutrients become more bio-available in processed foods, the quantity of lycopene in canned and cooked tomatoes compared with fresh tomatoes being a well-known example.

Bottled and canned vegetables, pulses (legumes) and fruits. Are these really benign methods? It depends. When I am travelling and economizing, I buy spinach and beans canned in water and eat them in my hotel room, with fresh salad vegetables and fruits. Bottled or canned fruits are less good choices, because these often include sugar as a preservative and sweetener, and this migrates into the fruit; besides, fruits are always available in whole form. Use common sense. If you buy and store bottled and canned food, as my family does, avoid products using substantial amounts of added sugar, salt, or unspecified oil, and drain the liquid.

Nuts and seeds, and plant oils. Sure you should enjoy nuts and seeds: they are rich in many vitamins and minerals, and in essential fats. And sure, add the plant oils you find most delicious, and don't get too concerned about their fatty acid profiles. If you prefer (extra-virgin) olive oil, fine. If you like nut oils, enjoy these. A tip from cook and dietitian Gerry Kasten of Vancouver: prefer oils with a relatively short shelf life, keep the bottles in a cool dark place, and decant them into small bottles before use. If, like me and other enthusiasts for African-influenced Brazilian cuisine, you are crazy for the flavours of coconut and other palm oils, especially delicious used with fish dishes, enjoy. But don't count these when following this rule.

Balance between vegetables, fruits and pulses (legumes). Many dieting books, and also 'eat for health' books, get prescriptive and detailed about relative amounts of raw versus cooked vegetables, or about types of vegetable (green leafy, cruciferous, allium, etc.), or proportions as between vegetables, fruits and pulses (legumes). Good advice is to enjoy

a wide variety and all sorts of colours, and to experiment.

Methods of preservation, processing, and preparation. Most of the problematic and even malign methods such as salting, salt-pickling, smoking, 'refining', use of chemical additives, hydrogenation, hydrolysation, frying, and use of direct flame, apply mostly to animal foods. Also see chapter 4 and golden rule 4.

Nourishment. If you avoid animal foods that's fine, as long as you prefer whole, fresh plant foods. The diets of wholefood vegans, who consume wholegrain and minimally processed cereals (grains) as well as fresh vegetables, pulses (legumes) and fruits, but no foods of animal origin – meaning, no milk and other dairy products, or eggs – are not lacking in any known nutrients, with the probable exception of vitamin B_{12}. However, this rule is not advocating veganism, nor for that matter vegetarianism.

Smoothies. Yes, I know that it's nutritionally better to eat fruits whole and to munch their dietary fibre rather than have the blades of a machine do this for you. But liquidized to the consistency of yoghurt, mixtures of fruits, together with added goodies like ginger and cinnamon, are much, much more delicious. Nor have I noticed any energy switchback effects.

Safety. Some fungi are poisonous; you need to soak red kidney beans before cooking; peanuts could possibly be contaminated with aflatoxins; and so forth and so on. 'Safe' does not mean always totally and completely safe. Nothing worthwhile in life is absolutely safe.

Golden rule 4

Methods of cooking. In general, and as with other food processes, the 'lighter' the method of cooking, the better. Frying adds fat and so increases the energy-density of food. Cooking in direct flame creates substances known to be carcinogenic when tested on animals. The re-use of cooking fat also creates carcinogens. You certainly should not eat burned or charred food. Many people think microwaving is a good choice; my hunch is that one day it will turn out to be a bad choice.

Plant and animal foods. Most conventional nutrition teaching is heavily biased in favour of foods of animal origin, for example claiming the supremacy or essentiality of cow's milk, meat and eggs for children, and animal foods in general as superior sources of vitamin A. Such ideas are wrong. It is also wrong to teach the nutritional superiority of radical vegetarian diets. A vegan diet can be constructed from sandwiches of white bread, margarine and sugar, and sugared soft drinks and gin. Industrialized food systems are distorted in favour of foods of animal origin, but the main issue with all foods is the nature, type and degree of processing.

Meat, poultry, fish and animal food in general. My own position is identical with that of Colin Tudge: enjoy meat, fish, seafood, and other animal foods, respectfully and sparingly.

Milk (meaning, cow's milk). Together with eggs (usually meaning hen's eggs) milk has been seen as almost an ideal food, especially for children. It is a better choice than sugared soft drinks for sure, but otherwise in general I disagree. There is a lot of politics involved in the promotion of milk and dairy products, and their inclusion as one of the basic food groups. They are pushed in countries that tend to have dairy surpluses, and when exported, for example in the form of dried milk, disrupt traditional food systems. Claims that the calcium in milk and dairy products is needed to guard against brittle bone

disease are implausible: such diseases are rare in parts of the world where active people consume little if any such foods, besides which other foods are good sources of calcium. My advice is to consume foods and drinks derived from cattle sparingly.

Industrially produced animal food. This is a difficult issue. At least, I find it difficult. Clearly, the ways in which animals are treated when factory farmed is abominable, dangerous in their effects and potential effects on human health, and also environmentally outrageous as well as unsustainable. See the work of Tony McMichael, Michael Pollan, Orville Schell and Eric Schlosser, as well as that of Peter Singer. If you do not accept that industrially produced animal food can be 'fresh', or have decided not to consume it anyway, I support you. But my decision here is not to go that far: rather it is to give everybody who is following these rules time to become more conscious of the issues and of how they want to respond. In answer to your question, yes I do eat some industrially produced animal food. Not much, and whenever I think about this I feel uneasy.

Animal foods and disease. Targeting relatively whole and fresh forms of animal food as major causes of heart disease in particular has proved to be a mistake; and the evidence that foods high in dietary cholesterol are a problem only for this reason is now generally agreed to be shaky. Avoid processed foods that are high in animal fats, saturated fats, and trans-fatty acids, and also in 'refined' starches, added sugars, and cosmetic and other chemical additives.

Golden rule 5

Nutrition science and feasting. Why do experts on food, nutrition and health have practically nothing to say about feasting? You might think from this that they are a glum lot, but that's not my experience. International nutrition science conferences are replete with magnificent buffets, private dinners and receptions, and usually include a gala banquet or two. It's just that feasting seems not to enter into nutrition scientists' professional thinking. This is odd, and I think also a pity, because the omission seems puritanical. Is there some kind of turf agreement as a result of which food culture and the social enjoyment of food is agreed to be off-limits for scientists? Occasionally I have read the work of behavioural scientists whose speciality is food, and they too give a puritanical impression; I can't remember papers on feasting, but I have read plenty on the dread effects of gorging and bingeing, and anorexia-bulimia cycling. Maybe enjoying ourselves, being hard to quantify, is therefore not thought to be scientific.

Food writers and feasting. For the social and cultural joys of feasting, rely on food writers, and some social scientists and anthropologists. Once in London I helped to organize a joint meeting of the Nutrition Society and the Guild of Food Writers on Mediterranean food, which culminated in a splendid supper created by Prue Leith's team, served in the marquee restaurant then overlooking the Serpentine in London's Hyde Park. We all were I think nourished at least as much by the feast in good company as we were by the research papers presented during the day.

Golden rule 6

Radical fasting. After you have followed the seven (or six) golden rules, including abstinence from some foods and drinks, and observed the effects, and become interested, I recommend regular fruit-only fasts or water-only fasts. For the first two or three days you are likely to be ravenous. But then the body gets the message of no food, and

thereafter you are not hungry. This alone is a very interesting experience. Thereafter you are likely to become super-aware of your sensations and observations and not to be interested in or even to notice food. A normally nourished person can stay with water-only fasting for more than a month, and the books say that the body signals need for food with a return of appetite. My own limit so far has been a couple of weeks, but this was simply because part of the discipline of fasting is to decide in advance when to break the fast, and to stay with that decision. I did not feel any need to stop. Consult your physician or relevantly qualified professional before starting a radical fast, but if you are in ordinary good health don't be put off. I also suggest that you try a week's fast, because radical fasts are most interesting after you stop feeling hungry and get through feeling tired. Then your body gets the message. Please remember though that radical fasting will not result in reduction of weight. This will rebound after the fast has ended.

Golden rule 7

Energy density. The idea of 'energy density' applied to food and drink is not new, but fairly recently has become rightly seen as vital for health and wellbeing and also weight reduction. This is because of the rapid rise in sugary and fatty processed foods and drinks, including convenience, fast, and junk foods and drinks; the parallel rapid rise of weight increase, overweight, and obesity; and the work above all of Barbara Rolls. Her *Volumetrics Eating Plan* includes long lists of the energy density of foods, and if you want a lot of detail is the best source.

Energy density and drinks. It is sometimes said that while many foods are energy-dense, drinks are not, on the grounds that drinks are mostly water and therefore, in terms of weight, deliver less energy than almost all foods. Sweetened drinks, for example, contain 35-40 calories per 100 millilitres, which is roughly the same as most vegetables. In my opinion this reasoning is piffle. The concept of energy density should be applied separately to the main types of food, and also to drinks.

Quality. Scientists avoid concepts like 'quality' that can't be measured – unless these are reduced to a measurable definition. So what is quality? In *Zen and the Art of Motorcycle Maintenance* Robert Pirsig says: 'Quality. You know what it is, yet you don't know what it is … when you try to say what the quality is, apart from the things that have it, it all goes poof! … Obviously some things are better than others, but what's the *betterness*?' A book waits to be written on the quality of foods and drinks. Meanwhile, following Robert Pirsig's 'you know what it is' … Chocolate with a higher cocoa content is higher quality – suggesting that quality is to do with being more genuine. The flesh of free-range chicken is higher quality than that of battery chicken – suggesting that quality is to do with the animal's way of life and also nutritional content. Fruits fresh from the tree or bush are higher quality than fruits that have been treated to survive international travel – suggesting that quality is to do with a sense of communion with the earth, and also sensory delight. Single malt whisky is higher quality than blended whisky – suggesting that quality is to do with care and skill in the making. And so on.

Processed foods making health claims. It may seem odd to avoid processed foods and drinks that make health claims. The first reason is that this rule recommends fresh foods. The second reason is – sorry to say – that many if not most health claims, while legal and indeed usually approved by regulatory authorities, and even endorsed by health organizations, are deceptive. Prod-

ucts 'fortified' with vitamins and minerals are often basically junky. Products relatively low in fat are often either still fatty, or relatively high in sugar – and so on. A tip is to notice what the products are not making health claims about. Michael Pollan recommends total avoidance of all processed foods making health claims; I think this is too stringent.

Alcoholic drinks. Remember the 'drinking man's diets' mentioned in chapter 2? How come that Luigi Cornaro, Jean Anthelme Brillat-Savarin and William Banting – who from self-experiment and observation knew as much as anybody about the effect of foods and drinks on body weight in those days before physicians and researchers got in on the act – include substantial amounts of alcoholic drinks in their prescriptions to live long, shed weight, and be healthy? Here is a clue. Brillat-Savarin says 'shun beer as if it were the plague'. Banting identifies beer (and also milk, sugar and butter) as 'insidious enemies'. Cornaro, being Italian, drank only wine. Nutrition students, and dieters, learn that carbohydrates and protein supply roughly 4 calories per gram, whereas fat weighs in at 9 calories and alcohol at 7 calories a gram. So obviously people who want to shed weight should cut down dietary fat and cut out alcohol. So you might think. However, as you now know from chapter 3, a calorie is not a calorie, if this means that all nutrients are metabolized equivalently according to their energy value. Sure, alcohol is a concentrated source of energy. Indeed, heavy drinkers are liable to crash cars, punch friends, talk rot, lose jobs, go nuts, die young, and also are more likely to develop various serious diseases. Absolutely alcohol is often addictive. But of themselves it may be only those alcoholic drinks that also contain sugar that make you fat. Here's the story. The body cannot store alcohol. Light to moderate drinkers usually consume alcohol as well as a full amount of food and other drink. As the word *aperitif* indicates, alcohol stimulates appetite, and so people who consume alcoholic drinks *as well as* full diets are liable to gain extra weight. But people who consume alcohol *instead of* food and other drinks shed weight. This has been known for over 30 years. So following the rules here and also consuming moderate amounts of some alcoholic drinks *instead of* significant amounts of sugary or fatty foods may actually help weight control. That's the theory, which as far as I know has not been tested recently. Check it out for yourself, if you like alcoholic drinks and are a moderate drinker.

References: books, reports

In alphabetical order of authors. Publishing details are usually of first edition. Also see the references for chapters 2–5.

Harry Benjamin. The methods of nature cure: fasting. [Chapter 7]. *Everybody's Guide to Nature Cure*. London: Health for All, 1936.

Jean Anthelme Brillat-Savarin. *The Physiology of Taste. Or, Meditations on Transcendental Gastronomy.* M F K Fisher (trs). Washington DC: Counterpoint, 1999. First published in French, 1825.

Christopher Connolly, Hetty Einzig. *The Fitness Jungle.* London: Century, 1986.

Luigi Cornaro. *The Art of Living Long.* Milwaukee, WI: Butler, 1905. Also known as *The Temperate Life.* First published in Italian, 1558.

Allen Cott. *Fasting: the Ultimate Diet.* London: Bantam, 1975.

Elizabeth David. *Mediterranean Food.* London: Penguin, 1955.

Boyd Eaton, Marjorie Shostak, Melvin Konner. The first fitness formula. [Chapter 7]. *The Paleolithic Prescription. A Program of Diet and Exercise and a Design for Living.* New York: Harper and Row, 1988.

Paul Ehrlich. *Human Natures. Genes, Cultures, and the Human Prospect.* London: Penguin, 2002.

Food and Agriculture Organization of the United Nations. *Human Energy Requirements.* Report of a Joint FAO/WHO/UNU expert consultation. FAO food and nutrition technical report series 1. Rome: FAO, 2004.

Joel Fuhrman. *Fasting and Eating for Health. A medical doctor's program for conquering disease.* New York: St Martin's Press, 1995.

Galen. *Hygiene (De Sanitate Tuenda).* Translated by R M Green. Springfield, IL: Charles Thomas. 1951.

Siegfried Giedion. Mechanization encounters the organic. [Part IV] *Mechanization Takes Command.* New York: Oxford University Press, 1948.

Jane Grigson. *Jane Grigson's Vegetable Book.* London: Penguin, 1980.

Kirsten Hartvig, Nic Rowley. *You Are What You Eat.* London: Piatkus, 1996.

Hippocrates. *Regimen I.* Translated by W H S Jones. Cambridge MA: Harvard University Press, 1953.

Robert Hutchison. The History of Dietetics. In: Mottram V, Graham G (eds). *Hutchison's Food and the Principles of Dietetics.* Ninth edition. London: Edward Arnold, 1940. First published in *The Practitioner*, 1934.

Martin Katahn. *The 200 Calorie Solution.*

How to Burn an Extra 200 Calories a Day and Stop Dieting. New York: Norton, 1982.

Frances Moore Lappé. *Diet for a Small Planet*. New York: Ballantine, 1982. First published 1971.

Mark Lynas. *Six Degrees. Our Future on a Hotter Planet*. London: Fourth Estate, 2007.

Robert McCarrison. *Nutrition and Health*. Cantor Lectures delivered at the Royal Society of Arts in London in 1936, published by Faber and Faber in a revised and enlarged edition in 1953, and then later by the McCarrison Society. Obtainable at: www.mccarrisonsociety.co.uk.

Tony McMichael. *Planetary Overload. Global Environmental Change and the Health of the Human Species*. Cambridge: University Press, 1993.

Tony McMichael. *Human Frontiers, Environments, and Disease. Past Patterns, Uncertain Futures*. Cambridge: University Press, 2001.

Elizabeth Lambert Ortiz. *The Book of Latin American Cooking*. London: Penguin, 1985.

Marion Nestle. *Food Politics*. Berkeley CA: University of California Press, 2002.

Marion Nestle. *What To Eat*. New York: Farrar, Straus, Giroux, 2006.

Carlo Petrini. *Slow Food Nation. Why Our Food Should Be Good, Clean, and Fair*. New York: Rizzoli, 2007. First published in Italian, 2005.

Michael Pollan. *In Defense of Food*. An Eater's Manifesto. New York: The Penguin Press, 2008.

Claudia Roden. *A Book of Middle Eastern Food*. London: Penguin, 1970.

Barbara Rolls. *The Volumetrics Eating Plan*. New York: Harper, 2005. See also www.VolumetricsEatingPlan.com.

Orville Schell. *Modern Meat. Antibiotics, Hormones, and the Pharmaceutical Farm*. New York: Random House, 1984.

Eric Schlosser. *Fast Food Nation. What the All-American Meal is Doing to the World*. Boston MA: Houghton Mifflin, 2001.

Peter Singer, Jim Mason. *The Way We Eat. Why Our Food Choices Matter*. Emmaus, PA: Rodale, 2006.

Colin Spencer. *Vegetarianism: a History*. London: Grub Street, 2000.

Colin Tudge. *So Shall We Reap*. London: Allen Lane, 2003.

UK Department of Health. *At Least Five a Week. Evidence on the Impact of Physical Activity and its Relationship to Health*, Chief Medical Officer's Report. Obtainable at: www.dh.gov.uk/en/PublicationsandStatistics.

US Department of Health and Human Services. *Physical Activity and Health*. A report of the Surgeon General. Washington DC: DHHS, 1996.

US Department of Health and Human Services/ US Department of Agriculture. Dietary Guidelines for Americans 2005. Washington DC: USDHHS/USDA, 2005. Obtainable at: www.healthierus.gov/dietary guidelines.

Margaret Visser. Fasting. In: *The Way We Are*. London: Viking, 1995.

Bernhard Watzl, Claus Leitzmann. *Bioaktive Substanzen in Lebensmitteln*. Stuttgart: Hippokrates, 1999.

World Cancer Research Fund/ American Institute for Cancer Research. *Food, Nutrition, Physical Activity, and the Prevention of Cancer: a Global Perspective.* Washington DC: AICR, 2007.

World Health Organization. *Diet, Nutrition and the Prevention of Chronic Diseases.* Report of a joint WHO/FAO expert consultation. WHO technical report series 916. Geneva: WHO, 2003.

References: papers, features

In alphabetical order of authors. Also see the references for chapters 2–5.

Anderson E. Traditional medical values of food. In: Counihan C, van Esterik P (eds). *Food and Culture.* London: Routledge, 1997.

Åstrand P-O. General discussion. In: *Nutrition and Physical Activity* (ed Blix G). Symposia of the Swedish Nutrition Foundation V. Stockholm: Almqvist and Wiksell, 1967.

Bassett D, Schneider P, Huntington G. Physical activity in an older order Amish community. *Medicine and Science in Sports and Exercise* 2004; 36: 79–85.

Cannon G. Why the Bush administration and the global sugar industry are determined to demolish the 2004 WHO global strategy on diet, physical activity and health. *Public Health Nutrition* 2004; 7(3): 769–80.

King N. The relationship between physical activity and food intake. *Proceedings of the Nutrition Society* 1998; 57: 77–84.

Lynas M. How only carbon rationing can save the world. *New Statesman,* 23 October 2006.

Martins C, Robertson D, Morgan L. Effects of exercise and restrained eating behaviour on appetite control. *Proceedings of the Nutrition Society* 2008; 67: 28–41.

Nordqvist C. British wrong to think moderate exercise is better than vigorous exercise. *Medical News Today,* 10 October 2007.

Prentice A, Jebb S. Fast foods, energy density and obesity: a possible mechanistic link. *Obesity Reviews* 2003; 4: 187–94.

Saris W, Blair S, van Baak M, Eaton SB, Davies P, Di Pietro L, Fogelholm M, Rissanen A, Schoeller D, Swinburn B, Westerterp K, Wyatt H. How much physical activity is enough to prevent unhealthy weight gain? Outcome of the 1st IASO Stock conference. Obesity Reviews 2003; 4: 101–14.

Walsh B. Back to the tap. *Time,* 17 August 2007.

Warburton D, Nicol C, Bredin S. Health benefits of physical activity - the evidence. *Canadian Medical Association Journal* 2006; 174(6): 801–09.

THANKS

What we think, say and write comes partly from what we sense, partly from what we are shown, and also from what's in the air. Sometimes insights are original. Most work is a synthesis of that of others, or builds on what others have experienced or discovered. Lists like this are always inadequate.

The first people to thank are those from the past or who I have not met, whose writings have impressed me. Some I have not mentioned in the text or the notes. Twenty of these are Fernand Braudel, Manuel Castells, Mike Davis, Jared Diamond, René Dubos, Paul Farmer, Paul Feyerabend, Tim Flannery, Siegfried Giedion, Susan George, Ivan Illich, Lynn Margulis, Mary Midgley, Joseph Needham, Michael Pollan, Amartya Sen, John Seymour, Tzvetan Todorov, Alan Watts, Daniel Yergin.

Among the acquaintances, colleagues and friends, dead and alive, whose writings also influence me, twenty are Alan Davidson, Denis Burkitt, Michael Crawford, Edward Goldsmith, Jane Grigson, Kirsten Hartvig, Marshall McLuhan, T C McLuhan, Tim Lang, Tony McMichael, Leonardo Mata, Michael Murphy, Marion Nestle, Nic Rowley, Rupert Sheldrake, Hugh Sinclair, Colin Spencer, Hugh Trowell, Colin Tudge, Ricardo Uauy. This does not mean that they agree with what I say, nor do I always agree with them.

Writers on and from Brazil who have guided me include Leonardo Boff, Bartolomé de las Casas, Gilberto Freire, Paulo Freire, John Hemming, Eduardo Galeano, Darcy Ribeiro, Peter Robb, Nancy Scheper-Hughes.

Some passages in this book have been developed from papers and other contributions published since 2002 in *Public Health Nutrition*, *Asia Pacific Journal of Clinical Nutrition* and other journals; in my 2003 book *The Fate of Nations*; and from presentations and workshops since 1999 in Guatemala City, Porto Alegre, Brasília, Recife, Lake Como (a Bellagio meeting), Vienna, Melbourne, Auckland, Johannesburg (on the occasion of the Earth Summit), Acapulco, London, Bristol, Giessen (the inaugural New Nutrition Science meeting), Durban (the International Conference on Nutrition), Barcelona (the first World Conference on Public Health Nutrition), Hangzhou, Hobart, Santiago, and São Paulo.

The people who have guided me by their responses and in workshop discussions and agreements are too numerous to thank here. You know who you are! Special thanks are owed to Colin Campbell and Michael Latham for their invitations to lecture twice at Cornell University in 1992, and then, for meetings since 1999 (in chronological order) to: Rafael Flores, Noel Solomons; Sonia Slavutsky, Clara Brandão, Lia Giraldo; Barry Popkin; Ibrahim Elmadfa; Kevin Jackson, Cathy McDonald, Mark Wahlqvist; Pekka Puska, Derek Yach; George Davey Smith; Elvira Kratz, Claus Leitzmann; Esté Vorster; Joy Ngo de la Cruz, Lluis Serra-Majem; Duo Li; Claire Hewat, Julie Hulcombe, Mark Lawrence, Judy Seal,

Andrew Sinclair; Eva Hertrampf, Marcela Reyes; Antonio Lucio, Indra Nooyi, Jonathan Weiner, Derek Yach.

Thanks also to the many people who have contributed to and worked on expert reports published by the World Health Organization, the Food and Agriculture Organization of the United Nations, World Cancer Research Fund International/American Institute for Cancer Research, the UK Department of Health, the US National Research Council, the Royal College of Physicians of London, and other authoritative sources, whose research and conclusions have guided me. Some are thanked individually above and below.

Like party invitations, acknowledgements are hard to get right. Everybody listed below is thanked. Some, including friends and colleagues, will know how much they have helped me. Others who I have not met have informed and guided me with their published work. With some exceptions, I have mentioned people just once. None has any responsibility for what I have written. So, thank you . . .

Energy balance, physical activity: Marian Apfelbaum, Per-Olof Åstrand, Marleen van Baak, George Bray, Kenneth Cooper, John Durnin, Jack Farquhar, Anna Ferro-Luzzi, Robert Fogel, Keith Frayn, John Garrow, William Haskell, James Hill, Jules Hirsch, Philip James, Susan Jebb, Rudolph Leibel, Jerry Morris, Ralph Paffenbarger, Eric Ravussin, Prakash Shetty, James Stubbs, John Waterlow, Peter Wood, Margriet Westerterp-Plantenga, Arvid Wretlind.

Food, nutrition, food culture, food and agriculture policy. Douglas Black, Norman Blacklock, Richard Body, Junshi Chen, John Cummings, Hans Kolbein Dahle, Elizabeth David, Alan Davidson, Hans Engylst, Cutberto Garza, Stuart Gillespie, C Gopalan, Jane Grigson, John Gummer, Lawrence Haddad, Kenneth Heaton, Mark Hegsted, Elisabet Helsing, David Horrobin, Alan Jackson, Tom Jaine, Francis Avery Jones, Laurence Kolonel, Richard Lacey, Michael Latham, Felicity Lawrence, Michael Lipton, Alan Long, Jim Mann, Tore Midtvedt, Carlos Monteiro, José Dutra de Oliveira, Michael Oliver, Mercedes de Onis, Gabrielle Palmer, Barry Popkin, John Potter, Srinath Reddy, Elio Riboli, John Rivers, Claudia Roden, Geoffrey Rose, Nevin Scrimshaw, Aubrey Sheiham, Atul Singhal, David Southgate, M S Swaminathan, Boyd Swinburn, Stewart Truswell, César Victora, John Vidal, Walter Willett, Arthur Wynn, Margaret Wynn, John Yudkin.

And now my thanks to people who have supported me at times in my life and in various enterprises, which have influenced the thinking and work that has gone into this book:

The human potential movement: Graham Alexander, John Falkiner, Tim Gallwey, Arianna Huffington, Bob Kriegel, Tony Morgan, Mark Shapiro, John Whitmore, and especially Ben Cannon.

Citizen running and physical activity projects: Will Chapman, Ted Charlesworth, David Denison, Steven Downes, Malcolm Emery, Andy Etchells, James Godber, Tom McNab, David Player, John Ridgway, Bev Risman, Sylvester Stein, Kevin Sykes, and especially Simon Morris.

The Sunday Times, The Times, The Observer: Don Berry, David Driver, Norman Harris, Magnus Linklater, John Lovesey, Nick Mason, Nick Wapshott, and especially Harry Evans.

Guild of Food Writers, Soil Association, McCarrison Society, Caroline Walker Trust, National Food Alliance (now Sustain), Food Commission, International Baby Food Action Network, Center for Science in the Public Interest: Colin Spencer; Patrick Holden, Julian Rose, Lawrence Woodward; Lillian Schofield, Andrew Strigner, Walter Yellowlees; Jonathan Aitken, David Dickinson, Maggie Sanderson, Richard Watt; Tim Lang, Jeanette Longfield, Mike Rayner, Jack Winkler; Sue Dibb, Tim Lobstein; Gabrielle Palmer, Annelies Allain, Marina Rea, Patti Rundall; Michael Jacobson, Bruce Silverglade.

World Cancer Research Fund / American Institute for Cancer Research: Kelly Browning, Deirdre McGinley-Gieser, Jeff Prince, Kathy Ward, especially my colleague and director of the 2007 WCRF/AICR report Martin Wiseman, and above all my colleague, friend and boss Marilyn Gentry.

Public Health Nutrition: Gill Watling, Agneta Yngve, Roger Hughes, and especially Barrie Margetts.

World Health Policy Forum: Max Pettoello-Mantovani, and the Baroness Mariuccia Zerilli-Marimò.

World Health Organization: Robert Beaglehole, Gro Harlem Brundtland, David Nabarro, Chizuru Nishida, Pekka Puska, Derek Yach.

United Nations System Standing Committee on Nutrition: Ted Greiner, Lida Lhotska, Harriet Kuhnlein, George Kent, Arne Oshaug, Sonya Rabeneck, Judith Richter, David Sanders, Roger Shrimpton, Elisabeth Sterken, Flavio Valente.

Brazil federal government: Denise Coitinho, Elisabetta Recine, José Serra, João Yunes.

Within Brazil: Clara Brandão, José Dutra de Oliveira, Eduardo and Eloisa Manzano, Carlos Monteiro, Inês Rugani, Flavio Valente, César Victora. Also many people in government, civil society organisations and the community, in the Federal District and the states and municipalities of Ceará, Minas Gerais, Pará, Pernambuco, Rio Grande do Sul, Tocantins. Above all, Raquel Bittar.

The New Nutrition Science project: Christopher Beauman, Ibrahim Elmadfa, Elvira Kratz, Mark Lawrence, Uwe Spiekermann, Esté Vorster, Mark Wahlqvist, and above all Claus Leitzmann.

This and the first version of Dieting Makes You Fat: Richard Cable, Carolyn Thorne, Ian Allen, Vickie Boff, Gareth Fletcher, Han Ismail, Clare Pierotti, Deborah Rogers, Anthony Cheetham, Susan Lamb, Christopher Pick, Rob Shreeve, Kathy Crilley; and above all Gail Rebuck and Ben Mason.

This second version of Dieting Makes You Fat has been written first and foremost with the support of my first co-author and friend Hetty Einzig. We agreed that a new book was needed, and she has supported me throughout, from writing the new proposal to the final editing a year later, both done in her London home. Joan Bakewell, Claus Leitzmann and Barrie Margetts made many helpful comments on drafts. Above all thanks to Eugenie Verney who edited all of the final drafts and made many proposals for additions and revisions that have improved the text and saved me from error. Remaining mistakes are mine.

Love to my immediate family in Britain, including my stepmother Elise and her husband John who died in 2007; my son Ben who died in 2006, Melissa, and their lovely

children Francesca and Elizabeth; my son
Matt, Loll, and their grown-up and accom-
plished daughters Flo and Issey; and my
daughter Lou.

Love also to the two people central in both
my professional and personal life who have
shown me the way, my past wife Caroline
Walker who died in 1988; and my wife
Raquel Bittar de Oliveira, also the mother of
Taná and our son Gabriel – to whom both
love always – who has proved to this
Englishman that there is in word and indeed
a world elsewhere.

INDEX